PHYSICAL ACTIVITY IN DIVERSE POPULATIONS

The health benefits associated with regular physical activity are now widely recognized. This book examines how social determinants such as race, ethnicity, socioeconomic status, sexual orientation and disability can impact on physical activity and its associated health outcomes. It explores the social, cultural, political and environmental factors that influence engagement in physical activity in a range of diverse populations and presents evidence-based, culturally appropriate strategies for targeting and promoting physical activity participation.

Each chapter considers how the social determinants that impact on health are formed by the environments in which people live, work, learn and play. Incorporating a series of original case studies, this book analyzes physical activity behaviors in groups such as:

• African Americans, Latinos, Asian Americans and Native Americans
• military veterans and physically disabled populations
• low-income populations
• rural populations
• LGBT populations.

It also includes a variety of useful features such as key terms, summary points and critical thinking questions, as well as a chapter on international perspectives.

Physical Activity in Diverse Populations: Evidence and Practice is vital reading for any course touching on social factors in physical activity behavior.

Melissa Bopp is an associate professor of kinesiology at Pennsylvania State University, USA. Her research expertise includes community-based strategies for promoting physical activity. She has worked extensively with underserved populations in a variety of settings. She has been teaching undergraduate and graduate students about health disparities in underserved populations for more than 10 years.

PHYSICAL ACTIVITY IN DIVERSE POPULATIONS

Evidence and Practice

Edited by Melissa Bopp

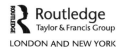
Routledge
Taylor & Francis Group

LONDON AND NEW YORK

First published 2018
by Routledge
2 Park Square, Milton Park, Abingdon, Oxon OX14 4RN

and by Routledge
711 Third Avenue, New York, NY 10017

Routledge is an imprint of the Taylor & Francis Group, an informa business

British Library Cataloguing-in-Publication Data
A catalogue record for this book is available from the British Library

Library of Congress Cataloging-in-Publication Data
A catalog record for this book has been requested

ISBN: 978-1-138-67456-1 (hbk)
ISBN: 978-1-138-67457-8 (pbk)
ISBN: 978-1-315-56126-4 (ebk)

Typeset in ApexBembo
by Apex CoVantage, LLC

To all of the knowledgeable, insightful and generous
authors who contributed to this text.
To my mentors who instilled a passion in me for
examining health disparities.
To my students whose drive for knowledge helped
me to envision this book.
To my family for their love and support throughout
the process of building this text.

CONTENTS

List of figures, tables and boxes   *ix*
List of abbreviations   *xii*
List of contributors   *xiii*

1   Introduction to physical activity and health disparities   1
    Melissa Bopp

2   Introduction to race, ethnicity, and related theories
    of disparities   13
    Scherezade K. Mama, Deborah H. John
    and Nishat Bhuiyan

3   Development of culturally appropriate strategies for
    promoting physical activity   26
    Sandra Soto, Adrian Chavez, Jessica Haughton
    and Elva M. Arredondo

4   Physical activity among African Americans   45
    Melicia C. Whitt-Glover, Ogechi Nwaokelemeh,
    Amanda A. Price and Jammie M. Hopkins

5   Physical activity among Latinos   62
    David X. Marquez, Susan Aguiñaga, Priscilla Vásquez,
    Isabela Gouveia Marques and Maricela Martinez

6 Physical activity among Asian Americans   84
   Edith W. Chen, Grace J. Yoo, Elaine A. Musselman
   and Jane Jih

7 Physical activity among Native Americans   102
   Heather J. A. Foulds

8 Physical activity among Native Hawaiians and
   Pacific Islanders   123
   Cheryl L. Albright, Marjorie M. Mau, Lehua B. Choy
   and Tricia Mabellos

9 Physical activity among low-income populations   143
   Wendell C. Taylor

10 Physical activity among rural populations   159
    Deborah H. John and Katherine B. Gunter

11 Physical activity among lesbian, gay, bisexual and
    transgender populations   180
    Danielle R. Brittain and Mary K. Dinger

12 Physical activity among military veterans   200
    David E. Goodrich and Katherine S. Hall

13 Physical activity among physically disabled populations   226
    Robert B. Shaw and Kathleen A. Martin Ginis

14 Physical activity among diverse populations internationally   244
    Justin Richards, Adewale Oyeyemi and Adrian Bauman

15 Future directions for addressing physical activity
    in diverse populations   273
    Melissa Bopp

Index   *283*

FIGURES, TABLES AND BOXES

Figures

1.1	Social determinants of health	6
1.2	Social ecological framework	8
3.1	Example of surface- and deep-level strategies used in *Fe en Acción*	30
3.2	Example of surface- and deep-level strategies used in *Fe en Acción*	31
4.1	AACORN's Expanded Obesity Research Paradigm	48
6.1	Regular physical activity for adults, ages 18–44, by race and Asian ethnicity in California	86
6.2	Regular physical activity for Californian adults, ages 65–85, by race and Asian ethnicity	88
6.3	Regular physical activity for Californian adults, ages 18–44, by race and gender	90
7.1	Sports and activities such as lacrosse (A) and snowshoeing (B) are derived from traditional Native American games and activities	106
8.1	Geographic regions in the South Pacific for Native Hawaiians and Pacific Islanders	123
8.2	Native Hawaiian, Other Pacific Islander percentages of Hawai'i population	124
8.3	BRFSS 2011 data – percent meeting national guidelines for physical activity by race and sex	128
8.4	Percent meeting recommended physical activity levels by race in Hawai'i	128
9.1	Percentage of adults who met federal guidelines for aerobic physical activity, by poverty status	146

11.1   Median percentage of adolescents by sexual orientation
        participating in moderate to vigorous physical activity   184
11.2   Rates of participation in moderate to vigorous physical
        activity and muscle strengthening among college students
        by sexual orientation   185
12.1   Prevalence rates of health conditions in nonveterans versus
        veterans who do or do not use VHA services   207
14.1   Prevalence of people insufficiently active by country   247
14.2   Prevalence of people insufficiently active by World Bank
        income status   248
14.3   Prevalence of people insufficiently active by WHO region   250
15.1   Prevalence of no leisure-time physical activity among adults
        by race/ethnicity, education level, and disability status, 2012 278
15.2   Prevalence of meeting guidelines for aerobic physical
        activity among adolescents, 2011   279

Tables

1.1   Methods of measuring physical activity   3
1.2   Social determinants of health examples   7
2.1   Theories of health disparities related to physical activity and
        conceptual frameworks used for community-level interventions   14
2.2   Stages of change and physical activity intervention examples   18
3.1   Examples of surface structure strategies   33
3.2   Process of development and adaptation of culturally
        sensitive/competent intervention   35
5.1   Barriers and strategies to physical activity for Latinos   67
5.2   Social support   72
7.1   The prevalence of health disparities among Native
        American populations   104
9.1   Federal TRIO Programs current-year low-income levels   144
10.1   Rural Active Living Research Call to Action Areas of Focus   174
11.1   Barriers to physical activity among LGBT populations   188
12.1   Surface and deep structure dimensions for culturally
        sensitive interactions with veterans   203
12.2   Health and sociocultural factors affecting physical activity
        prescription in veterans   205
12.3   Clinical and cultural considerations for physical activity
        interventions to veterans   216
13.1   Types of interventions and the determinants of physical
        activity they influence   231
14.1   Common physical activity correlates and determinants globally   252
14.2   Unique physical activity correlates and determinants according
        to country income   255

14.3   Application of the "Seven Best Investments for Physical
         Activity" in community settings and low- and
         middle-income countries   261

Boxes

1.1   Putting it into practice: the social ecological model   9
2.1   Ecologic Model of Physical Activity   15
4.1   Evidence-based practice: Instant Recess®   53
5.1   Evidence for practice: Faith in Action   77
6.1   Evidence-based practice: Asian and Pacific Islander Obesity
       Prevention Alliance tackles obesity by improving neighborhoods   94
7.1   Evidence-based practice: Aboriginal RunWalk Program   115
8.1   Evidence for practice: a physical activity intervention in
       Hawai'i using hula dancing   134
9.1   Evidence for practice: low-income, predominantly Hispanic
       communities promoting physical activity in parks   152
10.1   Evidence for practice: generating rural options through
       community partnerships   167
11.1   Evidence-based practice: Healthy Weight in Lesbian and
       Bisexual Women: Striving for a Healthy Community   190
12.1   Evidence-based practice: Team Red, White & Blue (RWB)
       integrates military veterans with local communities through
       physical and social activity   214
13.1   Evidence-based practice: active accessible living in Canada's
       Okanagan Valley   237
14.1   Evidence-based practice: Kau Mai Tonga uses netball to reduce
       the burden of non-communicable diseases and address broader
       social inequities   265

ABBREVIATIONS

ACSM:	American College of Sports Medicine
AHA:	American Heart Association
BMI:	Body Mass Index
BRFSS:	Behavioral Risk Factor Surveillance System
CDC:	Centers for Disease Control and Prevention
CHD:	Coronary heart disease
CVD:	cardiovascular disease
NHANES:	National Health and Nutrition Examination Survey
NHIS:	National Health Interview Survey
SES:	socioeconomic status
USDHHS:	US Department of Health and Human Services
WHO:	World Health Organization

CONTRIBUTORS

Susan Aguiñaga
University of Illinois at Chicago

Cheryl L. Albright
University of Hawai'i at Manoa

Elva M. Arredondo
San Diego State University

Adrian Bauman
University of Sydney

Nishat Bhuiyan
Pennsylvania State University

Melissa Bopp
Pennsylvania State University

Danielle R. Brittain
Colorado School of Public Health at the University of Northern Colorado

Adrian Chavez
Institute of Behavioral and Community Health

Edith W. Chen
California State University, Northridge

Lehua B. Choy
University of Hawai'i at Manoa

Mary K. Dinger
Colorado School of Public Health at the University of Northern Colorado

Heather J. A. Foulds
University of Saskatchewan

David E. Goodrich
Ann Arbor VA Healthcare System

Isabela Gouveia Marques
University of Illinois at Chicago

Katherine B. Gunter
Oregon State University

Katherine S. Hall
Durham Veterans Affairs Medical Center-GRECC, Duke University

Jessica Haughton
Institute of Behavioral and Community Health

Jammie M. Hopkins
Morehouse School of Medicine

Jane Jih
University of California, San Francisco

Deborah H. John
Oregon State University

Tricia Mabellos
University of Hawai'i at Manoa

Scherazade K. Mama
Pennsylvania State University

David X. Marquez
University of Illinois at Chicago

Kathleen A. Martin Ginis
University of British Columbia, Okanagan Campus

Maricela Martinez
University of Illinois at Chicago

Marjorie M. Mau
University of Hawai'i at Manoa

Elaine A. Musselman
San Francisco State University

Ogechi Nwaokelemeh
Westmont College

Adewale Oyeyemi
University of Maiduguri

Amanda A. Price
Winston-Salem State University

Justin Richards
University of Sydney

Robert B. Shaw
University of British Columbia, Okanagan Campus

Sandra Soto
San Diego State University/University of California, San Diego

Wendell C. Taylor
The University of Texas Health Science Center School of Public Health

Priscilla Vásquez
University of Illinois at Chicago, Institute for Minority Health Research

Melicia C. Whitt-Glover
Gramercy Research Group

Grace J. Yoo
San Francisco State University

1

INTRODUCTION TO PHYSICAL ACTIVITY AND HEALTH DISPARITIES

Melissa Bopp

Modern medical technology combined with organized public health efforts have led to the greatest advances in human life span, health-related quality of life and an expanded understanding of factors that influence morbidity and mortality. Collectively, as a species we have never been healthier than we are today. These gains in population level health, however, are not equally distributed across the populace. Many population groups across the globe experience poorer health outcomes and experience higher rates of chronic diseases compared with the majority.

The importance of physical activity

Current recommendations for physical activity indicate that adults should engage in 150 minutes a week of moderate-intensity aerobic physical activity or 75 minutes of vigorous intensity aerobic activity (or a combination of the two). Strength training is also recommended twice a week. For youth, 60 minutes of moderate to vigorous physical activity daily is recommended. This dose of physical activity is associated with lower morbidity and mortality, most notably a decreased risk of CVD, certain forms of cancer, diabetes, obesity, mental illness and premature mortality. Regular physical activity participation has many positive health outcomes including improved cardiovascular and muscular fitness, body composition, improved psychological well-being and longevity (Physical Activity Guidelines Advisory Committee 2008). Despite these known benefits, globally, physical inactivity (a lack of physical activity) is a noted public health problem (Kohl *et al.* 2012). The World Health Organization (WHO) estimates that 3.2 million deaths a year are attributable to insufficient physical activity (World Health Organization 2010). Estimates of the economic burden associated with a lack of physical activity related to premature morbidity and mortality have been estimated at $53.8 billion (USD) worldwide in 2013 (Ding *et al.* 2016).

WHO's Global Recommendations on Physical Activity for Health highlight the importance of scientifically informed strategies for addressing low rates of participation in physical activity. These recommendations would include population-level surveillance on the rates of participation, documenting influences on physical activity behavior and using evidence-based practices for targeting inactivity. The U.S. Department of Health and Human Service's Healthy People Initiative, along with many other international organizations, highlight the importance of multi-level approaches to address the full breadth of the influences on physical activity participation (U.S. Department of Health and Human Services (USDHHS) 2012).

Measuring physical activity

Measuring physical activity behavior can often be challenging and complex. It is important to understand how health and wellness professionals measure this behavior to better understand how physical activity is related to health outcomes (e.g. decreased disease risk), which groups of the population are more at risk for being inactive and understanding if a program or intervention was successful at improving physical activity participation. There are four main components of physical activity that can be measured:

1   Frequency: How many times per week physical activity is performed.
2   Intensity: Refers to the level of effort associated with doing the activity. This can be relative to the individual (e.g. % of aerobic capacity) or absolute (e.g. amount of energy used by the body during the activity). This is the most difficult component to measure.
3   Time/Duration: The number of minutes of physical activity.
4   Type: This can refer to aerobic or strength/resistance training, or can also refer to the context in which the physical activity is occurring (e.g. occupational activity, leisure time, household, transportation).

For health-related outcomes, the most important components of physical activity are frequency, intensity and time, the product of which is the volume of physical activity, which is most relevant for understanding benefits. There are a number of important considerations when selecting a measurement tool for physical activity. First, it is important to reflect on the fact that physical activity is a behavior, and like most behaviors, there is a lot of variability in an individual's physical activity participation hour-to-hour, day-to-day, week-to-week or even season-to-season. Measurement tools should do their best to capture typical behavior in a reliable, consistent manner. When deciding on measurement tools, a few considerations are necessary:

•   Population: Ensure that the tool is appropriate for the group who would be using it. This could include reading level, ability to recall information or types and intensities of activities.

- Feasibility: Consider whether the tool is costly, how many individuals will be measured, or how long it will take to complete the measurement process.
- Acceptability: Determine if the tool is user-friendly and individuals would be alright with completing the measurement process. This could consider time burden, what individuals would need to do to complete the process (e.g. complete a paper survey vs. wear a measurement device).
- Reliability: The measurement tool should give reliable and consistent results each time it is used under similar measurement conditions.

There are two main categories of physical activity measurement tools: subjective and objective. Both categories have a number of different tools, all with pros and cons. Table 1.1 outlines different measurement tools.

TABLE 1.1 Methods of measuring physical activity

Tool	Description	Pros	Cons
Subjective			
Recall Measure (e.g. retrospective survey)	Individuals are asked to remember how much physical activity they participated in over a certain time period (e.g. last month, typical week).	Low cost, can document types of activity, easy to administer, acceptable to participants.	Problems with accurately recalling information, subject to bias, may not capture all forms of activity.
Diaries/Logs (e.g. prospective methods)	Individuals are asked to write down or note all the activity they do over a period of time.	Low cost, can document types of activity, easy to administer.	May be tedious or burdensome, could cause behavior change (reactive).
Subjective			
Pedometer (step counter)	Small device worn on the waistband in line with the hip. Lever arm records vertical movement and a total step count for a time period can be recorded.	Relatively low cost, easy to use with simple instructions, removes problems with recall.	Could cause behavior change (reactive), depends on individual wearing device correctly, doesn't capture intensity of activity and can't measure strength training, swimming, bicycling.
Accelerometers	Small device worn on the hip, wrist or ankle. Measures acceleration of the body across all planes of movement. Stores information for processing.	Not reactive (no feedback mechanisms), can accurately measure intensity, duration, frequency, limited burden to participants.	Expensive, can't measure strength training, swimming.

(*Continued*)

TABLE 1.1 (Continued)

Tool	Description	Pros	Cons
Commercially available physical activity monitors	Wearable devices that assess the users' physical activity (e.g. steps, caloric expenditure).	Easy to use, high acceptability from participants.	Expensive, reliability and accuracy varies across models, could cause behavior change (reactive), may not assess certain types of activities, depending on models.

Physical inactivity and sedentary behavior

Physical inactivity (not being active enough to meet recommendations) and sedentary behavior (any waking activity with an energy expenditure less than 1.5 METS and in a sitting or reclining posture) have increasingly been the focus of more research (Sedentary Behavior Research Network 2017, World Health Organization 2010). As noted previously, WHO (2015) has indicated that physical inactivity is the fourth leading cause of death globally, tied closely to its relationship with many chronic diseases. Although inactivity is related to physical activity, it is important to recognize that they are different things. Throughout this text we may describe physical activity or inactivity in a given population and it is important to interpret them appropriately. It is important to know what factors are related to engaging in a behavior (physical activity) as well as what is related to *not* engaging in a behavior (physical inactivity) as they provide an indication of what to target to make improvements. There a wide range of strategies used to combat these issues that have a strong evidence base (Kohl *et al.* 2012). The study of sedentary behavior has grown exponentially over the past 20 years, likely related to the increase in sitting-based leisure-time activity (television viewing, video games, computer use). The American Heart Association has reviewed the evidence in terms of the negative health impact of sedentary time on cardiovascular morbidity and mortality and has noted an increase in CVD risk associated with more sedentary time (Young *et al.* 2016). One of the significant challenges associated with understanding how sedentary time is related to negative health outcomes is measurement. As noted, it is difficult to measure physical activity and beyond that, measuring a behavior that takes up several hours in a day presents some significant challenges in terms of accurate recall. Objective measures (e.g. accelerometers) may be better for determining time spent in sedentary activities; however, further research is needed to establish best practices for measurement.

Although inactivity and sedentary time are not exactly the opposite of physical activity, they are a part of the larger picture of an individual's overall health and well-being. Throughout this book, we will outline how physical activity is impacted by race, ethnicity, income, location, sexual orientation or ability level. However emerging research is also suggesting that there are differences in sedentary time based on these factors as well. For example, a study by Whitt-Glover and colleagues (2009) noted differences in the amount of sedentary time among youth by race, income and gender, though the relationship was different in children compared with adolescents. Research among adults living in New York City noted sit time was related to income and education levels (Yi *et al.* 2015). As the detrimental health effects of sedentary time and inactivity are further documented, the impact of many of these factors on this behavior will be essential.

Health disparities and equity

Health disparities refer to the differences in the burden of disease and opportunity to engage in behaviors to optimize one's health (e.g. physical activity) (Issac 2013). Disparities can occur across a number of factors, including race, ethnicity, education level, income or socioeconomic status, sexual orientation, disability, veterans' status, or geographic location (e.g. urban or rural). Many of the disparities that exist are related to some of the historical and current social, economic and environmental resources that can impact health. For example, individuals living in rural communities often have higher rates of obesity than those living in urban areas. This is possibly linked to fewer resources for physical activity and poor access to grocery stores that sell fresh fruits and vegetables at a reasonable cost. The lack of environmental resources to engage in healthy behaviors (i.e. regular exercise and eating healthy) has led to higher obesity prevalence. In the United States and other countries with a very diverse population, health disparities are a noteworthy issue as direct and indirect medical expenses are an increasingly larger portion of the countries' economy. USDHSS's Healthy People Initiative has included goals and objectives aimed at reducing disparities and inequities. Additionally, Healthy People aims to work toward health equity, which is "the attainment of the highest level of health for all people" (U.S. Department of Health and Human Services 2010). Achieving health equity is a long-range goal to eliminate many of the health disparities facing underserved populations. It is important to note that many of the disparities facing underserved groups are not only in the higher prevalence rate of a disease (e.g. CVD or diabetes) but also within the health behaviors that can contribute to the development of a disease (e.g. physical inactivity or smoking). This text will address the notable health disparities and inequities associated with physical inactivity across race, ethnicity, income, sexual orientation, disability level, veterans' status, income level and geographic location.

The social determinants of health

The most modern movements in public health include recognizing the many factors that influence an individual's health. The social determinants of health refer to the conditions of one's environment where you live, work, learn and play that can impact your health, well-being, quality of life and health behaviors. They are closely tied to health disparities and achieving health equity in that they are the factors that influence an individual's or population's health. Some of these determinants could include access to a health–equality education, nutritious food and culturally sensitive healthcare providers. The USDHHS model of the social determinants of health is

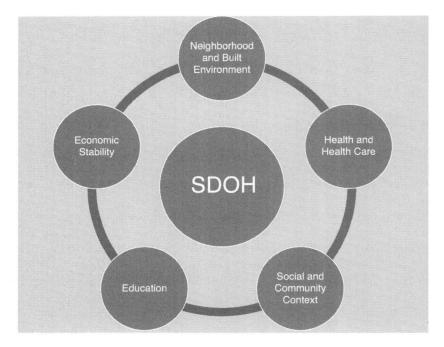

FIGURE 1.1 Social determinants of health

Source: U.S. Department of Health and Human Services (USDHHS) (2012), www.usa.gov/government-works

shown in Figure 1.1. The five determinant areas highlight the different types of factors that can impact health or engagement in healthy behaviors. Examples of each are shown in Table 1.2. The model provides us with a framework, or an organized way of understanding, researching and measuring how many factors external to the individual can influence their health. By better understanding these factors, health professionals can help to address health disparities and develop effective programs and policies to eliminate them.

For example: Consider Jasmine, a 32-year-old single mother of two children, ages 4 and 2. Jasmine has a job at a local hospital working in the laundry room, her job is not full-time and she also watches her neighbor's children after school to earn some extra money. She lives in an apartment with her children in a neighborhood near the hospital so that she can walk to work but there is a high crime rate, no parks or playgrounds, and lots of busy streets. Under the social determinants of health model in Figure 1.1, Jasmine has a number of factors that influence her and her children's health and opportunities to engage in healthy behaviors. She lacks economic stability because of her part-time position and having to take on multiple jobs restricts her time to engage in healthy behaviors (i.e. physical activity). Her part-time position is also associated with a lack of health insurance, reducing her access to preventive health services and regular health care. Jasmine is unable to pay

TABLE 1.2 Social determinants of health examples

Determinant Area	Examples
Neighborhood and Built Environment	• Access to healthy foods
	• Having safe places to be physically active
	• Crime and violence
Health and Health Care	• Having access to health care and primary care services
	• Having healthcare providers supportive of preventive health behaviors
Social and Community Context	• Facing discrimination based on age, sex, race, sexual orientation, etc.
	• Social cohesion in one's community or neighborhood
Education	• Access to high-quality education at all levels
Economic Stability	• Poverty and employment
	• Food security

Source: U.S. Department of Health and Human Services (USDHHS) 2012

for quality early childhood education for her children while she's at work and must rely on family members to look after them. She doesn't feel safe walking with her kids in her neighborhood and doesn't often take them outside to play; they spend more time in front of the television instead of being active. Many of these outside factors influence Jasmine's health status, stress level and opportunity to engage in healthy behaviors that could prevent chronic disease.

The social determinants of health framework has also been emphasized by WHO, highlighting the need for improved policies to address the factors related to the determinants, including socioeconomic and political contexts which impact health equity (World Health Organization 2015). Across the globe inequities by many factors exist in terms of chronic disease morbidity and mortality as well as rates of physical inactivity. Many countries, including the United States, the United Kingdom, Australia, Canada, New Zealand and a number of European countries have identified social determinants as key factors impacting the health of their population and have developed policies or strategies to attempt to address the resulting inequities (World Health Organization 2014).

Addressing health from many levels

To target the factors that influence health outcomes and behaviors in the population we need to consider many different factors. Models and frameworks that encompass social and ecological factors allow us to understand a wide range of influences on health behaviors, including physical activity, and allow us to organize our approach toward the problem of physical inactivity (McLeroy et al. 1988, Sallis et al. 2008). Social ecological frameworks examine factors from across levels, as

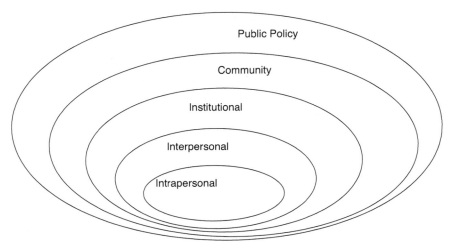

FIGURE 1.2 Social ecological framework
Source: McLeroy *et al.* (1988, p. 355)

shown in Figure 1.2. This framework goes from a narrow focus at the individual level to a very broad focus of policy. Within each level there are a number of factors to examine in more detail as they relate to physical activity.

> Intrapersonal: These individual-based factors could include demographics (e.g. age, sex, race/ethnicity), medical/health related, psychological (attitudes, beliefs, motivation) or previous history with physical activity.
>
> Interpersonal: This encompasses the social environment and an individual's social network. This could include friends, family, neighbors, coworkers and any other individuals that someone may interact with.
>
> Institutional: This includes any setting in the community; schools, worksites, faith-based organizations, seniors' centers, healthcare organizations, fitness facilities, etc. Settings typically include a physical space (e.g. a building), often include a social environment and may have environments and policies that could impact physical activity.
>
> Community: This is a much broader area and can be defined in a variety of different ways: geographically (e.g. an entire town) or by specific characteristics (e.g. the African American community of a city). Typically, many institutions are part of communities and there is a social environment, a physical environment and policies that could influence physical activity.
>
> Policy: Policies can be enacted at the local, state or national level and help to address physical activity through rules, laws or legislation. Policies can help in establishing programs, allocating resources, creating safe spaces to be active or enhancing opportunities for physical activity.

All of these levels have the potential to impact physical activity and provide a basis both for understanding physical activity participation as well as promoting active lifestyles.

This text will attempt to examine the interaction of physical activity and health with the social determinants of health by using a social ecological framework. This will allow us to examine issues from many levels and develop a better understanding of how health and physical activity are shaped in the many populations outlined throughout this text. Chapter 2 will outline some other approaches to health disparities in more detail.

BOX 1.1   PUTTING IT INTO PRACTICE: THE SOCIAL ECOLOGICAL MODEL

Consider Sam, a divorced, 45-year-old man who lives in a rural community and does shift work at a manufacturing plant. Sam is currently overweight and not very active. We can use a social ecological framework to both understand why Sam isn't active and help develop strategies to increase his activity.

Intrapersonal: Sam used to play sports when he was younger in school but doesn't anymore. He currently lacks motivation toward becoming active and feels self-conscious about going to fitness facilities because he is overweight. He also does not have a lot of extra money each month to pay membership fees. Strategies: Look for opportunities to be active away from the gyms to build up his confidence.

Interpersonal: Sam's brothers are also not very active and spend a lot of time watching television instead of being active. Many of his coworkers are also inactive and unhealthy; they often speak about how they enjoyed activity when they were younger but can't be bothered to do anything now. Strategies: Use local exercise groups as a chance to meet others who are active.

Institutional: At his workplace Sam has access to a worksite wellness program but he does not participate since his shift typically doesn't allow him to. At his last physical his physician indicated that he needed to be more active since his blood pressure and lipids were increasing. Strategies: At the local church, community members can gather for a walking club in the mornings, Sam could join in there.

Community: Sam's community is very rural and there are not a lot of places nearby to be active. The small downtown area has some sidewalks and is pleasant to walk through but outside of town there are no sidewalks for the roads and traffic travels very fast and it is dangerous to walk. Strategies: When heading into town to do errands, Sam could park a few blocks away and get in some walking.

Policy: Recently a policy was passed at the school district level that allows for schools to stay open after hours and on the weekend to provide community members with access to school grounds, gym space and equipment for exercise. Strategies: He could start stopping by to get in some activity on the way home from work.

Application in different populations

The ideas (social determinants of health) and framework (social ecological model) out-lined in this chapter provide the foundation for the discussion of how physical activity and health are impacted among all of the population groups included in this text. These include discussions of race and ethnicity (African Americans, Latinos, Asian Americans, Native Americans, Native Hawaiian and Pacific Islanders), income (low socioeconomic status), location (rural), sexual orientation (lesbian, gay, bisexual and transgender), mili-tary veterans' status, disabled individuals and international populations.

In the United States, the National Physical Activity Plan was developed with the specific purpose of developing a set of programs, policies and initiatives targeting physi-cal activity in all population segments (National Physical Activity Plan 2016). The plan serves as a blueprint for the development of a culture that supports and encourages physical activity across multiple sectors. These sectors (Business and Industry, Com-munity Recreation, Fitness and Parks, Education, Faith-based Settings, Healthcare, Mass Media, Public Health, Sport, and Transportation, Land Use and Community Design) collectively offer opportunities for increasing population-level physical activity partici-pation. This plan is in line with the previously outlined social ecological model and many of the sector strategies are outlined throughout this text as possible approaches for improving physical activity in the different populations featured.

Key terms

The following terms are found throughout the text. A broad definition is offered to provide some context for the chapters.

Barrier: A factor that may impede an individual from participating in a behavior.

Cultural competency: Includes attitudes, beliefs and behaviors that enable an individual to work in a cross-cultural situation.

Ethnicity: Refers to a cultural or ethnic group that individuals identify with or belong with. Typically is a measure of cultural affiliation rather than race or ancestry.

Facilitator: A factor that may encourage or motivate an individual to participate in a behavior.

Intervention: The act of intervening on a behavior in order to change it (e.g. physical inactivity).

Morbidity: This is another term for illness and typically refers to prevalence of a particular disease or condition in a population (e.g. diabetes).

Mortality: Another term for death due to a specific cause within a population (e.g. lung cancer deaths among African Americans).

Race: Refers to the biological characteristics that make a population group similar or may include a social definition where individuals self-identify as a particular racial group.

Randomized controlled trial: The gold standard for research studies; includes measurement of outcomes of interest before and after the trial and a control group with a different (or no) treatment from the experimental group.

Socioeconomic status (SES): Commonly conceptualized as a measure of class and includes income, education and occupation.

Implications for practice

Throughout this chapter, we have outlined the importance of physical activity and how it is measured, defined health disparities and inequities, identified the social determinants of health and discussed a framework for addressing the problem of inactivity. This content will serve as a foundation for further examining the diverse populations outlined in this text and other groups that may be encountered through health and wellness initiatives. As the general population of the United States and other countries become increasingly more diverse, it is important for health and wellness professionals to be comfortable, confident and culturally competent when working with all groups within the population to promote and maintain physical activity and overall health.

Summary points

- There are a number of significant physical and mental health benefits associated with regular physical activity participation.
- Physical activity can be measured in a number of different ways.
- Health disparities are an important public health issue and are related to physical inactivity–related chronic disease morbidity and mortality.
- The social determinants of health refer to the conditions of one's environment where you live, work, learn and play that can impact your health, well-being, quality of life and health behaviors.
- Social ecological frameworks examine factors from across levels from a narrow focus at the individual level to a very broad focus of policy.

Critical thinking questions

1   What are some important considerations for measuring physical activity?
2   What are health disparities? Provide an example.
3   What are the different types of factors that can impact health or engagement in healthy behaviors?
4   Why would the social ecological model be useful for helping to address disparities in physical activity participation in different population groups?

References

Ding, D., Lawson, K. D., Kolbe-Alexander, T. L., Finkelstein, E. A., Katzmarzyk, P. T., Van Mechelen, W., Pratt, M. and Lancet Physical Activity Series 2 Executive Committee. (2016). The economic burden of physical inactivity: A global analysis of major non-communicable diseases. *Lancet*, 388: 1311–1324.

Issac, L. A. (2013). Defining Health and Health Care Disparities and Examining Disparities across the Life Span. *In:* Laveist, T. A. & Issac, L. A. (eds.) *Race, Ethnicity and Health.* 2nd ed. San Francisco: Jossey-Bass.

Kohl, H. W., 3rd, Craig, C. L., Lambert, E. V., Inoue, S., Alkandari, J. R., Leetongin, G. and Kahlmeier, S. (2012). The pandemic of physical inactivity: Global action for public health. *Lancet,* 380: 294–305.

McLeroy, K. R., Bibeau, D., Steckler, A. and Glanz, K. (1988). An ecological perspective on health promotion programs. *Health Education Quarterly,* 15: 351–377.

National Physical Activity Plan. (2016). *National Physical Activity Plan* [Online]. Available: www.physicalactivityplan.org/index.php (Accessed August 8 2016).

Physical Activity Guidelines Advisory Committee. (2008). *Physical Activity Guidelines Advisory Committee Report, 2008.* Washington, DC: US Department of Health and Human Services.

Sallis, J. F., Owen, N. and Fisher, E. B. (2008). Ecological Models of Health Behavior. *In:* Glanz, K., Rimer, B. K. & Viswanth, K. (eds.) *Health Behavior and Health Education: Theory, Research and Practice.* 4th ed. San Francisco: Jossey-Bass.

Sedentary Behavior Research Network. (2017). *What is sedentary behavior* [Online]. Available: www.sedentarybehaviour.org/what-is-sedentary-behaviour/ (Accessed January 13 2017).

U.S. Department of Health and Human Services. (2010). HHS Action Plan to Reduce Racial and Ethnic Health Disparities. Washington, DC: Office of Minority Health, USDHHS.

U.S. Department of Health and Human Services (USDHHS). (2012). *Healthy people 2020* [Online]. Available: www.healthypeople.gov/2020/default.aspx (Accessed June 20 2012).

Whitt-Glover, M. C., Taylor, W. C., Floyd, M. F., Yore, M. M., Yancey, A. K. and Matthews, C. E. (2009). Disparities in physical activity and sedentary behaviors among US children and adolescents: Prevalence, correlates, and intervention implications. *Journal of Public Health Policy,* 30 Suppl 1: S309–S334.

World Health Organization. (2010). *Global Recommendations on Physical Activity for Health.* Geneva, Switzerland: World Health Organization.

World Health Organization. (2014). *Review of Social Determinants and the Health Divide in the WHO European Region: Final Report.* Copenhagen: World Health Organization Regional Office for Europe.

World Health Organization. (2015). *Health in the post-2015 development agenda: Need for a social determinants of health approach* [Online]. Available: www.who.int/social_determinants/advocacy/UN_Platform_FINAL.pdf?ua=1 (Accessed April 5 2016).

Yi, S. S., Bartley, K. F., Firestone, M. J., Lee, K. K. and Eisenhower, D. L. (2015). Self-reported sitting time in New York City adults, the physical activity and transit survey, 2010–2011. *Preventing Chronic Disease,* 12: E85.

Young, D. R., Hivert, M. F., Alhassan, S., Camhi, S. M., Ferguson, J. F., Katzmarzyk, P. T., Lewis, C. E., Owen, N., Perry, C. K., Siddique, J., Yong, C. M., Physical Activity Committee of the Council on Lifestyle and Cardiometabolic Health, Council on Clinical Cardiology, Council on Epidemiology and Prevention, Council on Functional Genomics and Translational Biology and Stroke, C. (2016). Sedentary behavior and cardiovascular morbidity and mortality: A science advisory from the American Heart Association. *Circulation,* 134: e262–e279.

2

INTRODUCTION TO RACE, ETHNICITY, AND RELATED THEORIES OF DISPARITIES

Scherezade K. Mama, Deborah H. John and Nishat Bhuiyan

An examination of disparities in health or health behavior between population groups that are defined along a shared characteristic, such as race, ethnicity, education level, income or socioeconomic status, sexual orientation, disability, veteran status, or geographic location, is best guided by theory, models and frameworks. This chapter provides a guiding framework for examining physical activity in the many populations discussed in this text. The first half of this chapter describes theories that have been developed to explain health disparities, predict health outcomes, or change health behaviors, such as physical activity. The second half of this chapter explores systems theories and determinants of health status among several population groups, which are explored in more detail throughout this book.

Theories of health disparities related to physical activity

A behavioral theory is a set of interrelated concepts that present a systematic view of behavior by specifying relationships among variables in order to explain and predict the behavior (Glanz *et al.* 2002). Theories help you understand a behavior and to design and evaluate health behavior and health promotion interventions based on that understanding (National Cancer Institute 2005). Behavioral theories can be explanatory or change theories. An *explanatory* theory helps describe why a particular problem or disparity exists and guides the search for modifiable factors. A *change* theory guides the development and evaluation of interventions to change behavior.

Although explanatory and change theories have different foci, one on describing *why* a problem exists (e.g. physical inactivity) and the other on *how* to intervene on a problem (e.g. promoting physical activity), they are complementary. Thus, we will explore examples of both in this chapter. We will organize our approach within the social ecological model, as outlined in Chapter 1. These theories are categorized as biological and physiological theories, psychosocial and behavioral theories, and socio-environmental theories, as described in the following sections and shown in Table 2.1.

TABLE 2.1 Theories of health disparities related to physical activity and conceptual frameworks used for community-level interventions

Theories

Biological and physiological theories

Psychosocial and behavioral theories of health

    Individual or intrapersonal level

        Transtheoretical Model

        Theory of Planned Behavior

    Interpersonal level

        Social Cognitive Theory

    Socioenvironmental theories of health disparities

        Risk Exposure Theory

        Resource Deprivation Theory

Conceptual frameworks

Community-Based Participatory Research

Diffusion of Innovation Theory

Community Readiness Model

Biological and physiological theories of health disparities

Biological and physiological theories of health disparities suggest possible ways that biological factors or genetics may explain health disparities among different identity groups. Existing research suggests that biological factors or genetics influence health disparities directly or through interactions with the environment (LaVeist 2005). The direct influence of biological factors or genetics on health outcomes suggests that there are biological or genetic differences among population groups that lead to increased risk of disease. For example, research suggests that African American adults are more insulin resistant than their non-Hispanic white counterparts and have upregulated beta cell function, resulting in increased insulin secretion and development of type 2 diabetes mellitus (Hasson *et al.* 2015). However, there have been mixed findings on the actual contribution of racial differences to insulin secretion and disparities in type 2 diabetes, which suggest that gene-environment interactions may be more likely to explain health disparities.

Socioecological models, like the Ecologic Model of Physical Activity (see Box 2.1), suggest that sociocultural, environmental, or lifestyle factors may explain differences rather than true biological factors or genetics. Recent epigenetic work in the cancer field suggests that the environment can cause changes in behavior that increase or decrease the expression of genes or particular traits via DNA methylation (Phillips 2008). For example, Jean Baptiste Lamarck posited that the giraffe developed its long neck from the "inner need" to stretch and reach leaves higher up on trees. Similarly, cancer researchers suggest that modifiable factors, like physical activity and nutrition, and non-modifiable factors, like age, race/ethnicity and gender, influence epigenetic modifications and result in disease (Bishop and Ferguson 2015). Although there is growing evidence for the link between gene–environmental interactions and physical activity (Hibler 2015), there is limited research on differences by population groups. This is a promising new area of research that may identify population groups at high risk for disease for whom physical activity interventions may alter their risk and related health disparities.

BOX 2.1   ECOLOGIC MODEL OF PHYSICAL ACTIVITY (EMPA)

Rebecca Lee and Catherine Cubbin

Lee and Cubbin (2009) proposed that the physical activity context should be examined through an ecologically grounded social justice lens. They hypothesized that external forces – social injustices and environmental inequities – shape socially disadvantaged individuals' ability to meet physical activity recommendations differently compared to socially advantaged individuals. These external forces also differentially shape interactions with physical activity opportunities at every environmental level, including micro-, meso-, exo-, and macro-environments.

For example, the micro-level closest to the individual includes the day-to-day living, learning, working, and playing contexts. The most frequently reported barriers to physical activity at the micro-level are time and inconvenience (Centers for Disease Control and Prevention 2011). While these intrapersonal factors can be examined using the psychosocial theories described in Chapter 2 and interventions developed to increase self-efficacy to overcome barriers and provoke behavior change, applying a justice lens will reveal the reality of disparate conditions that individuals have to overcome to be similarly physically active. Consider time a barrier to physical activity reported by working women. Single women with children, who also have long commutes to work, work long hours for low wages, and, at a workplace without resources to be physically active, will have more time and schedule constraints for physical activity. They will have to personally exert more effort to overcome those scheduling barriers than men, single women without children, or married women with children. Inequitable distribution of physical activity resources or supports in the micro-environments of diverse individuals contribute to physical activity disparities among diverse individuals.

The meso- and exo-environments connect an individual's micro-environments and include both physical and social contexts. The physical commute or commuting environment between home and work or school is an example of the meso-environment. The social environmental linkage between a parent's workplace and their child's school is an example of the exo-environment. Commuting between home and work represents an environmental factor that may affect physical activity differently for rural populations, populations of color, and those with low socioeconomic status. Active transportation, including walking and biking to or from work or school, is less likely in rural places with greater distance between destinations. Lower socioeconomic status, urban residents who use public transit for commuting are subject to transit schedules and spend time inactively waiting or riding. This counteracts the active time spent walking to and from the transit stops before and after their workday. Besides increasing sedentary time, vehicular commuting also limits time for shared physical activities between parents and children or within social groups.

Social interactions and connectedness are theorized to be key supportive mechanisms for overcoming individual and environmental barriers to physical activity. School and workplace contexts, which are resourced differently among schools and worksites, have the capacity to directly and indirectly influence physical activity values, motives, and patterns of individuals in families. Students who attend schools in higher socioeconomic status neighborhoods with high-quality physical education programs may also participate in recreational physical activities on school fields, and higher socioeconomic status students may have parents who participate in workplace-based physical activities and who support recreational physical activity as a valued family norm. In contrast, students who attend under-resourced schools in lower socioeconomic status neighborhoods may not be exposed to a structured physical education program, may not have opportunities, real or perceived, to safely participate in before and after school physical activity programs, and may have a parent or parents who work long hours, rarely participate in leisure-time physical activity, and have few resources to enable physical activity involvement for the family.

The macro-environmental level represents influences that are most distant to the individual's everyday experience, yet influence inequitably across groups. National and state policies, such as those requiring physical education in schools, are only effective when implemented and resourced equitably among schools. National initiatives like the U.S. Surgeon General's *Step It Up* 2015 Call to Action (U.S. Department of Health and Human Services 2015) centers walking and neighborhood walkability as a key public health strategy for increasing physical activity in all people at all ages and life stages. Despite the recognition that individuals make the decision to walk, *Step It Up* contends that all people have the right to make easy, safe choices and to have easy access to safe walking programs and walkable features supported by policies that encourage walking and community walkability. It will be interesting to observe the physical activity impact of a national call to action when examined through a social justice lens for physical activity equity at every ecological level.

Psychosocial and behavioral theories of health disparities

Psychosocial and behavioral theories of health disparities suggest possible ways that individual-level and interpersonal factors may explain health behaviors, like physical activity, and contribute to health disparities among different identity groups.

Individual or intrapersonal level

Theories and models targeting the individual or intra- (within) person level often seek to modify individual characteristics that influence physical activity, such as knowledge, attitudes, beliefs, motivation, self-concept, past experience, and skills. One theory used to explain behavior change that is commonly applied to physical activity is the Transtheoretical Model. This model recognizes that changing unhealthy behaviors, like physical inactivity or sedentary behavior, is challenging and occurs as a process and in stages rather than as a one-time event (Glanz and Bishop 2010, Prochaska and Velicer 1997).

The five stages, as originally described by Prochaska and DiClemente (1983), are precontemplation, contemplation, preparation, action, and maintenance. Termination was later added as a sixth stage of change (Prochaska and Velicer 1997). Descriptions of each stage of change and examples of physical activity intervention strategies applied to each stage are presented in Table 2.2. The Transtheoretical Model refutes the "one-size-fits-all" philosophy and, instead, argues that interventions should be tailored based on an individual's stage of readiness to change.

Another theory used to explain behavior change that has been applied to physical activity research is the Theory of Planned Behavior. This theory suggests that behavior is a result of intention, which is influenced by an individual's attitudes toward the behavior, subjective norms about the behavior, and their perceived behavioral control over the behavior or their confidence in their ability to change (self-efficacy) (Ajzen and Driver 1991, National Cancer Institute *et al.* 2005). The Theory of Planned Behavior takes into account an individual's social context or environment and recognizes that there are conditions outside of an individual's control that may restrict them from engaging in a behavior, like physical activity. This theory is useful for understanding behaviors of diverse individuals by accounting for salient beliefs, including cultural or normative beliefs, about a behavior and perceived behavioral control or self-efficacy. However, the Theory of Planned Behavior does not take into account individual personality variables, demographic differences, or exposure to environmental variables. The Transtheoretical Model and Theory of Planned Behavior also fail to account for various other intrapersonal factors, such as motivation, competence, and health beliefs. Therefore, a combination of these theoretical models and or other models described within this chapter may be more predictive and useful for developing physical activity programs and interventions.

TABLE 2.2 Stages of change and physical activity intervention examples

Stage of Change and Description	Physical Activity Intervention Example
Precontemplation No intention to take action in the near future (within the next 6 months).	Educate individuals on the consequences of physical inactivity and sedentary lifestyles; encourage individuals to begin thinking and talking about their unhealthy behaviors.
Contemplation Thinking about changing behavior within the next 6 months.	Discuss the pros and cons of becoming physically active or starting a new exercise routine; encourage individuals to work through costs and benefits and the ambivalence contributing to procrastination; encourage individuals to become emotionally invested in the problem of physical inactivity.
Preparation Intends to take action to change behavior in the immediate future (within the next month); has a plan of action and may have taken some small steps toward action (e.g., joined a class, consulted a health professional, bought a self-help book or downloaded an app).	Enroll emotionally charged individual in an action-oriented physical activity program; provide with a calendar of physical activity sessions, so that they may add them to their calendar and plan their exercise routine.
Action Has made specific overt change in their lifestyles within the past 6 months.	Individuals are engaged in regular exercise and are meeting physical activity recommendations for important health benefits (150 minutes of moderate-intensity aerobic activity every week and muscle-strengthening activities on 2 or more days a week).[b]
Maintenance Has maintained healthy lifestyle changes for over 6 months; striving to prevent relapse.	Foster individual's self-efficacy to continue their regular exercise routine; provide booster sessions from 6 months up to 5 years.
Termination[a] No temptation to relapse; healthy behavior becomes automatic (total self-efficacy).	Not realistic for most physical activity interventions, where the goal is to promote a lifetime of maintenance.

a Not realistic for most people, and, therefore, has not been emphasized in the Transtheoretical Model and in physical activity research.
b Physical Activity Guidelines Advisory Committee (2008). *Physical Activity Guidelines Advisory Committee Report, 2008*, Washington, DC, U.S. Department of Health and Human Services.

Interpersonal level

Theories and models targeting the interpersonal level often seek to influence individuals' situational environments, including people within their environment, such as their family, friends, coworkers, health care professionals, and so on. Social

Cognitive Theory has been used to explain the dynamic, interactive relationships among personal factors, such as those described in the previous section, physical and social environmental factors external to the individual, and health behavior (Bandura 1977, 1986). One of the most frequently applied theories of health behavior, Social Cognitive Theory has been widely used to both explain and guide health behavior change (Baranowski *et al.* 2002). The core determinants of behavior suggested by this theory influence an individual's learning to engage in healthful or health risk behaviors (Bandura 2004).

Although there are a number of core determinants in the Social Cognitive Theory, behavioral capabilities, outcome expectancies, observational learning, and self-efficacy are the key constructs in this theory that have been explored and help explain how people both initiate and maintain physical activity and reduce sedentary behaviors over time (Fjeldsoe *et al.* 2013, Sharpe *et al.* 2008, Stahl *et al.* 2001, Van Dyck *et al.* 2011). Behavioral capability refers to an individual's knowledge and skill or ability to perform a behavior and is obtained through skills training and mastery experiences. For example, teaching an individual how to use a treadmill and allowing them to test the treadmill increases their behavioral capability to walk on the treadmill. Outcome expectancies or outcome expectations are the anticipated outcomes of a particular behavior. Examples of outcome expectancies related to physical activity may include increased endurance or stamina while performing physical activity, weight loss, and improved cardiovascular function and health. Observational learning, also referred to as peer or social modeling, describes how the behavior of others may influence an individual's behavior. For example, having others who look similar, such as family members, friends, or co-workers or others in a similar situation (e.g., an expecting mother or new mother) who are engaging in physical activity and achieving success (e.g., able to maintain a regular physical activity routine) can promote or aid physical activity adoption and maintenance. Lastly, perceived self-efficacy is the most widely studied and understood construct in the Social Cognitive Theory and describes an individual's confidence or beliefs about their ability to engage in a valued behavior (Bandura 1994).

Although the Social Cognitive Theory is the most widely used theory to explain and change health behaviors, it has its limitations. Because the model uses an all in the "kitchen sink" approach, it is difficult to tease out the effects of any one construct on behavior change. It is also difficult to measure constructs of the theory, like behavioral capability, which combines knowledge and skills, which raises concerns about reliability. Additional research is needed and underway to understand which Social Cognitive Theory constructs explain versus predict health behaviors, like physical activity.

Socioenvironmental theories of health disparities

Socioenvironmental or contextual theories of health disparities suggest possible ways social factors or environmental exposures may contribute to health disparities and poor health outcomes among identity groups. These theories emphasize the community context in which people live, learn, work, play, and visit. Although community places are often designated in geographic or spatial terms, communities may also be described by other criteria, like race/ethnicity, culture, or another collective social identity (National Cancer Institute *et al.* 2005).

Risk Exposure Theory and Resource Deprivation Theory were developed to explain the higher prevalence of disease and death in racial/ethnic minority communities. Risk Exposure Theory states that a high prevalence of social and environmental health risks results in higher exposure to these risks, contributing to increased risk of morbidity and mortality (LaVeist 2005). Resource Deprivation Theory states that low presence or access to resources that support health and healthy lifestyles also contributes to increased risk of morbidity and mortality. Together, these theories suggest that individuals or identity groups with high exposure to social and environmental health risks and low access to resources that support a healthy lifestyle have the highest prevalence of disease and death, which adds to health disparities. An example of these theories applied to physical activity would be the presence of increased crime, poor pedestrian environments, and poor access to and quality of physical activity resources, like parks and community centers, in low socioeconomic status neighborhoods or communities where racial/ethnic minorities live, learn, work, and recreate. Previous research suggests that, even when physical activity resources and favorable built environments are available, exposure to the social environment in certain communities may deter individuals from being physically active (Salvo *et al.* 2014, Steinmetz-Wood and Kestens 2015).

Conceptual frameworks for community-level interventions

Both Risk Exposure Theory and Resource Deprivation Theory seek to explain physical activity or inactivity behavior as a consequence of socioenvironmental exposures. Conceptual frameworks, like the Social Ecological Model (see Figure 1.2) or Diffusion of Innovation Theory, and participatory approaches, like Community-Based Participatory Research, have utility for shaping socioenvironmental interventions that aim to incidentally change health behaviors like physical activity. Community-Based Participatory Research uses a collaborative approach to behavior change by equitably involving all stakeholders in the research process, from conception through implementation and evaluation (Israel *et al.* 2013, Minkler and Wallerstein 2008). This community-level approach is often guided by behavioral theories, such as the Social Cognitive Theory, to account for and address multiple levels of influence on a health problem or behavior. Community-based participatory approaches begin with the community's identified issues and seek to empower communities to set priorities and drive change. Because participatory discovery and action research approaches start by engaging the community in identifying the community's issues and priorities, resulting programs and interventions are more relevant to the community and sustainable. Churches and faith-based organizations have been identified as key partners in the effort to promote health and reduce health disparities (Campbell *et al.* 2007) among diverse congregations. Research suggests that physical activity interventions that partner with faith-based organizations using a participatory approach have been successful for promoting physical activity and changing health behaviors in ethnic minority communities (Coughlin and Smith 2016, Fawcett *et al.* 2013, Wilcox *et al.* 2013). These approaches are outlined in more detail in Chapter 3.

The premise of the Diffusion of Innovation Theory is that it is not enough to simply understand and change health behavior, but that an emphasis must also be placed on disseminating successful interventions among hard-to-reach populations in an effort to reduce health disparities (Rogers 1995). Diffusion theory centers on the conditions that increase or decrease the likelihood that an innovative intervention or program will be adopted by members of a given culture or community. Adoption of a new idea is facilitated by social interaction through interpersonal networks. The theory considers that innovations are not adopted by all individuals in a social system at the same time. Thus, like participatory approaches and ecological models, Diffusion of Innovation Theory is a complementary socioenvironmental theory to the psychosocial and behavioral theories and models discussed previously, and it has been used to increase the number of individuals exposed to evidenced-based behavior change interventions in an effort to promote health and reduce health disparities.

Socioenvironmental or contextual theories of health disparities suggest that changing the context is key to reducing health disparities and assuring equitable access to healthy lifestyle resources and supports for all individuals, groups, and communities. The Community Readiness Model is a theoretical framework for determining a community's stage of readiness to take action to address a health priority (Edwards *et al.* 2000). Community readiness is determined according to nine stages (no awareness, denial or resistance, vague awareness, preplanning, preparation, initiation, stabilization, confirmation/expansion, and high level of community ownership) and six dimensions (community knowledge of issue, current efforts, community knowledge of efforts, leadership, current resources, and community climate). The model operates on the premises that a community's stage of readiness is issue-specific and varies among dimensions of readiness and stakeholder groups within a community. The rate of progress is determined by the community dimension operating at the lowest stage of readiness to change (Edwards *et al.* 2000). The Community Readiness Model is a participatory approach to changing the context that has raised awareness of socioenvironmental inequities that contribute to disparities in health and health behaviors among population groups and impact the health of all people within a community. These three frameworks provide opportunity for developing and delivering intervention programs that promote physical activity, using many of the tailored strategies that Chapter 3 outlines in greater detail.

Social systems and categories of difference

The theories and conceptual frameworks described previously help illustrate how social and environmental determinants contribute to the health status and health behaviors of individuals. They also help us understand how disparities in health and health behaviors form among population groups. These are explored in greater detail in subsequent chapters. However, this section briefly presents systems theories and social determinants of health, and how social determinants intersect with the system of privilege and oppression to influence health status and health behaviors.

Historically, systems theories organize social institutions (e.g., science) and sectors (e.g., the health sector) within an interlocking hierarchical structure that is set up to maintain social order. Power, privilege, and social status are produced and reproduced within the system and are based on social identity and group membership. The *interlocking systems of oppression* theory states that socially constructed categories, such as race and ethnicity, socioeconomic status, and gender, are collectively meaningful when examining and challenging power, privilege, and social status within social institutions. Thus, in order to understand and improve individuals' health status and health behaviors, it is important to recognize the multiple and intersecting categories of difference. These categories of difference additively contribute to differences in power and privilege between and within racial and ethnic groups. For example, African American women and Asian American men experience power and privilege differently due to differences in both their race *and* gender.

Interlocking systems of oppression theory explains that sexism, racism, classism, heterosexism, ableism, ageism, and other –isms are experienced, resisted, and reproduced on three levels: personal biographies, group cultural or symbolic context, and social systems or institutions. These levels are similar to those described in the social ecological model in Chapter 1 and are sites of privilege and prejudice (Collins 1993). The personal biographies level, similar to the intrapersonal level, has to do with individual differences or one's unique personal biography, comprising experiences, biology, motivations, emotions, abilities, talents, and social identities, including gender, race or ethnicity, and social class. The group cultural or symbolic context acknowledges the impact of cultural beliefs that give meaning to individual biographies. Last, the social systems or institutions level, which encompasses the personal biographies and the group cultural or symbolic context, frames the systematic ways social institutions (e.g., medicine, education, the media, industry, government) are structured in order to maintain power and privilege of the dominant or socially advantaged group (Collins 1993). All three levels serve to maintain the dominant order and perpetuate hierarchies that intersect and interact by one's social identities and group memberships, or their categories of difference.

When the intersectional social inequalities described previously are paired with systematic exposure to negative socioenvironmental factors, it leads to tremendous inequalities in the ability of individuals to meet minimal physical activity guidelines to protect health. Some environmental factors, such as unsafe neighborhoods, lack of access to physical activity resources, absence of a supportive built environment for active transportation, inaccessibility of health information, and geographic isolation, make physical activity harder for some groups than others. Adapting Braveman and Gruskin's (2003) definition of social justice, we can operationalize *socially just* physical activity to mean *the absence of systematic disparities in physical activity (or in the major determinants of physical activity) between social groups who have different levels of underlying social advantage or disadvantage.* This definition is rooted in the principle of fairness. **That is, in a just society, opportunities to be physically active are equally distributed as a right, not a privilege, for everyone.** It challenges the current physical activity system, which positions people who are more socially advantaged (due to the intersection of their gender, race or ethnicity, or socioeconomic status) to more easily be able to take advantages of opportunities to be physically active and meeting physical activity recommendations compared to those who are socially disadvantaged.

Conclusion

Attributes of people, including genetic, biological, physical, psychological, psychosocial, and demographic attributes, interplay with socioenvironmental, structural, physical, and political attributes of the behavioral environment, which is experienced and exercises pressure directly and indirectly in the places people live, learn, work, play, and visit. At every level of influence, theories have been applied to explain disparities, predict health outcomes, or change health behaviors, such as physical activity. Thus, it is important to understand theories that help explain health disparities, predict health outcomes, and change health behaviors in addition to being aware of how systems theories and determinants of health status intersect and interact to perpetuate health disparities and impact health status among different population groups.

Summary points

- Behavioral theories and conceptual frameworks help us understand how social determinants of health contribute to the health status and health behaviors of individuals.
- Behavioral theories, conceptual frameworks and change models, like Social Cognitive Theory, Transtheoretical Model, and Community Readiness Model are used to design and evaluate health behavior and health promotion interventions.
- Systems theories organize social institutions and sectors and help us understand how social determinants of health contribute to health disparities between and within different population groups.
- Behavioral theories and conceptual frameworks coupled with systems theories help us understand how health disparities are perpetuated among different population groups and how social determinants of health differentially impact population groups.

Critical thinking questions

1   How are biological and physiological theories, psychosocial and behavioral theories, and socioenvironmental theories similar? How are they different? Describe how these theories overlap and/or complement each other to impact physical activity in individuals.

2   How do conceptual frameworks for community-level interventions differ from behavior change theories? How are the two used together to change health behaviors and improve health status?

3   How do systems theories maintain social order? Provide an example.

References

Ajzen, I. and Driver, B. L. (1991). 'Prediction of leisure participation from behavioral, normative, and control beliefs: An application of the Theory of Planned Behavior.' *Leisure Sciences*, 13: 185–204.

Bandura, A. (1977). *Social Learning Theory*. Englewood Cliffs, NJ: Prentice Hall.

Bandura, A. (1986). *Social Foundations of Thought and Action*. Englewood Cliffs, NJ: Prentice Hall.

Bandura, A. (1994). 'Self-Efficacy.' *In*: Ramachaudran, V. S. (ed.) *Encyclopedia of Human Behavior*. New York, NY: Academic Press.

Bandura, A. (2004). 'Health promotion by social cognitive means.' *Health Education and Behavior*, 31: 143–64.

Baranowski, T., Perry, C. L. and Parcel, G. S. (2002). 'How Individuals, Environments, and Health Behavior Interact: Social Cognitive Theory.' *In*: Glanz, K., Rimer, B. K. and Lewis, F. M. (eds.) *Health Behavior and Health Education: Theory, Research, and Practice*. 3rd ed. San Francisco, CA: Jossey-Bass.

Bishop, K. S. and Ferguson, L. R. (2015). 'The interaction between epigenetics, nutrition and the development of cancer.' *Nutrients*, 7: 922–47.

Braveman, P. and Gruskin, S. (2003). 'Defining equity in health.' *Journal of Epidemiology and Community Health*, 57: 254–8.

Campbell, M. K., Hudson, M. A., Resnicow, K., Blakeney, N., Paxton, A. and Baskin, M. (2007). 'Church-based health promotion interventions: Evidence and lessons learned.' *Annual Reviews in Public Health*, 28: 213–34.

Centers for Disease Control and Prevention. (2011). *Overcoming Barriers to Physical Activity* [Online]. Atlanta, GA: Centers for Disease Control and Prevention. Available: www.cdc.gov/physicalactivity/basics/adding-pa/barriers.html (Accessed 15 May 2016).

Collins, P. H. (1993). 'Toward a new vision: Race, class, and gender as categories of analysis and connection.' *Race, Sex & Class*, 1: 25–45.

Coughlin, S. S. and Smith, S. A. (2016). 'A review of community-based participatory research studies to promote physical activity among African Americans.' *Journal of Georgia Public Health Association*, 5: 220–7.

Edwards, R. W., Jumper-Thurman, P., Plested, B. A., Oetting, E. R. and Swanson, L. (2000). 'Community readiness: Research to practice.' *Journal of Community Psychology*, 28: 291–307.

Fawcett, S. B., Collie-Akers, V., Schultz, J. A. and Cupertino, P. (2013). 'Community-based participatory research within the Latino health for all coalition.' *Journal of Prevention and Intervention in the Community*, 41: 142–54.

Fjeldsoe, B. S., Miller, Y. D. and Marshall, A. L. (2013). 'Social cognitive mediators of the effect of the MobileMums intervention on physical activity.' *Health Psychology*, 32: 729–38.

Glanz, K. and Bishop, D. B. (2010). 'The role of behavioral science theory in development and implementation of public health interventions.' *Annual Reviews in Public Health*, 31: 399–418.

Glanz, K., Rimer, B. K. and Lewis, F. M. (2002). 'Theory, Research, and Practice in Health Behavior and Health Education.' *In*: Glanz, K., Rimer, B. K. and Lewis, F. M. (eds.) *Health Behavior and Health Education: Theory, Research, and Practice*. 3rd ed. San Francisco, CA: Jossey-Bass.

Hasson, B. R., Apovian, C. and Istfan, N. (2015). 'Racial/ethnic differences in insulin resistance and beta cell function: Relationship to racial disparities in type 2 diabetes among African Americans versus Caucasians.' *Current Obesity Reports*, 4: 241–9.

Hibler, E. (2015). 'Epigenetics and colorectal neoplasia: The evidence for physical activity and sedentary behavior.' *Current Colorectal Cancer Reports*, 11: 388–96.

Israel, B., Eng, E., Schulz, A. and Parker, E. A. (2013). 'Introduction to the Methods for CBPR for Health.' *In:* Isreal, B., Eng, E., Schulz, A. and Parker, E. A. (eds.) *Methods for Community-Based Participatory Research for Health*. 2nd ed. San Francisco, CA: Jossey-Bass.

LaVeist, T. A. (2005). 'Theories of Racial/Ethnic Differences in Health.' *In: Minority Populations and Health: An Introduction to Health Disparities in the United States*. 1st ed. San Francisco, CA: Jossey-Bass.

Lee, R. E. and Cubbin, C. (2009). 'Striding toward social justice: The ecologic milieu of physical activity.' *Exercise and Sport Science Reviews*, 37: 10–17.

Minkler, M. and Wallerstein, N. (2008). 'Introduction to Community-Based Participatory Research: New Issues and Emphasis.' *In:* Minkler, M. and Wallerstein, N. (eds.) *Community-Based Participatory Research for Health: From Process to Outcomes*. 2nd ed. San Francisco, CA: Jossey-Bass.

National Cancer Institute, National Institutes of Health and U.S. Department of Health and Human Services. (2005). 'Theory at a Glance: A Guide for Health Promotion Practice.' 2nd ed. Bethesda, MD: National Cancer Institute, National Institutes of Health, U.S. Department of Health and Human Services.

Phillips, T. (2008). 'The role of methylation in gene expression.' *Nature Education*, 1: 116.

Prochaska, J. O. and DiClemente, C. C. (1983). 'Stages and processes of self-change of smoking: Toward an integrative model of change.' *Journal of Consulting and Clinical Psychology*, 51: 390–5.

Prochaska, J. O. and Velicer, W. F. (1997). 'The transtheoretical model of health behavior change.' *American Journal of Health Promotion*, 12: 38–48.

Rogers, E. M. (1995). *Diffusion of Innovations*. New York, NY: Free Press.

Salvo, D., Reis, R. S., Stein, A. D., Rivera, J., Martorell, R. and Pratt, M. (2014). 'Characteristics of the built environment in relation to objectively measured physical activity among Mexican adults, 2011.' *Preventing Chronic Disease*, 11: E147.

Sharpe, P. A., Granner, M. L., Hutto, B. E., Wilcox, S., Peck, L. and Addy, C. L. (2008). 'Correlates of physical activity among African American and White women.' *American Journal of Health Behavior*, 32: 701–13.

Stahl, T., Rutten, A., Nutbeam, D., Bauman, A., Kannas, L., Abel, T., Luschen, G., Rodriquez, D. J., Vinck, J. and Van Der Zee, J. (2001). 'The importance of the social environment for physically active lifestyle: Results from an international study.' *Social Science Medicine*, 52: 1–10.

Steinmetz-Wood, M. and Kestens, Y. (2015). 'Does the effect of walkable built environments vary by neighborhood socioeconomic status?' *Preventive Medicine*, 81: 262–7.

U.S. Department of Health and Human Services. (2015). *Step It Up! The Surgeon General's Call to Action to Promote Walking and Walkable Communities*. Washington, DC: U.S. Department of Health and Human Services, Office of the Surgeon General.

Van Dyck, D., De Greef, K., Deforche, B., Ruige, J., Tudor-Locke, C. E., Kaufman, J. M., Owen, N. and De Bourdeaudhuij, I. (2011). 'Mediators of physical activity change in a behavioral modification program for type 2 diabetes patients.' *International Journal of Behavioral Nutrition and Physical Activity*, 8: 105.

Wilcox, S., Parrott, A., Baruth, M., Laken, M., Condrasky, M., Saunders, R., Dowda, M., Evans, R., Addy, C., Warren, T. Y., Kinnard, D. and Zimmerman, L. (2013). 'The Faith, Activity, and Nutrition program: A randomized controlled trial in African-American churches.' *American Journal of Preventive Medicine*, 44: 122–31.

3

DEVELOPMENT OF CULTURALLY APPROPRIATE STRATEGIES FOR PROMOTING PHYSICAL ACTIVITY

Sandra Soto, Adrian Chavez, Jessica Haughton and Elva M. Arredondo

Understanding culture and health

The impact and sustainability of health promotion efforts are enhanced when the cultural characteristics of a target group are taken into account and integrated into the framework of an intervention, service, or system (Conn *et al.* 2014, Nierkens *et al.* 2013). Culture includes complex and multi-dimensional constructs that refer to socially derived beliefs, symbols, institutions, values, rules, practices, communication patterns, and familial roles, among others that are learned and shared inter-generationally (Barrera *et al.* 2013, Kreuter *et al.* 2003). Another important characteristic of culture is that it changes over time in response to new experiences and contexts (Kreuter *et al.* 2003, Marsiglia and Booth 2015). For example, culture may change when individuals immigrate from their country of origin to a new country or reside in a new environment or country for an extended period of time (e.g., acculturation). Culture is also known to influence health behaviors and individuals' response to health promotion strategies (Kreuter and McClure 2004, Marsiglia and Booth 2015). Therefore, it is important for public health practitioners and researchers to understand the role of culture as it relates to physical activity and to have a toolbox of strategies that will enable cultural integration into physical activity interventions. In this chapter, we define culture and describe its influence on physical activity behaviors, as well as provide suggestions for how to develop culturally competent/sensitive interventions.

Culture and physical activity

Culture represents the manner in which individuals perceive the world, their attitudes, beliefs, values toward behaviors, and decisions to behave in certain ways (e.g., engage in physical activity; Fernando 2010). Race/ethnicity, gender roles, social class (e.g., SES), and religious traditions are important contributors to culture (Betancourt and López 1993). Given that culture is difficult to define and measure (Fernando 2010), many researchers use race/ethnicity or other cultural characteristics as a proxy for culture. In a qualitative study among English-speaking middle-aged women representing four racial/ethnic backgrounds (i.e., White, African American, Latina, and Asian), participants engaged in an online forum (e.g., focus groups) to discuss their attitudes toward physical activity (Im *et al.* 2013). Four key differences were found between the groups of women. First, White women aspired to engage in daily physical activity, whereas minority women identified more barriers and family obligations that prohibited them from engaging in routine physical activity. Second, White participants preferred organized fitness classes and gyms, whereas minority participants were satisfied with engaging in physical activity through non-structured methods (e.g., walking outdoors). Third, using physical activity as a means to achieve a slim body type was common among White and Asian participants. On the contrary, African American and Latina participants explained that their culture had different ideals for women's body types that allowed them to be less self-conscious about exercising in public or made it easier for them to undervalue physical activity. Lastly, White participants had a more individualized perspective on their engagement in physical activity than minority women. Specifically, White participants believed the decision to be active was theirs alone, whereas minority women had a more collectivist view and believed they had to weigh the responsibility to their families in their decision to be active. This last finding is prevalent in the literature among minority women (Vrazel *et al.* 2008). In addition to household responsibilities, minority women, in particular, Latinas, also rely on spousal support for their decision to engage in physical activity (Vrazel *et al.* 2008). Among Latinos, the influential role of husbands on their wives' engagement in physical activity has roots in the traditional cultural characteristics of patriarchal authority and *marianismo*. Patriarchal authority refers to the traditional role of men as the decision-makers for the family (Cantu and Fleuriet 2008), whereas *marianismo* refers to women's priority for providing and caring for their families over their own needs (D'Alonzo 2012). Gender roles can also define the types of activity and whether or not women engage in physical activity. Latina women, for example, have been discouraged from engaging in certain sports (e.g., basketball) and activities (e.g., bike riding) because it is believed that these activities can be harmful to their reproductive health (Im *et al.* 2010, Juarbe *et al.* 2003). Throughout this text we will highlight differences in physical activity participation and influences by gender because of these well-documented roles. Chapters 4 through 8 highlight some of these concepts by racial or ethnic group.

Social class is another important contributor to culture, which can also influence engagement in physical activity. Indicators of individual and neighborhood SES (e.g., income, household wealth, education, occupation prestige) are aspects of social class. As illustrated by Kraus *et al.* (2011) social class influences individuals' preferences and behaviors through the neighborhoods they live in, the schools they attend, the foods they consume, and the types of recreation they engage in.

Researchers have found that individuals of lower SES or living in lower SES neighborhoods are less likely to engage in moderate or vigorous physical activity than individuals of higher SES or living in higher SES neighborhoods (Giles-Corti and Donovan 2002, Parks *et al.* 2003). For example, women living in low SES neighborhoods reported engaging in fewer moderate activities than women living in moderate SES neighborhoods (Lee *et al.* 2007). Additionally, women living in high SES neighborhoods reported engaging in more vigorous activities than women in moderate SES neighborhoods. The authors suggested that higher-quality resources in moderate to high SES neighborhoods (e.g., less litter and graffiti) may promote engagement in moderate and vigorous activities. The authors also found that women in low SES neighborhoods reported overall greater energy expenditure than other women, suggesting that women in low SES neighborhoods may expend energy through daily activities (e.g., household chores, walking for transportation) rather than through structured exercise. It is important to note that these findings were present regardless of women's race/ethnicity. Therefore, although race/ethnicity and SES may overalap (Williams *et al.* 2010), social class plays its own, independent role in physical activity. Chapter 9 addresses many of these issues pertaining to social class.

The relationship between culture and physical activity can be complex and the nature of this relation will be unique to the target population. As a result, it would be valuable for public health professionals to consider how culture may impact physical activity behaviors in the design and implementation of culturally competent/sensitive physical activity interventions (Yancey *et al.* 2006). The following sections will provide a definition for cultural competency/sensitivity and provide examples of how culturally competent/sensitive physical activity promotion strategies can be developed or adapted.

Approaches for developing culturally competent and sensitive interventions

Cultural competency and sensitivity

Numerous terms, including *culturally adapted, appropriate, based, competent, informed, matched, relevant, responsive, sensitive, targeted,* and *tailored,* are used to describe the incorporation of cultural characteristics of the target population into health promotion strategies (Conn *et al.* 2014, Cross 1989). For the purpose of this text, we will use the term *culturally competent/sensitive* to describe the extent to which congruent behaviors, attitudes, and policies of a specific cultural group are used in a respectful and skillful manner to promote physical activity (Barrera *et al.* 2013, Cross 1989, Nierkens *et al.* 2013). In other words, to deliver a program that is culturally competent/sensitive, public health professionals should be knowledgeable about the cultural factors at play with regard to physical activity and the preferences and barriers to engaging in a health program of a particular cultural group (Brach and Fraserirector 2000).

Cultural targeting and tailoring

Cultural targeting and tailoring are two distinct concepts, though they are often used interchangeably (Kreuter *et al.* 1999). The two concepts are similar in that they both refer to the use of strategies to adapt an intervention to the values and beliefs of a specific group or individual (Kreuter *et al.* 2003). In the case of cultural targeting, an intervention is adapted to match a group's culture, whereas, in the case of tailoring, an intervention is adapted to a specific individual.

Interventions can effectively *target* a group that is well defined. For example, intervention strategies can target a previously inactive group by implementing feasible activities such as walking groups or beginner-level group exercise classes. A physical activity intervention may also target specific cultural groups by incorporating common cultural themes into intervention strategies. An example of how this may be accomplished among African Americans or Latinos is by including a religious component in the intervention. While using broad generalizations about a cultural group is not advised, this approach may be successful given a relatively homogenous group (e.g., Latina mothers, church-going African Americans; Kreuter *et al.* 2003). However, even within a homogenous cultural group, variability will exist between individuals of that group. For instance, among a group of Asian mothers, some individuals will have young children in the home, whereas others will have adult children who no longer live at home. Although the levels of family responsibility will vary between individuals, all members of the cultural group will understand the important cultural concept of collectivism and family responsibility. Another example of targeting a well-defined group is when an intervention is designed for a specific heritage subgroup (e.g., Puerto Ricans, Cubans, Mexicans) rather than an entire racial/ethnic group (e.g., Latinos). *Tailoring* requires assessing an individual's characteristics such as family responsibility or religiosity to identify how an existing intervention can be further modified to better suit a specific individual (Kreuter *et al.* 2003).

The purpose of cultural targeting and tailoring is to develop an intervention that is more acceptable by the target population and thus more effective in promoting physical activity. Kreuter and colleagues (2003) stress that although we do not know which approach is more effective in delivering a successful intervention (targeting versus tailoring), emphasis should be on using a combination of targeting and tailoring to the degree indicated by the needs of the target population. Some of the populations outlined in this text (e.g., military veterans, rural populations, LGBT populations) have considerably less history of culturally targeted and tailored strtageies, but many of the same ideas and principles apply here as well.

Deep- and surface-level approaches

Strategies to enhance cultural competency/sensitivity of an intervention have traditionally been divided into two overarching categories: surface structure strategies and deep structure strategies (Resnicow *et al.* 1999). Surface structure strategies refer to matching the intervention content to the observable characteristics of the target group. Deep structure strategies involve engaging the beliefs, attitudes, and norms of the target group to promote a behavior (Resnicow *et al.* 1999). Where surface structure strategies are primarily used to make the target group feel comfortable and familiar with the program or materials, deep structure strategies aim to engage the core values and beliefs of the target audience to move them toward behavior change (Kreuter *et al.* 2003, Resnicow *et al.* 1999). For example, surface structure strategies for a physical activity intervention targeting Latina women would be teaching group classes in Spanish and using Spanish-language music. An example of a deep structure strategy for this same target population would be integrating messages about the importance of taking care of one's own health to better care for one's family. Figures 3.1 and 3.2 illustrate both deep- and surface-level strategies used in the physical activity intervention, *Fe en Acción* (Faith in Action; Arredondo *et al.* 2015).

Surface structure strategies

Surface structure strategies include translating content to native language, involving research personnel who represent members of the target population, conducting recruitment and intervention activities in community locations, and using images that the target population may identify with (Resnicow *et al.* 1999).

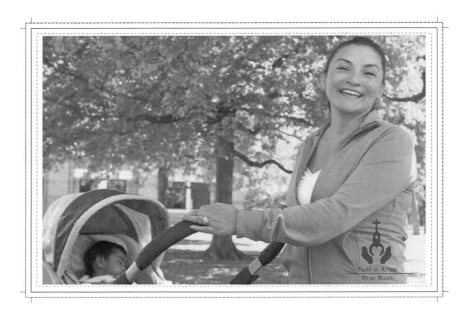

FIGURE 3.1 Example of surface- and deep-level strategies used in *Fe en Acción*

¡Clases gratuitas que ahora se ofrecen en su iglesia!
Free classes now being offered at your church!

SAN DIEGO STATE UNIVERSITY
Research Foundation
9245 SKY PARK CT STE 221
SAN DIEGO CA 92123-4311

Grupos de caminata / Walking Groups

día / day hora / time lugar / place

Clases de actividad física / Physical activity classes

día / day hora / time lugar / place

Para más información, póngase en contacto con:
For more information, call:

**¡Por favor, lleva zapatos y ropa cómodos y lleva agua para tomar!*
**Please wear comfortable clothing and shoes and bring water!*

FIGURE 3.1 Continued

Superando los obstáculos de la actividad física

A veces permitimos que otras cosas nos impidan ser activos.
¡Aquí presentamos algunas maneras prácticas para superar estos obstáculos!

Pequeños pasos hacia el bienestar
Hoy me comprometo a:

- ☐ Planear tiempo en mi semana para hacer actividad física.
- ☐ Invitar a un amigo a que me acompañe en mi actividad física.
- ☐ Ir a una aminata con mis hijos
- ☐ Otros:___________

"Pues Dios no nos ha dado un espíritu de cobardía y timidez, sino de poder, de amor y de dominio propio."
2 Timoteo 1:7

Obstáculo	Consejo
No hay tiempo	Planee tiempo para ser activo. Identifique bloques de 30 minutos durante su semana para ser activo.
Falta de energía	Haga actividad física cuando se sienta con más energía.
Falta de equipo	Elija actividades que no necesiten equipo: caminar, trotar, y bailar.
Falta de apoyo	Invite a sus amigos y familiares a que hagan ejercicio con usted. Planee actividades sociales que involucren ejercicio, por ejemplo, torneos de futbol y jugar en el parque.
No hay quien cuide a los niños	Haga ejercicio con sus hijos. Vaya a una caminata o juegue deportes con su familia.

Adaptado de: Centros para el Control y la Prevención de Enfermedades—División de Nutrición, Actividad Física y Obesidad http://www.cdc.gov/physicalactivity/everyone/health/index.html

FIGURE 3.2 Example of surface- and deep-level strategies used in *Fe en Acción*

	Barrier	Tip
	Not enough time	Plan time to be active. Schedule 30-minute time slots during your week to be active.
	Not enough energy	Do physical activity when you feel most energetic.
	No exercise equipment	Choose activities that need no equipment: walking, jogging, and dancing.
	No support	Invite friends and family members to exercise with you. Plan social activities involving exercise. For example, soccer games and playing at the park.
	No childcare	Exercise with the kids. Go for a hike or play sports with your family.

Overcoming barriers to physical activity

Sometimes we let other things prevent us from being active. Here are some practical ways to overcome these barriers!

Small Step to Wellness
Today I commit to:
☐ Plan time in my week for physical activity
☐ Invite a friend to join me in physical activity
☐ Take my kids on a walk
☐ Other:_____

"For God has not given us a spirit of fear and timidity, but of power, love, and self-discipline."
2 Timothy 1:7

Adapted from: Centers for Disease Control and Prevention—Division of Nutrition, Physical Activity and Obesity http://www.cdc.gov/physicalactivity/everyone/health/index.html

FIGURE 3.2 Continued

Kreuter and colleagues (2003) proposed organizing surface structure strategies into four categories: (a) peripheral, (b) evidential, (c) linguistic, and (d) constituent-involving (Table 3.1). These four strategies are examples of how to *target* an intervention to a cultural group. *Peripheral strategies* include design characteristics such as titles, colors, and images that overtly portray relevance to the group's cultural identification: the use of colors that represent cultural heritage (e.g., colors of a flag), the use of images that resemble individuals of the target population, and the use of an intervention title that clearly defines the target group. *Evidential strategies* involve the use of statistics and epidemiology data that are specific to the target group. For example, including the rates of physical inactivity among LGBT populations in the material shared with intervention participants matching those demographic characteristics. *Linguistic strategies* involve translation of material to the target group's preferred communication dialect. Linguistic strategies can include language translation, but can also incorporate the use of slang and jargon familiar to the target group (e.g., words used among Puerto Rican versus Cuban individuals). Last, *constituent-involving strategies* involve the use of members from the target population in the development and delivery of physical activity programs (Kreuter *et al.* 2003). Constituent-involving strategies could include hiring professionals who are members of the target group or hiring community health workers or lay health advisors to lead intervention activities such as physical activity classes (e.g., Haughton *et al.* 2015).

TABLE 3.1 Examples of surface structure strategies

Strategy	Examples
Peripheral	• Title of the intervention • Colors of materials • Images in materials
Evidential	• Frequency, proportion, and other epidemiologic statistics specific to the target group
Linguistic	• Translation of materials • Delivery of intervention in preferred language of target group • Use of slang or jargon familiar to the target group

Constituent-involving	• Involving members of the target population in the:
	  • Development of the intervention
	  • Recruitment of participants
	  • Implementation of the intervention
	  • Evaluation of the intervention

Source: Kreuter *et al.* (2003, p. 135)

Deep structure strategies

Deep structure strategies aim to incorporate unobservable attributes matched to the target population such as beliefs, attitudes, norms, and cultural practices into physical activity promotion efforts (Resnicow *et al.* 1999). Incorporating deep structure strategies into the development or adaptation of an intervention may require formative work (e.g., focus groups with the target population), including members of the cultural group in the design of the intervention, and soliciting feedback from the target group throughout the development process. Examples of using deep structure strategies for a cultural group that holds collectivist values and frequently cites family responsibilities as a barrier to engaging in physical activity are to provide childcare during intervention activities, include family members in intervention activities, and present physical activity and health as a family responsibility.

To maximize cultural competency/sensitivity, the development and adaptation of physical activity interventions should incorporate both surface and deep structure strategies (Resnicow *et al.* 1999). The extent to which these strategies are incorporated will depend on the needs of the target population, goals of the intervention, resource constraints, and whether an intervention will be developed or adapted (Okamoto *et al.* 2014).

Deciding between developing or adapting an intervention

When developing a physical activity program for a cultural group, public health professionals typically have the choice between developing a new intervention designed specifically for their target population and adapting an already existing intervention. Throughout this text, the implications for developing programs for specific populations highlight the unique challenges for each group. While no guidelines have been reported on how to decide between developing or adapting an intervention, several factors should be considered. Typically, an idea for an intervention comes from reviewing the needs of a population by reviewing the literature and collecting information from community members and organization leaders. If the idea for the intervention is novel and has not previously been tested in other populations, the only option will be to develop a new intervention. On the other hand, if there is an existing intervention, important factors to consider are the availability of resources and relationships with community partners to develop or adapt an intervention. For example, if an existing physical activity intervention is church-based (e.g., many of its components are tied to the church and religious teachings), a current relationship with churches or religious communities may make it easier to successfully implement the intervention. If a health practitioner or researcher has established relationships with local recreation centers, but no relationships with churches or religious leaders, they may decide to either identify a different physical activity intervention to adapt, develop relationships with churches and religious leaders so that they can adapt the intervention, or develop a new intervention using the resources and community relationships they currently have. Ultimately, the decision to develop or adapt an intervention will need to be made on a case-by-case basis by a team of practitioners or researchers who must weigh the pros and cons of each choice within the context of the available resources and partnerships. Sometimes the decision does not have to be one or the other, but can be a combination of an adaptation and the development of a new physical activity intervention. For example, the randomized controlled trial for Latinas, *Fe en Acción* (Faith in Action; Arredondo *et al.* 2015), was the first faith-based physical activity intervention designed for a Latino community. Before *Fe en Acción*, most faith-based physical activity interventions were developed for African American communities (Bopp *et al.* 2009, Duru *et al.* 2010, Wilcox *et al.* 2007, Wilcox *et al.* 2010, Yanek *et al.* 2001, Young and Stewart 2006). Instead of adapting one of these previous interventions for Latinas, the developers of the *Fe en Acción* study chose to conduct focus groups with Latinas to ask them about their interest in the strategies used in many of the faith-based interventions for African American women (e.g., involving church leaders, participating in group exercise). In addition to weaving in strategies used in previous faith-based interventions for African Americans, the developers of the *Fe en Acción* study integrated the *promotora* model into the intervention, a strategy that is known to help promote behavior change among Latinos (Haughton *et al.* 2015). In the case of the *Fe en Acción* study, the developers chose to adapt strategies used in previous successful interventions in their development of a new intervention.

Steps to develop or adapt culturally competent/sensitive physical activity promotion interventions

Whether a new intervention will be developed or an existing one will be adapted, it is important to consider using a methodology or framework that can serve as a guide throughout the development or adaptation process. Several frameworks have been developed to guide the adaptation of existing physical activity programs (Barrera and Castro 2006, Kumpfer *et al.* 2008, McKleroy *et al.* 2006, Wingood and DiClemente 2008). These frameworks share similarities in their approach, which can be used as a general guide for developing or adapting culturally competent/sensitive physical activity interventions. The intervention development or adaptation process involves (a) identifying the target group, method of delivery, and determining community readiness; (b) identifying goals of the intervention; (c) determining how these goals will be measured; (d) developing or adapting the intervention; and (e) pilot testing and refining the intervention. In the case of adapting a previously developed intervention, there are additional steps that must be considered. For example, identifying how the new target group differs from the original group is recommended early in the process of an intervention adaptation. Furthermore, formative research can be used to make decisions regarding how and which aspects of the original intervention will be adapted without compromising its effects. Table 3.2 illustrates the steps to be considered in the development and adaptation of a physical activity intervention.

TABLE 3.2 Process of development and adaptation of culturally sensitive/competent intervention

Process Components	Development/Adaptation
Identify a target group	• Specify the population that the intervention will target
Characterize the target group, method of delivery, and determine community readiness	• Use formative research to characterize the target group, explore acceptable methods of intervention delivery, and identify community readiness for the intervention by evaluating interest and availability of resources
Identify goals of the health promotion intervention	• Review current physical activity guidelines for the target population
	• Collect information regarding the target population's current activity levels either by directly assessing physical activity or by reviewing the literature
Measurement considerations	• Assess construct validity and reliability
	• Ensure that all constructs being measured are relevant to target population
Develop the intervention	• Include members of the target population in the research team
	• Include methodology features to facilitate intervention participation (e.g., recruitment from community sites)
	• Match intervention characteristics with the target group

(*Continued*)

TABLE 3.2 (Continued)

Process Components	Development/Adaptation

If adapting an intervention: Identify sources of mismatch with a pre-existing intervention	• Potential sources of mismatch between the pre-existing and adapted intervention are:
	    • Target group characteristics
	    • Program delivery staff
	    • Community factors

If adapting an intervention: Determine which aspects of the intervention to adapt	• Review the original intervention for components that should and components that should not be modified to maintain efficacy
Pilot test the intervention	• Run one or multiple small-scale studies to test their feasibility and/or test components or the entire study • Obtain participants' perceptions of the pilot study(ies)
Refine the intervention	• Make modifications based on results from pilot studies and information gathered from participants of the pilot studies

Sources: Barrera and Castro (2006), Kumpfer *et al.* (2008), McKleroy *et al.* (2006), Wingood and DiClemente (2008)

Identifying and characterizing the target group, method of delivery, and determining community readiness

When identifying a target group, it is important to identify common characteristics, such as general cultural values to allow for adequate targeting of the intervention. For example, in the *Fe en Acción* study, the target population was low-active, church-going, adult Latinas living in San Diego County. This approach allowed for the intervention to focus on several important cultural factors shared by group members (i.e., ethnicity, gender, and religion). Castro and colleagues (2004) identified three factors that should be well characterized prior to the development or adaptation of an intervention: (a) target group characteristics (e.g., language preference, SES, urban-rural context); (b) program delivery staff (e.g., type of staff delivering the intervention, level of cultural competency of staff); and (c) community factors (e.g., level of readiness of community partners). These factors can be identified in several ways. Surveys allow for the quantitative assessment of characteristics among a group of individuals; however, they lack information on *why* individuals behave in certain ways. Focus groups and one-on-one interviews, on the other hand, can provide rich information on a given topic. For instance, focus groups and interviews can explore why individuals of a particular group prefer to receive an intervention in a certain way (e.g., in person) and by whom (e.g., a veteran who is from their community). This information can be helpful in designing an intervention that will be acceptable to the target population. One-on-one interviews, as well as meetings with potential community partners, can also help determine community partner readiness by evaluating interest and availability of resources (e.g., space for intervention activities). Conducting these interviews and meetings can help identify and select the most enthusiastic and ready community partners for the intervention, improving the chances of successful intervention implementation. Speaking with community partners also has the benefit of identifying potential barriers and challenges that can be addressed prior to implementing the intervention in that setting. For example, in the *Fe en Acción* study, researchers met with church leaders in the target area and shared ideas for the intervention. Church leaders then provided feedback and helped to increase the likelihood of success of the intervention by identifying potential challenges to implementation that were addressed prior to beginning the intervention.

Identifying goals of the health promotion intervention

Physical activity promotion interventions aim to increase physical activity in various ways (e.g., increase in daily steps, leisure-time activity, moderate-to-vigorous intensity physical activity, or the number of participants who meet the CDC's guidelines for physical activity as outlined in Chapter 1). It is important to establish physical activity goals in the context of the target population and to ensure that the goals are attainable and impactful. In addition to reviewing current recommendations for the target group, goal-setting will also require collecting information about the target group's current level of physical activity and/or reviewing relevant epidemiology reports of the prevalence of physical activity among the target population. This information can assist in developing realistic physical activity goals.

Physical activity measurement considerations

General methods of measuring physical activity are outlined in Chapter 1; however careful consideration of the measures assessing the impact of physical activity interventions is needed when developing or adapting a physical activity intervention. Measures that do not account for cultural influences of a particular group are problematic in a number of ways (Arredondo *et al.* 2012, Warnecke *et al.* 1997). These types of measures are not likely to capture the construct of interest and encounter challenges in construct validity and reliability. Consequently, they are not likely to detect intervention changes and are prone to alienate the target population (e.g., asking about activities that are not relevant). For example, many physical activity measurement tools assess leisure-time activities that may be more relevant to White, middle- and upper-class groups but omit an assessment of other forms of activity (e.g., household chores) that may be more relevant to minority, lower-econmic class groups (Im *et al.* 2013, Lee *et al.* 2007). The Global Physical Activity Questionnaire (GPAQ) measures three domains of activity: occupational, transport-related, and leisure-time (Armstrong and Bull 2006). In recognition of the additional types of activity Latinas engage in throughout the day at home, the GPAQ was modified for the *Fe en Acción* study by adding a domain to measure household activity. When a measurement tool does not apply to the target population or the target population does not interpret questions the way they were intended, error in the measure is introduced. This can result in missing data, making it difficult to detect physical activity changes following program implementation. Reducing measurement error improves the sensitivity in which true health behavior patterns are captured.

Developing and adapting culturally competent and sensitive physical activity promotion strategies

The development of a new intervention or adaptation of a previous one should carefully consider how to integrate culturally sensitive/competent strategies. A content analysis revealed three categories of strategies used to enhance the cultural sensitivity/competence of physical activity interventions (Conn *et al.* 2014). First, practitioners or researchers can include members of the target population on the intervention team (e.g., co-investigator, recruiter, community partner). These staff members may be involved in any phase of the intervention, from development to implementation and evaluation. Second, several methodological features can be included to facilitate intervention participation. These features include recruiting from and conducting intervention activities at familiar, community sites (e.g., churches), measuring culturally related constructs (e.g., familism), and designing interventions that minimize the cost of participation (e.g., offering childcare during intervention activities). Third, intervention characteristics can be matched with the target group, primarily through the use of six strategies:

1 Seeking input from the target group during the design of the intervention;
2 Linking the target group's values to the intervention (e.g., family, spirituality);
3 Providing intervention material in the native language of the target group and delivered by native speakers;
4 Selecting intervention content, images, and media to match the target group (e.g., using images that resemble target population);
5 Incorporating physical activity that is culturally matched to the target population (e.g., dancing for Latina populations); and
6 Linking culturally relevant barriers to physical activity within the intervention (e.g., situate interventions in close proximity to low-income populations).

Although these categories primarily reflect surface structure rather than deep structure strategies, the authors suggested that deep structure strategies are likely frequently used, though not typically reported in the literature (Conn *et al.* 2014). In designing the *Fe en Acción* study, many of the strategies listed previously were used. Members of the target population and church leaders provided feedback on intervention content and activities, biblical passages and prayers were incorporated into the curriculum, intervention materials were provided in Spanish and delivered by Spanish-speaking *promotoras*, handouts had images of Latino families and women, physical activity opportunities included Latin dance styles (e.g., merengue, bachata), and cultural barriers and myths about physical activity were discussed during intervention activities.

When *adapting* an existing intervention, the goal is to develop a culturally equivalent intervention for the target group (Castro *et al.* 2004). For example, if a public health practitioner wanted to adapt the *Fe en Acción* study, which was conducted within Catholic churches, to participants who attend Protestant churches, the goal would be to alter the aspects of the intervention that do not conform to Protestant values so that the adapted intervention is well accepted by members of the new cultural group. Two issues are of primary concern when adapting an intervention: (a) ensuring that the efficacy of the adapted intervention is comparable to the efficacy of the original intervention, and (b) ensuring adequate participation and retention in the adapted intervention as compared to the original intervention (Lau 2006). A recommended method of ensuring adequate efficacy and participation in the adapted intervention is to identify, evaluate, and address the sources of mismatch between the original intervention's target population and the new target population (Castro *et al.* 2010). For example, if the original intervention targeted middle-class individuals, assumptions were likely made about the resources available to that population (e.g., the ability to a pay for a local gym or access to safe neighborhood parks). However, these assumptions may not hold if the adapted intervention will target individuals of a lower social class. The same three factors that should be well characterized prior to developing an intervention were also identified as common sources of mismatch by Castro *et al.* (2004): (a) group characteristics (e.g., language, SES, urban-rural context), (b) program delivery staff (e.g., staff delivering intervention, level of cultural competency of staff), and (c) community factors (e.g., community readiness for the intervention).

Pilot testing and refining culturally competent and sensitive physical activity promotion strategies

Pilot testing is a valuable strategy in the development or adaptation of a culturally competent/sensitive intervention. A pilot study is a small-scale study used to assess the feasibility of conducting a study or to test components or the entirety of an intervention prior to conducting a large-scale intervention (Thabane *et al.* 2010). All of the frameworks that guide the development or adaptation of existing physical activity programs include a pilot testing phase (Barrera and Castro 2006, Kumpfer *et al.* 2008, McKleroy *et al.* 2006, Wingood and DiClemente 2008), suggesting the importance of using pilot studies to ensure that the intervention components are well received and show a potential for a positive impact. Following pilot testing of the intervention, additional qualitative and quantitative information may be gathered to examine participants' experience in the intervention and their opinions on the aspects of the intervention that were or were not well received. The information learned from running the pilot study(ies) and from obtaining participants' perceptions are then used to refine the intervention to better suit the cultural group. During the development of the *Fe en Acción* study, intervention components were pilot tested with members of the target population. Physical activity workshops were taught to a group of Latina churchgoing women. Following each session, the women provided feedback, both written and through focus groups, on ways to improve the intervention. Their feedback included suggestions on terminology, images used in intervention materials, class length, and how to increase participation. Findings from the pilot tests were used to refine the large-scale community intervention.

An important unanswered question in the field of cultural adaptation is the extent to which adapted interventions compare to interventions that have not been adapted or have only minimally been adapted in their efficacy among the target group (Castro *et al.* 2010, Conn *et al.* 2014, Whitt-Glover and Kumanyika 2009). In their systematic review of physical activity interventions for African Americans, Whitt-Glover and Kumanyika (2009) identified only 3 out of 43 studies that compared a culturally adapted intervention to the same intervention with no adaptation (Fitzgibbon *et al.* 2005, Newton and Perri 2004, Yanek *et al.* 2001). The studies did not detect statistically significant changes in physical activity between the culturally adapted and the same intervention without any adaptation. The potential reasons for the null findings vary across studies but include the possibility that the intervention was not sufficiently adapted (Newton and Perri 2004) and that the interventions were too similar to have a differential effect on physical activity. In a church-based study comparing a standard physical activity intervention to an identical intervention with additional spiritual messages and content, the standard intervention was "contaminated" when prayer, scripture, and gospel music was incorporated into every session of the intervention, effectively eliminating the differences between the interventions (Yanek *et al.* 2001). Until further research is conducted, we will not know if and to what extent adapted interventions impact the efficacy of physical activity interventions compared to unadapted interventions.

Conclusion

Despite a lack of empirical evidence from which to draw conclusions, it is likely that physical activity promotion strategies targeting diverse groups can benefit from incorporating cultural characteristics of the target group. Given the wide variety of differences between cultural groups, it would be beneficial for public health professionals to develop the skills necessary to improve the likelihood of delivering an intervention that is well accepted, well attended, and effective in its goal to change physical activity behaviors. In this chapter, we outlined a framework for development and adaptation of culturally competent/sensitive physical activity promotion strategies. This framework relies on defining a specific culturally homogenous group, collecting information about this group, using that information to identify goals of the intervention, and if adapting an intervention, identifying mismatches between the original and current target group. The framework finally recommends pilot testing and refining the intervention through multiple iterations if necessary until the goals of the intervention are achieved.

Summary points

• Culture includes complex and multi-dimensional constructs that influence behaviors and an individual's acceptance of and response to health promotion strategies.

• Physical activity is highly influenced by culture, especially race/ethnicity and gender roles.

• Cultural competency/sensitivity describes the extent to which congruent behaviors, attitudes, and policies of a specific cultural group are used in a respectful and skillful manner to promote physical activity.

• Surface structure strategies refer to matching the intervention content to the observable characteristics of the target group, whereas deep structure strategies involve engaging the beliefs, attitudes, and norms of the target group with the physical activity intervention.

• The intervention development process involves identifying the target group, collecting information about the group, setting goals, determining how these goals will be measured, developing or adapting the intervention, and pilot testing and refining the intervention.

• The intervention adaptation process also includes identifying how the new target group differs from the original group and making decisions about how and which aspects of the original intervention will be adapted without compromising its effects.

Critical thinking questions

1   Describe the benefits of implementing deep structure over surface structure strategies to enhance the cultural competency/sensitivity of an intervention.

2   How can sources of mismatch between the original and target population characteristics jeopardize the success of an adapted intervention?

3   Explain why even though there is not enough evidence to show that adapted interventions have more success than those that are not adapted, public health professionals should still make the effort to develop culturally competent/sensitive interventions.

References

Armstrong, T. and Bull, F. (2006) 'Development of the world health organization Global Physical Activity Questionnaire (GPAQ).' *Journal of Public Health*, 14: 66–70.

Arredondo, E.M., Haughton, J., Ayala, G.X., Slymen, D.J., Sallis, J.F., Burke, K., Holub, C., Chanson, D., Perez, L.G. and Valdivia, R. (2015) 'Fe en Acción/Faith in Action: Design and implementation of a church-based randomized trial to promote physical activity and cancer screening among churchgoing Latinas.' *Contemporary Clinical Trials*, 45: 404–415.

Arredondo, E.M., Mendelson, T., Holub, C., Espinoza, N. and Marshall, S. (2012) 'Cultural adaptation of physical activity self-report instruments.' *Journal of Physical Activity and Health*, 9: S37.

Barrera, M. and Castro, F.G. (2006) 'A heuristic framework for the cultural adaptation of interventions.' *Clinical Psychology: Science and Practice*, 13: 311–316.

Barrera, M., Jr., Castro, F.G., Strycker, L.A. and Toobert, D.J. (2013) 'Cultural adaptations of behavioral health interventions: A progress report.' *Journal of Consulting and Clinical Psychology*, 81: 196.

Betancourt, H. and López, S.R. (1993), 'The study of culture, ethnicity, and race in American psychology.' *American Psychologist,* 48(6): 629.

Bopp, M., Wilcox, S., Laken, M., Hooker, S.P., Parra-Medina, D., Saunders, R., Butler, K., Fallon, E.A. and McClorin, L. (2009) '8 steps to fitness: A faith-based, behavior change physical activity intervention for African Americans.' *Journal of Physical Activity & Health*, 6: 568–577.

Brach, C. and Fraserirector, I. (2000) 'Can cultural competency reduce racial and ethnic health disparities? A review and conceptual model.' *Medical Care Research and Review*, 57: 181–217.

Cantu, A.G. and Fleuriet, K.J. (2008) 'The sociocultural context of physical activity in older Mexican American women.' *Hispanic Health Care International*, 6: 27–40.

Castro, F.G., Barrera, M., Jr. and Holleran Steiker, L.K. (2010) 'Issues and challenges in the design of culturally adapted evidence-based interventions.' *Annual Review of Clinical Psychology*, 6: 213–239.

Castro, F.G., Barrera, M., Jr. and Martinez, C.R., Jr. (2004) 'The cultural adaptation of prevention interventions: Resolving tensions between fidelity and fit.' *Prevention Science*, 5: 41–45.

Conn, V.S., Chan, K., Banks, J., Ruppar, T.M. and Scharff, J. (2014) 'Cultural relevance of physical activity intervention research with underrepresented populations.' *International Quarterly of Community Health Education*, 34: 391–414.

Cross, T.L. (1989) *Towards a Culturally Competent System of Care: A Monograph on Effective Services for Minority Children Who Are Severely Emotionally Disturbed.* Washington, DC: Georgetown University, Child Development Center.

D'Alonzo, K.T. (2012) 'The influence of marianismo beliefs on physical activity of immigrant Latinas.' *Journal of Transcultural Nursing: Official Journal of the Transcultural Nursing Society/Transcultural Nursing Society*, 23: 124–133.

Duru, O.K., Sarkisian, C.A., Leng, M. and Mangione, C.M. (2010) 'Sisters in motion: A randomized controlled trial of a faith-based physical activity intervention.' *Journal of the American Geriatrics Society*, 58: 1863–1869.

Fernando, S. (2010) *Mental Health, Race and Culture*, New York, NY: Palgrave Macmillan.

Fitzgibbon, M.L., Stolley, M.R., Ganschow, P., Schiffer, L., Wells, A., Simon, N. and Dyer, A. (2005) 'Results of a faith-based weight loss intervention for black women.' *Journal of the National Medical Association*, 97: 1393–1402.

Giles-Corti, B. and Donovan, R.J. (2002) 'Socioeconomic status differences in recreational physical activity levels and real and perceived access to a supportive physical environment.' *Preventive Medicine*, 35: 601–611.

Haughton, J., Ayala, G.X., Burke, K.H., Elder, J.P., Montanez, J. and Arredondo, E.M. (2015) 'Community health workers promoting physical activity: Targeting multiple levels of the social ecological model.' *The Journal of Ambulatory Care Management*, 38: 309–320.

Im, E., Ko, Y., Hwang, H., Chee, W., Stuifbergen, A., Walker, L. and Brown, A. (2013) 'Racial/ethnic differences in midlife women's attitudes toward physical activity.' *Journal of Midwifery & Women's Health*, 58: 440–450.

Im, E., Lee, B., Hwang, H., Yoo, K.H., Chee, W., Stuifbergen, A., Walker, L., Brown, A., McPeek, C. and Miro, M. (2010) ' "A waste of time": Hispanic women's attitudes toward physical activity.' *Women & Health*, 50: 563–579.

Juarbe, T.C., Lipson, J.G. and Turok, X. (2003) 'Physical activity beliefs, behaviors, and cardiovascular fitness of Mexican immigrant women.' *Journal of Transcultural Nursing: Official Journal of the Transcultural Nursing Society/Transcultural Nursing Society*, 14: 108–116.

Kraus, M.W., Piff, P.K. and Keltner, D. (2011) 'Social class as culture the convergence of resources and rank in the social realm.' *Current Directions in Psychological Science*, 20: 246–250.

Kreuter, M.W., Lukwago, S.N., Bucholtz, R.D., Clark, E.M. and Sanders-Thompson, V. (2003) 'Achieving cultural appropriateness in health promotion programs: Targeted and tailored approaches.' *Health Education & Behavior: The Official Publication of the Society for Public Health Education*, 30: 133–146.

Kreuter, M.W. and McClure, S.M. (2004) 'The role of culture in health communication.' *Annual Review of Public Health*, 25: 439–455.

Kreuter, M.W., Strecher, V.J. and Glassman, B. (1999) 'One size does not fit all: The case for tailoring print materials.' *Annals of Behavioral Medicine*, 21: 276–283.

Kumpfer, K.L., Pinyuchon, M., Teixeira de Melo, A. and Whiteside, H.O. (2008) 'Cultural adaptation process for international dissemination of the strengthening families program.' *Evaluation & the Health Professions*, 31: 226–239.

Lau, A.S. (2006) 'Making the case for selective and directed cultural adaptations of evidence based treatments: Examples from parent training.' *Clinical Psychology: Science and Practice*, 13: 295–310.

Lee, R.E., Cubbin, C. and Winkleby, M. (2007) 'Contribution of neighbourhood socioeconomic status and physical activity resources to physical activity among women.' *Journal of Epidemiology and Community Health*, 61: 882–890.

McKleroy, V.S., Galbraith, J.S., Cummings, B. and Jones, P. (2006) 'Adapting evidence-based behavioral interventions for new settings and target populations.' *AIDS Education and Prevention*, 18: 59.

Marsiglia, F.F. and Booth, J.M. (2015) 'Cultural adaptation of interventions in real practice settings.' *Research on Social Work Practice*, 25: 423–432.

Newton, R. and Perri, M.G. (2004) 'A randomized pilot trial of exercise promotion in sedentary African-American adults.' *Ethnicity and Disease*, 14: 548–557.

Nierkens, V., Hartman, M.A., Nicolaou, M., Vissenberg, C., Beune, E.J., Hosper, K., Valkengoed, I.G. van and Stronks, K. (2013) 'Effectiveness of cultural adaptations of interventions aimed at smoking cessation, diet, and/or physical activity in ethnic minorities: A systematic review.' *PloS One*, 8: e73373.

Okamoto, S.K., Kulis, S., Marsiglia, F.F., Steiker, L.K.H. and Dustman, P. (2014) 'A continuum of approaches toward developing culturally focused prevention interventions: From adaptation to grounding.' *The Journal of Primary Prevention*, 35: 103–112.

Parks, S.E., Housemann, R.A. and Brownson, R.C. (2003) 'Differential correlates of physical activity in urban and rural adults of various socioeconomic backgrounds in the United States.' *Journal of Epidemiology and Community Health*, 57: 29–35.

Resnicow, K., Baranowski, T., Ahluwalia, J.S. and Braithwaite, R.L. (1999) 'Cultural sensitivity in public health: Defined and demystified.' *Ethnicity & Disease*, 9: 10–21.

Thabane, L., Ma, J., Chu, R., Cheng, J., Ismaila, A., Rios, L.P., Robson, R., Thabane, M., Giangregorio, L. and Goldsmith, C.H. (2010) 'A tutorial on pilot studies: The what, why and how.' *BMC Medical Research Methodology*, 10: 1.

U.S. Department of Health and Human Services, Office of Disease Prevention and Health Promotion (2008) *2008 Physical Activity Guidelines for Americans*, Washington, DC: USDHHS.

Vrazel, J.E., Saunders, R.P. and Wilcox, S. (2008) 'An overview and proposed framework of social-environmental influences on the physical-activity behavior of women.' *American Journal of Health Promotion*, 23: 2–12.

Warnecke, R.B., Johnson, T.P., Chavez, N., Sudman, S., O'Rourke, D.P., Lacey, L. and Horm, J. (1997) 'Improving question wording in surveys of culturally diverse populations.' *Annals of Epidemiology*, 7: 334–342.

Whitt-Glover, M.C. and Kumanyika, S.K. (2009) 'Systematic review of interventions to increase physical activity and physical fitness in African-Americans.' *American Journal of Health Promotion*, 23: S33–S56.

Wilcox, S., Laken, M., Bopp, M., Gethers, O., Huang, P., McClorin, L., Parrott, A.W., Swinton, R. and Yancey, A. (2007) 'Increasing physical activity among church members: Community-based participatory research.' *American Journal of Preventive Medicine*, 32: 131–138.

Wilcox, S., Laken, M., Parrott, A.W., Condrasky, M., Saunders, R., Addy, C.L., Evans, R., Baruth, M. and Samuel, M. (2010) 'The Faith, Activity, and Nutrition (FAN) program: Design of a participatory research intervention to increase physical activity and improve dietary habits in African American churches.' *Contemporary Clinical Trials*, 31: 323–335.

Williams, D.R., Mohammed, S.A., Leavell, J. and Collins, C. (2010) 'Race, socioeconomic status, and health: Complexities, ongoing challenges, and research opportunities.' *Annals of the New York Academy of Sciences*, 1186: 69–101.

Wingood, G.M. and DiClemente, R.J. (2008) 'The ADAPT-ITT model: A novel method of adapting evidence-based HIV interventions.' *Journal of Acquired Immune Deficiency Syndromes (1999)*, 47: S40–S46.

Yancey, A.K., Ory, M.G. and Davis, S.M. (2006) 'Dissemination of physical activity promotion interventions in underserved populations.' *American Journal of Preventive Medicine*, 31: 82–91.

Yanek, L.R., Becker, D.M., Moy, T.F., Gittelsohn, J. and Koffman, D.M. (2001) 'Project Joy: Faith based cardiovascular health promotion for African American women.' *Public Health Reports (Washington, DC: 1974)*, 116: 68–81.

Young, D.R. and Stewart, K.J. (2006) 'A church-based physical activity intervention for African American women.' *Family & Community Health*, 29: 103–117.

4

PHYSICAL ACTIVITY AMONG AFRICAN AMERICANS

Melicia C. Whitt-Glover, Ogechi Nwaokelemeh, Amanda A. Price and Jammie M. Hopkins

Understanding the African American population

Physical activity is an important health-related behavior that has been associated with prevention and treatment of chronic disease, decreased mortality, and improved quality of life as outlined in Chapter 1 (Physical Activity Guidelines Advisory Committee 2008). Despite the known benefits of physical activity many population subgroups, including African Americans, consistently report low levels of physical activity. Consequently, population subgroups with low levels of physical activity also report the highest levels of chronic diseases (e.g., hypertension, obesity, cardiovascular disease, type 2 diabetes) that could be ameliorated by physical activity participation. This chapter describes physical activity prevalence among African Americans using data from national sources. The chapter also provides an overview of factors that are associated with physical activity participation among African Americans, and a review of research on physical activity promotion strategies among African Americans. The chapter concludes with a discussion of implications and potential next steps for continuing to address and promote physical activity among African Americans.

Demographic characteristics

African Americans are a diverse ethnocultural group of individuals with complete or partial ancestry from any of the Black racial groups of Africa. African Americans are the third largest racial and ethnic group in the United States, comprising 14% (42.0 million) of the U.S. population (U.S. Bureau of the Census 2011). African American populations are geographically concentrated in the South (55%), Midwest (18%), Northeast (17%), and West (10%) regions of the United States (U.S. Bureau of the Census 2011). African American populations tend to cluster in majority

Black urban and rural counties in the South, and within metropolitan statistical areas outside of the South (U.S. Bureau of the Census 2011). As it pertains to educational attainment, significantly fewer African Americans graduate from college (19.8%) compared to Whites (30.3%) and the national average (29.9%) (U.S. Bureau of the Census 2012). In 2009, median incomes of African American households ($38,409) were significantly lower than Whites ($62,545) and all families ($60,088) (U.S. Bureau of the Census 2012). African Americans are disproportionately impacted by poverty (25.8% below poverty level) compared to Whites (12.3%) and the national average (14.3%) (U.S. Bureau of the Census 2012). Life expectancy for both African American men (72.0 years) and women (78.1 years) lags behind the national average of 76.4 and 81.2 years, respectively (Arias 2016).

Health disparities and inequities among the African American population

African Americans are disproportionately impacted by a number of health concerns and chronic diseases across the lifespan, particularly disparities that could be positively impacted by increased levels of physical activity. Despite significant reductions in rates overall over the last two decades, African American men and women had the highest prevalence of hypertension among all racial and ethnic groups at 42.4% and 44.0%, respectively (National Center for Health 2016). In 2010, the age-standardized prevalence of medically diagnosed diabetes was significantly higher among African Americans (11.3%) than Whites (6.8%) and Asians (7.9%) (Centers for Disease Control and Prevention 2013b). In 2011–2014, obesity prevalence for children and adolescents aged 2–19 years was significantly higher among African Americans (19.5%) than Whites (14.7%) and Asians (8.6%) (National Center for Health 2016). African Americans have the highest age-adjusted adult obesity rate (48.1%) of all major race/ethnicity groups in the United States (Ogden *et al.* 2015). Mental health disparities also persist among African Americans. African Americans are 20% more likely to experience serious mental health problems than the general population (Mental Health America 2016, U.S. Department of Health and Human Services Office of Minority Mental Health 2016).

Physical activity among African Americans

National statistics describing the prevalence of physical activity among people in the U.S. are collected using several datasets, including the Youth Risk Behavior Surveillance System (YRBSS; middle and high school students only), BRFSS, NHANES, and NHIS. All four surveys rely on self-report to obtain data on physical activity prevalence. NHANES also collects accelerometer data on a subsample of respondents to obtain an objective measure of physical activity. YRBSS data from 2015 showed that 14.3% of students across the nation reported not meeting the guideline for > 60 minutes of activity on at least one day during the seven days preceding the survey; Black males and females were more likely than their counterparts in other racial/ethnic subgroups to report not meeting the recommendation (Kann *et al.* 2016). Interestingly, data from NHANES 2011–2012 showed no racial/ethnic differences in children (6–11 years) or adolescents (12–19 years) achieving the recommended > 1 hour of physical activity (Haughton *et al.* 2016). In the same dataset, however, non-Hispanic Black children and adolescents were significantly *less* likely to achieve the recommended < 2 hours of daily screen time. Although not one of the resources that provide national estimates of physical activity, the National Heart, Lung, and Blood Institute Growth and Health Study prospectively followed 1,213 Black and 1,166 White girls from the ages of 9–10 to the ages of 18–19 and showed a shocking *100% decline in physical activity for Black girls* over the 10-year study period (Kimm *et al.* 2002).

By adulthood disparities in physical activity levels begin to emerge. Data from the 2009–2011 NHIS showed that non-Hispanic Black and non-Hispanic White men were more likely than men from other race/ethnic groups to meet both the aerobic activity and muscle strengthening guidelines (Centers for Disease Control and Prevention 2013). In contrast, non-Hispanic Black women were less likely than non-Hispanic White women to meet the guidelines. Data from the 2011 BRFSS indicated that less than half of non-Hispanic Blacks (45.5%) reported meeting aerobic activity guidelines compared to 53.9% of non-Hispanic Whites, 45.8% of Hispanics, and 51.6% of other races (2013a). Results from NHANES were similar. Troiano et al. examined objectively measured PA in U.S. adults based on the 2003–2004 NHANES (Troiano *et al.* 2008). The study included a representative sample of 4,867 adults with four or more days of accelerometer wear time. Accelerometer-measured activity was substantially lower than self-reported data across all age categories; among adults, adherence to the activity recommendations (30 min/day) was less than 5%. Mexican American men and women had significantly greater activity counts and highest duration of moderate to vigorous physical activity than non-Hispanic Whites and Black men and women. A follow-up study of NHANES data from 2003–2004 and 2012–2013 suggested that the higher physical activity levels among Mexican Americans may be due to occupational activity (Gay and Buchner 2014). As adults age, disparities in physical activity continue; NHANES accelerometer data for adults > 60 years show that older African American adults report lower levels of physical activity than other racial/ethnic subgroups (Evenson *et al.* 2012).

While data on disparities between groups is important, it is also necessary to understand differences in physical activity *within* groups. Few papers have been published assessing differences in physical activity patterns within African Americans. Whitt-Glover and colleagues used BRFSS, NHANES, and NHIS data to understand differences in self-reported physical activity prevalence within African Americans (Whitt-Glover *et al.* 2007). The proportion of African American adults who reported meeting physical activity recommendations ranged from 24% to 36%. Across all three surveys, women consistently reported less physical activity than men. Physical activity levels also tended to increase with income and employment status, and to decrease as BMI levels increased.

Common barriers and facilitators to physical activity for African Americans

Understanding variables from multiple levels that influence behavior can provide cues for individual- and community-level strategies for successfully and positively impacting behavior. As outlined in Chapter 1, the social determinants of health include intrapersonal, interpersonal, institutional, community, and policy-level factors that influence a person's willingness and ability to engage in behaviors. The African American Collaborative Obesity Research Network (AACORN) has developed an exemplar paradigm for use in addressing weight and related behaviors, including physical activity, in African American communities that incorporates aspects of the social determinants of health (Kumanyika *et al.* 2007). The paradigm suggests that a broad approach that is informed by knowledge of life in African American communities is needed to create holistic approaches that embrace and reflect social and cultural perspectives of the community (Figure 4.1). The middle of the AACORN paradigm, labeled "Expanded Knowledge Domains," suggests that cultural and psychosocial processes, historical and social contexts, and physical and economic environments all influence behaviors that can impact energy balance. Several variables within these domains have been associated, both positively and negatively, with physical activity participation in African Americans (Joseph *et al.* 2015).

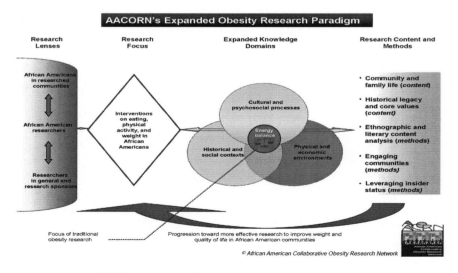

FIGURE 4.1 AACORN's Expanded Obesity Research Paradigm

Historical and social contexts and cultural and psychosocial processes

Historical and social contexts refer to a group's shared history and the impact on current behaviors, the influence of social institutions within communities, and strengths within communities. Cultural and psychosocial processes refer to a group's shared social values and beliefs, coping strategies, and trust within and outside the group. Because the two domains are so closely related, we discuss them together in this chapter. These domains also relate to intrapersonal, interpersonal, and community-level factors within the social determinants of health.

Data suggest that sociocultural knowledge and beliefs within the African American community about physical activity, health, and self-care may influence physical activity participation (Airhihenbuwa et al. 2000, Boyington et al. 2008, Hall et al. 2013, Kumanyika et al. 2007, Siddiqi et al. 2011, Thompson and Barksdale 2010, Woolford et al. 2016). For example, attitudes toward sports participation, hair maintenance, and body size have been correlated to decreased physical activity participation among Black adolescents and adults. Qualitative studies suggest that some African Americans may value rest and sleep as more important than, or necessary for, engaging in physical activity (Airhihenbuwa et al. 1995). African Americans may also perceive/interpret the term "leisure" as laziness (Tudor-Locke et al. 2003). If leisure time has a negative connotation for a population subgroup, this could impact one's desire to engage in leisure-time activity and reporting of such activities on national physical activity surveys that inquire about leisure time.

Community involvement and social support have been shown to be positively associated with physical activity in African American communities (Boyington et al. 2008, Cogbill et al. 2011, Miller and Marolen 2012, Strong et al. 2013). Participants with greater social involvement report greater levels of physical activity (Cogbill et al. 2011, Strong et al. 2013). Knowing someone who exercises or seeing others exercising in one's community has been shown to impact physical activity levels, both positively and negatively (Ainsworth et al. 2003, Wilbur 2003, Young and Voorhees 2003). The positive correlation may be in part due to the influence of positive physical activity role models and exercise partners. Other psychological and behavioral variables such as positive physical activity self-efficacy, outcome expectations, and physical activity enjoyment have also been associated with increased motivation to be physically active (Bopp et al. 2006, Chang et al. 2008, Fleury and Lee 2006, Sanderson et al. 2003).

Female gender has been associated with lower physical activity participation in part due to competing caregiver responsibilities and a resultant lack of time to be physically active (Ainsworth et al. 2003, Bopp et al. 2007, Chang et al. 2008, Miller and Marolen 2012, Siddiqi et al. 2011, Young and Voorhees 2003). Family structure has been shown to impact African American physical activity participation. Being married or being in a relationship has been associated with higher levels of physical activity due to having someone to share caregiving duties (i.e., increased social support) (Ainsworth et al. 2003, Cogbill et al. 2011, Johnson et al. 2005, Young and Voorhees 2003). However, data suggest that having a family can also present a barrier to physical activity participation, particularly among women, due to family obligations like caring for children or grandchildren and perceptions of role responsibilities for women (Bopp *et al.* 2007, Sanderson *et al.* 2003). African Americans, particularly women, may view physical activity as a luxury rather than necessary for optimal health, and may consider spending time on physical activity to be selfish, particularly when one has caregiving or work responsibilities (Airhihenbuwa *et al.* 1995, Im *et al.* 2013). The notion of collectivism, which prioritizes the needs of the group over individuals within the group, is ingrained in African, African American, and Latino cultures. Collectivism would suggest that until everyone in a group is taken care of, people within the group should not engage in activities that would benefit only the individual (e.g., leisure-time physical activity).

Other personal demographic variables like BMI, age, education, employment, and income have also been shown to impact physical activity participation. Among African American women higher BMI has been associated with increased time in sedentary behavior while those that have lower BMI values have been more likely to meet physical activity recommendations (Bopp *et al.* 2007, Buchowski *et al.* 2010). Greater participation in physical activity has been associated with younger ages (Bopp *et al.* 2006, Sanderson *et al.* 2003). Higher education, income, and SES levels have all shown to be positively correlated to physical activity in African American communities (Affuso *et al.* 2011, Ainsworth *et al.* 2003, Bopp *et al.* 2006, Fleury and Lee 2006, Johnson and Nies 2005, Wilbur 2003). Perceived positive health status also has been shown to have facilitated increased physical activity participation while poor health conditions have been reported to be a barrier to physical activity in African American communities (Ainsworth *et al.* 2003, Bopp *et al.* 2007, Sanderson *et al.* 2003, Wilbur 2003).

In addition to the factors listed earlier, physical activity levels among youth are also impacted by parental behaviors and support, perceived lack of safety for girls, access to transportation to participate in extracurricular activities, social support, and concerns about personal appearance (Boyington *et al.* 2008, Lytle *et al.* 2009, McDonald 2008, Rees *et al.* 2006, Wilson *et al.* 2011).

Physical and economic environments

Physical and economic environments relate directly to the availability and quality of resources that are available for engaging in physical activity, including tangible resources that can be used for physical activity (e.g., parks, recreation centers, sidewalks) or financial resources that allow participation in physical activity (e.g., funds for gym memberships or sign-up fees and equipment to participate in activities). Data from the 2011–2012 National Survey of Children's Health found that non-Hispanic Black adolescents were less likely to live in neighborhoods that had characteristics that supported physical activity (Watson *et al.* 2016). A recent study of the distribution of physical activity resources in 7,319 U.S. census tracts showed a lower probability of having > 1 park or recreational facility in neighborhoods that had predominantly racial/ethnic minority residents (Jones *et al.* 2015). Interestingly, an inventory of 351 private recreation facilities and 465 public parks in Maryland found no significant impact of income or percent minority within the census tract on the availability of facilities which, the authors noted, is inconsistent with findings from previous studies (Abercrombie *et al.* 2008). A systematic review of the impact of the built environment on weight-related behaviors in African American adults found that light traffic, presence of sidewalks, and perceived safety from crime were associated with higher levels of physical activity (Casagrande *et al.* 2009). A review of studies published between 1990 and 2013 identified barriers to physical activity among African American women, which included safety concerns, lack of facilities, weather, lack of sidewalks, and lack of visible role models as environmental barriers associated with lower levels of physical activity (Joseph *et al.* 2015). A study of elementary school students found that perceived access to parks and related facilities was associated with reports of more frequent exercise (Carroll-Scott *et al.* 2013).

Intervention strategies

Because of low physical activity participation among African Americans, interventions focused on improving physical activity behaviors are critical for reducing obesity and chronic disease risk disparities. Several systematic reviews of the literature have been conducted to summarize studies promoting physical activity among African Americans and to identify promising strategies (Banks-Wallace and Conn 2002, Conn *et al.* 2012, Jenkins *et al.* 2015, Joseph *et al.* 2016, Taylor *et al.* 1998, Whitt-Glover *et al.* 2009, Whitt-Glover *et al.* 2014, Whitt-Glover and Kumanyika 2009). Typical study settings have included churches, primary care/healthcare facilities, community recreational facilities, home-based settings, university campuses, and telephone/Internet. Studies among African American adults primarily included middle-aged women (40–65 years) and rarely included younger adults < 40 years, older adults > 65 years, or men. Interventions were delivered by a mix of professionals, trained facilitators (e.g., trained community health workers), or automated systems. Interventions with weekly sessions involving education, motivation, or supervised exercise are the most common (Banks-Wallace and Conn 2002, Conn *et al.* 2012). Most studies focused on increasing walking as the primary focus of physical activity; additional intervention strategies also included group-based fitness/exercise classes, training studies to improve fitness, or resistance training/use of exercise machines. Most reviews generally reported a positive impact of intervention strategies on physical activity–related behaviors when comparing baseline measures with measures assessed immediately post-intervention. A review of studies to improve healthy eating, physical activity, or obesity in African American children and adolescents identified 17 studies conducted in pre-schools, elementary schools, and middle/secondary schools (Robinson *et al.* 2014). Of the studies, three showed improvements in physical activity through programs in schools delivered by classroom teachers or professional staff. Studies primarily focused on increasing physical activity within the school day and at home, and reducing screen time.

A review of outside-of-school time strategies for prevention and treatment of obesity also showed general positive findings on the impact of physical activity in studies that attempted a variety of after school and summer time programs (Barr-Anderson *et al.* 2014).

Some general limitations of studies focused on promoting physical activity among African Americans as noted in systematic reviews of the literature included:

- *Limited reporting of null or negative findings.* Most studies did not describe any negative impacts of intervention strategies on physical activity participation. Sometimes researchers and journal editors may favor publication of studies with positive results because those findings could be considered more interesting to readers; however, describing null or negative results could be helpful for understanding what does not work, and could help to develop future interventions.
- *Limited data specific to African Americans.* Many of the studies included in the systematic review of literature did not include single race samples or stratified analyses. Because African Americans are a high-risk population, it is important to understand which specific strategies are most successful at increasing and sustaining increases in physical activity in this high-risk population.
- *Lack of inclusion of African American men.* Only two studies identified focused on promoting physical activity among African American men, both of which showed statistically significant physical activity improvements (Newton *et al.* 2014). It is particularly important to increase focus on African American men given recent findings that, while obesity rates have stabilized in some populations, rates continue to increase among men and boys (Ogden *et al.* 2015).
- *Use of weak study designs.* Very few studies included in the systematic reviews involved strong study designs such as large-scale, randomized control trials (Conn *et al.* 2012, Coughlin and Smith 2016). The utilization of weaker research designs, small sample sizes, and self-reported measures of physical activity rather than objective measures are also cause for concern (Coughlin and Smith 2016, Whitt-Glover *et al.* 2009, Whitt-Glover *et al.* 2014, Whitt-Glover and Kumanyika 2009).
- *Limited assessment of long-term (e.g., > 1-year post-intervention) impact of the intervention on physical activity participation.* Of the promising physical activity improvement findings, few studies have included long-term follow-ups, making the lasting intervention effects unknown (Conn *et al.* 2012, Whitt-Glover *et al.* 2009). Marcus and colleagues have previously called for attention to long-term follow-up to fully understand the impact of physical activity interventions (Marcus *et al.* 2000). That few studies have included long-term follow-up may be related to how funding to conduct physical activity intervention research is distributed; many grant/contract opportunities do not allow sufficient time or funding for long-term follow-up.
- *Limited focus on physical activity as the sole behavior to change.* Physical activity is rarely the primary intervention focus, and is often included with dietary and

other healthy behavior (Banks-Wallace and Conn 2002, Whitt-Glover *et al.* 2009, Whitt-Glover and Kumanyika 2009). Focusing on changing more than one behavior at a time might be difficult for individuals attempting behavior change. Additionally, it might be difficult to tease out effects on a single behavior for intervention strategies that target multiple behaviors at once.

- *Lack of studies that systematically focus on impacting the factors shown to influence physical activity–related behaviors.* In the previous section, we highlighted historical/social contexts, cultural and psychosocial processes, and physical and economic environment factors that have been shown to impact participation in physical activity. Most interventions, however, focus primarily on providing education and encouragement to increase physical activity without addressing many of the factors that have been shown to influence participation.

There are a few promising practices that should be noted for improving physical activity in African Americans. Churches and faith-based institutions in African American communities have been pivotal in providing safe and accessible spaces for physical activity for community members (Bopp *et al.* 2012, Bopp *et al.* 2009, Whitt-Glover *et al.* 2012), and when these spaces are available and free for use, could increase physical activity within communities. Churches have been a common venue for chronic disease prevention programs among African Americans. A recent review identified 27 studies implemented in faith-based organizations focused on weight and related behaviors (Lancaster *et al.* 2014); 38% of the studies reported increases in physical activity among study participants. Interestingly, although research recommends that interventions should include both surface- and deep-level cultural tailoring (see Chapter 3 for further explanation of these concepts), many of the interventions conducted in churches are *faith-placed* (surface-level tailoring) rather than *faith-based*, and do not include faith themes (deep-level tailoring), an example of surface-level tailoring (Conn *et al.* 2012). Additional deep-level cultural tailoring could improve the effectiveness of faith-based physical activity interventions.

BOX 4.1   EVIDENCE-BASED PRACTICE: INSTANT RECESS®

One practice-based strategy for promoting physical activity that is gaining momentum is *Instant Recess®* (www.instantrecess.com) (Yancey 2010). Created by Dr. Antronette (Toni) Yancey, *Instant Recess* is an innovative, information technology–based solution for economically challenged school environments based on promising scientific evidence. The *Instant Recess* break concept is to provide opportunities for individuals to participate in 10-minute bouts of PA, in line with recommendation for U.S. youth and adults, anywhere, anytime, in any type of attire. The breaks consist of a series of basic aerobic dance, calisthenics, and sports movements with funny and self-explanatory titles, like the Hulk, the Hallelujah, and the Knee High. Simple, moderate-intensity, low-impact moves – aerobic, stretching, and resistance – are performed in 10-minute bouts to music one or more times a day in groups. The breaks have been medically designed for sedentary, overweight, or less fit youth and adults in ordinary street attire. The 10-minute time interval reflects the suggested interval for achieving current physical activity recommendations (Physical Activity Guidelines Advisory Committee 2008). *Instant Recess* is particularly targeted to largely unmotivated captive audiences (rather than willing volunteers) within environments with resource and space constraints (e.g., classrooms, board rooms, conferences). While these exercises can be performed individually, social interaction in groups is a necessary ingredient to maximize organizational return on investment. Breaks are available via DVD, audio CD, and online streaming and include music and call-out instructions, which takes the onus off the group leader to have to memorize and lead movements. *Instant Recess* has been implemented in a variety of settings, and participants experience immediate benefits in terms of improved group dynamics, productivity, feelings of well-being, self-confidence, skill development, and positive reinforcement that motivates them to be more active on other occasions and in other settings (LaBreche *et al.* 2016, Yancey *et al.* 2004, Yancey *et al.* 2009, Yancey *et al.* 2011). Implementation in school-based settings, in particular, has shown improvements in behavior and focus among students (Whitt-Glover *et al.* 2011, Whitt-Glover *et al.* 2013, Woods 2011).

Implications for practice

Data from national samples have highlighted low levels of participation in leisure-time physical activity and higher rates of participation in sedentary behavior among African Americans. Data also suggest that African Americans perceive that they participate in greater levels of physical activity associated with occupational and daily living tasks, and that leisure time is equated with laziness. There is limited information on the association between physical activities associated with occupation, transportation, and daily living and chronic disease outcomes. Leisure-time physical activity, which includes purposeful exercise to improve aspects of health, may have different effects on chronic disease outcomes directly (through the positive impact of exercise) and indirectly (through mental health/stress-reducing benefits derived from participating in "pleasurable" activities rather than activities that are necessary). There might also be linkages related to real or perceived ability to engage in leisure-time physical activities, including socioeconomic status, family structure, and neighborhood environment that might also impact health status. These areas deserve further exploration.

The previous sections highlighted correlates of and strategies that have been tested to increase physical activity participation among African Americans. Importantly, previous reviews of the literature have noted that most intervention studies have not systematically tested strategies to impact factors that are known to increase physical activity in African Americans. The AACORN paradigm is an example of how the factors, mentioned earlier, that influence physical activity can be incorporated into strategies to address physical activity in African Americans groups. For example, in addition to providing education in adults, a successful strategy for increasing physical activity might include incorporating the importance of family/ friends, caregiving duties, and safety into intervention strategies. Such incorporation might lead to strategies that include family-based physical activities or strategies that emphasize the importance of engaging in physical activity *in addition to* existing daily activities. Interestingly, a review of family-focused strategies to promote physical activity, diet, and weight control in African American girls identified 27 studies, most of which targeted parent-child pairs but used intervention strategies that did not truly incorporate family into all aspects of the intervention (Barr-Anderson et al. 2013). A conclusion from the study was that additional attention is needed to understand how to best involve family members in intervention strategies.

Future intervention strategies might also focus on the importance of leisure time for overall health in an effort to change perceptions that leisure is related to laziness. Identifying strategies to address physical activity that are free or low cost could alleviate any socioeconomic concerns. Soliciting input from members of the communities in which interventions would be implemented would be helpful for incorporating additional feedback, which is a constituent-involving strategy for cultural tailoring. Future interventions should continue to involve the community in the design and implementation process through CBPR and should aim to include randomized control trial designs, objective physical activity measures, and culturally tailored intervention components with long-term follow-ups to bolster intervention effectiveness and to improve our ability to compare interventions and draw meaningful conclusions. Furthermore, intervention and study methods should be thoroughly detailed in research reports for best practices to be determined. The AACORN paradigm is one example for addressing sedentary behavior in racial/ ethnic minority communities. Even if the AACORN paradigm is not used, what is evident is that regular participation in leisure-time physical activity is low in racial/ ethnic minority communities; morbidity and mortality associated with low levels of physical activity is also high in racial/ethnic minority communities. Identifying successful paradigms and strategies to address low levels of physical activity in high-risk communities is a critical need.

Summary points

- Participation in leisure-time physical activity is low, and participation in sedentary behavior in African American adults and children is high.
- Correlates of leisure-time physical activity and sedentary behavior are known and should be considered in strategies to address physical activity in African Americans.

- The AACORN paradigm offers a unique strategy for incorporating factors that influence health-related behaviors.
- Interventions focused on improving physical activity behaviors among African Americans are diverse in regard to setting, target populations, and methods employed.
- Several important limitations exist in the current body of literature.

Critical thinking questions

1   How do we best tailor our physical activity interventions to be salient to African Americans, in alignment with the AACORN paradigm? Which cultural, psychosocial, historical, social, and environmental factors can effectively translate into higher-quality, more impactful intervention strategies?
2   What unique strategies may be employed to engage African American subgroups who are underrepresented in intervention studies: younger adults < 40 years, older adults > 65 years, and men?
3   How may study designs be strengthened to improve scientific rigor and assess longer-term intervention impacts?

References

Abercrombie, L. C., Sallis, J. F., Conway, T. L., Frank, L. D., Saelens, B. E. and Chapman, J. E. (2008) 'Income and racial disparities in access to public parks and private recreation facilities'. *American Journal of Preventive Medicine*, 34: 9–15.

Affuso, O., Cox, T. L., Durant, N. H. and Allison, D. B. (2011) 'Attitudes and beliefs associated with leisure-time physical activity among African American adults'. *Ethnicity & Disease*, 21: 63–7.

Ainsworth, B. E., Wilcox, S., Thompson, W. W., Richter, D. L. and Henderson, K. A. (2003) 'Personal, social, and physical environmental correlates of physical activity in African-American women in South Carolina'. *American Journal of Preventive Medicine*, 25: 23–29.

Airhihenbuwa, C. O., Kumanyika, S. K., Agurs, T. D. and Lowe, A. (1995) 'Perceptions and beliefs about exercise, rest, and health among African-Americans'. *American Journal of Health Promotion*, 9: 426–9.

Airhihenbuwa, C. O., Kumanyika, S. K., Tenhave, T. R. and Morssink, C. B. (2000) 'Cultural identity and health lifestyles among African Americans: A new direction for health intervention research?'. *Ethnicity & Disease*, 10: 148–64.

Arias, E. (2016) Changes in life expectancy by race and Hispanic origin in the United States, 2013–2014. *NCHS Data Brief, No. 244*. Hyattsville, MD.

Banks-Wallace, J. and Conn, V. (2002) 'Interventions to promote physical activity among African American women'. *Public Health Nursing*, 19: 321–35.

Barr-Anderson, D. J., Adams-Wynn, A. W., Disantis, K. I. and Kumanyika, S. (2013) 'Family-focused physical activity, diet and obesity interventions in African-American girls: A systematic review'. *Obesity Reviews*, 14: 29–51.

Barr-Anderson, D. J., Singleton, C., Cotwright, C. J., Floyd, M. F. and Affuso, O. (2014) 'Outside-of-school time obesity prevention and treatment interventions in African American youth'. *Obesity Reviews*, 15 Suppl 4: 26–45.

Bopp, M., Lattimore, D., Wilcox, S., Laken, M., McClorin, L., Swinton, R., Gethers, O. and Bryant, D. (2007) 'Understanding physical activity participation in members of an African American church: A qualitative study'. *Health Education Research*, 22: 815–26.

Bopp, M., Peterson, J. and Webb, B. (2012) 'A comprehensive review of faith-based physical activity interventions'. *American Journal of Lifestyle Medicine*, 6: 460–78.

Bopp, M., Wilcox, S., Laken, M., Butler, K., Carter, R. E., McClorin, L. and Yancey, A. (2006) 'Factors associated with physical activity among African-American men and women'. *American Journal of Preventive Medicine*, 30: 340–6.

Bopp, M., Wilcox, S., Laken, M., Hooker, S. P., Parra-Medina, D., Saunders, R., Butler, K., Fallon, E. A. and McClorin, L. (2009) '8 steps to fitness: A faith-based, behavior change physical activity intervention for African Americans'. *Journal of Physical Activity and Health*, 6: 568–77.

Boyington, J. E., Carter-Edwards, L., Piehl, M., Hutson, J., Langdon, D. and Mcmanus, S. (2008) 'Cultural attitudes toward weight, diet, and physical activity among overweight African American girls'. *Preventing Chronic Disease*, 5: A36.

Buchowski, M. S., Cohen, S. S., Matthews, C. E., Schlundt, D. G., Signorello, L. B., Hargreaves, M. K. and Blot, W. J. (2010) 'Physical activity and obesity gap between black and white women in the southeastern U.S'. *American Journal of Preventive Medicine*, 39: 140–7.

Carroll-Scott, A., Gilstad-Hayden, K., Rosenthal, L., Peters, S. M., McCaslin, C., Joyce, R. and Ickovics, J. R. (2013) 'Disentangling neighborhood contextual associations with child body mass index, diet, and physical activity: The role of built, socioeconomic, and social environments'. *Social Science Medicine*, 95: 106–14.

Casagrande, S. S., Whitt-Glover, M. C., Lancaster, K. J., Odoms-Young, A. M. and Gary, T. L. (2009) 'Built environment and health behaviors among African Americans: A systematic review'. *American Journal of Preventive Medicine*, 36: 174–81.

Centers for Disease Control and Prevention. (2013) QuickStats: Percentage of Adults Aged ≥18 Years Who Met the Aerobic Activity and Muscle Strengthening Guidelines,* by Sex and Selected Race/Ethnicity: National Health Interview Survey, United States, 2009–2011. *National Health Interview Survey, 2009–2011.*

Centers for Disease Control and Prevention (2013a) 'Adult participation in aerobic and muscle-strengthening physical activities: United States, 2011'. *MMWR Morbidity and Mortality Weekly Report*, 62: 326–30.

Centers for Disease Control and Prevention (2013b) 'CDC Health Disparities and Inequalities Report: United States, 2013'. *MMWR Supplements*, 62: 1–187.

Chang, M. W., Nitzke, S., Guilford, E., Adair, C. H. and Hazard, D. L. (2008) 'Motivators and barriers to healthful eating and physical activity among low-income overweight and obese mothers'. *Journal of the American Dietetic Association*, 108: 1023–8.

Cogbill, S. A., Sanders Thompson, V. L. and Deshpande, A. D. (2011) 'Selected sociocultural correlates of physical activity among African-American adults'. *Ethnicity & Health*, 16: 625–41.

Conn, V., Phillips, L., Ruppar, T. and Chase, J.-A. D. (2012) 'Physical activity interventions with healthy minority adults: Meta-analysis of behavior and health outcomes'. *Journal of Health Care for the Poor and Underserved*, 23: 59–80.

Coughlin, S. S. and Smith, S. A. (2016) 'A review of community-based participatory research studies to promote physical activity among African Americans'. *Journal of the Georgia Public Health Association*, 5: 220–7.

Evenson, K. R., Buchner, D. M. and Morland, K. B. (2012) 'Objective measurement of physical activity and sedentary behavior among US adults aged 60 years or older'. *Preventing Chronic Disease*, 9.

Fleury, J. and Lee, S. M. (2006) 'The social ecological model and physical activity in African American women'. *American Journal of Community Psychology*, 37: 129.

Gay, J. L. and Buchner, D. M. (2014) 'Ethnic disparities in objectively measured physical activity may be due to occupational activity'. *Preventive Medicine*, 63: 58–62.

Hall, R. R., Francis, S., Whitt-Glover, M., Loftin-Bell, K., Swett, K. and McMichael, A. J. (2013) 'Hair care practices as a barrier to physical activity in African American women'. *JAMA Dermatology*, 149: 310–14.

Haughton, C. F., Wang, M. L. and Lemon, S. C. (2016) 'Racial/ethnic disparities in meeting 5-2-1-0 recommendations among children and adolescents in the United States'. *Journal of Pediatrics*, 175: 188–194.

Im, E. O., Ko, Y., Hwang, H., Chee, W., Stuifbergen, A., Walker, L. and Brown, A. (2013) 'Racial/ethnic differences in midlife women's attitudes toward physical activity'. *Journal of Midwifery & Women's Health*, 58: 440–50.

Jenkins, F., Jenkins, C., Gregoski, M. J. and Magwood, G. S. (2015) 'Interventions promoting physical activity in African American women: An integrative review'. *Journal of Cardiovascular Nursing*, 32(1): 22–29

Johnson, K. S., Elbert-Avila, K. I. and Tulsky, J. A. (2005) 'The influence of spiritual beliefs and practices on the treatment preferences of African Americans: A review of the literature'. *Journal of the American Geriatrics Society*, 53: 711–19.

Johnson, R. L. and Nies, M. A. (2005) 'A qualitative perspective of barriers to health-promoting behaviors of African Americans'. *ABNF Journal*, 16: 39–41.

Jones, S. A., Moore, L. V., Moore, K., Zagorski, M., Brines, S. J., Diez Roux, A. V. and Evenson, K. R. (2015) 'Disparities in physical activity resource availability in six US regions'. *Preventive Medicine*, 78: 17–22.

Joseph, R. P., Ainsworth, B. E., Keller, C. and Dodgson, J. E. (2015) 'Barriers to physical activity among African American women: An integrative review of the literature'. *Women & Health*, 55: 679–99.

Joseph, R. P., Keller, C., Affuso, O. and Ainsworth, B. E. (2016) 'Designing culturally relevant physical activity programs for African-American women: A framework for intervention development'. *Journal of Racial & Ethnic Health Disparities*.

Kann, L., Mcmanus, T., Harris, W. A., Shanklin, S. L., Flint, K. H., Hawkins, J., Queen, B., Lowry, R., Olsen, E. O., Chyen, D., Whittle, L., Thornton, J., Lim, C., Yamakawa, Y., Brener, N. and Zaza, S. (2016) 'Youth risk behavior Surveillance: United States, 2015'. *MMWR Surveillance Summaries*, 65: 1–174.

Kimm, S. Y., Glynn, N. W., Kriska, A. M., Barton, B. A., Kronsberg, S. S., Daniels, S. R., Crawford, P. B., Sabry, Z. I. and Liu, K. (2002) 'Decline in physical activity in black girls and white girls during adolescence'. *New England Journal of Medicine*, 347: 709–15.

Kumanyika, S. K., Whitt-Glover, M. C., Gary, T. L., Prewitt, T. E., Odoms-Young, A. M., Banks-Wallace, J., Beech, B. M., Halbert, C. H., Karanja, N., Lancaster, K. J. and Samuel-Hodge, C. D. (2007) 'Expanding the obesity research paradigm to reach African American communities'. *Preventing Chronic Disease*, 4: A112.

Lancaster, K. J., Carter-Edwards, L., Grilo, S., Shen, C. and Schoenthaler, A. M. (2014) 'Obesity interventions in African American faith-based organizations: A systematic review'. *Obesity Reviews*, 15 Suppl 4: 159–76.

LaBreche, M., Cheri, A., Custodio, H., Fex, C. C., Foo, M. A., Lepule, J. T., May, V. T., Orne, A., Pang, J. K., Pang, V. K., Sablan-Santos, L., Schmidt-Vaivao, D., Surani, Z., Talavou, M. F., Toilolo, T., Palmer, P. H. and Tanjasiri, S. P. (2016) 'Let's move for Pacific Islander communities: An evidence-based intervention to increase physical activity'. *Journal of Cancer Education*, 31: 261–7.

Lytle, L. A., Murray, D. M., Evenson, K. R., Moody, J., Pratt, C. A., Metcalfe, L. and Parra-Medina, D. (2009) 'Mediators affecting girls' levels of physical activity outside of school: Findings from the trial of activity in adolescent girls'. *Annals of Behavioral Medicine*, 38: 124–36.

Marcus, B. H., Dubbert, P. M., Forsyth, L. H., Mckenzie, T. L., Stone, E. J., Dunn, A. L. and Blair, S. N. (2000) 'Physical activity behavior change: Issues in adoption and maintenance'. *Health Psychology*, 19: 32–41.

McDonald, N. C. (2008) 'Critical factors for active transportation to school among low-income and minority students: Evidence from the 2001 National Household Travel Survey'. *American Journal of Preventive Medicine*, 34: 341–4.

Mental Health America. (2016) *Black & African American Communities and Mental Health* [Online]. Available: www.mentalhealthamerica.net/african-american-mental-health#Source 3 (Accessed November 11, 2016).

Miller, S. T. and Marolen, K. (2012) 'Physical activity-related experiences, counseling expectations, personal responsibility, and altruism among urban African American women with type 2 diabetes'. *Diabetes Education*, 38: 229–35.

National Center for Health. (2016) *Health, United States, 2015: With special feature on racial and ethnic health disparities.* Hyattsville, MD: National Center for Health Statistics (US).

Newton, R. L., Jr., Griffith, D. M., Kearney, W. B. and Bennett, G. G. (2014) 'A systematic review of weight loss, physical activity and dietary interventions involving African American men'. *Obesity Reviews*, 15 Suppl 4: 93–106.

Ogden, C. L., Carroll, M. D., Fryar, C. D. and Flegal, K. M. (2015) 'Prevalence of obesity among adults and youth: United States, 2011–2014'. *NCHS Data Brief*, 219: 1–8.

Physical Activity Guidelines Advisory Committee (2008). *Physical Activity Guidelines Advisory Committee Report, 2008.* Washington DC: US Department of Health and Human Services.

Rees, R., Kavanagh, J., Harden, A., Shepherd, J., Brunton, G., Oliver, S. and Oakley, A. (2006) 'Young people and physical activity: A systematic review matching their views to effective interventions'. *Health Education Research*, 21: 806–25.

Robinson, L. E., Webster, E. K., Whitt-Glover, M. C., Ceaser, T. G. and Alhassan, S. (2014) 'Effectiveness of pre-school- and school-based interventions to impact weight-related behaviours in African American children and youth: A literature review'. *Obesity Reviews*, 15 Suppl 4: 5–25.

Sanderson, B. K., Foushee, H. R., Bittner, V., Cornell, C. E., Stalker, V., Shelton, S. and Pulley, L. (2003) 'Personal, social, and physical environmental correlates of physical activity in rural African-American women in Alabama'. *American Journal of Preventive Medicine*, 25: 30–7.

Siddiqi, Z., Tiro, J. A. and Shuval, K. (2011) 'Understanding impediments and enablers to physical activity among African American adults: A systematic review of qualitative studies'. *Health Education Research*, 26: 1010–24.

Strong, L. L., Reitzel, L. R., Wetter, D. W. and Mcneill, L. H. (2013) 'Associations of perceived neighborhood physical and social environments with physical activity and television viewing in African-American men and women'. *Health Promotion*, 27: 401–9.

Taylor, W. C., Baranowski, T. and Young, D. R. (1998) 'Physical activity interventions in low-income, ethnic minority, and populations with disability'. *American Journal of Preventive Medicine*, 15: 334–43.

Thompson, W. M. and Barksdale, D. J. (2010) 'Physical inactivity in female African-American adolescents: Consequences, costs, & care'. *Journal of National Black Nurses' Association: JNBNA*, 21: 39–45.

Troiano, R., Berrigan, D., Dodd, K., Masse, L., Tilert, T. and Mcdowell, M. (2008) 'Physical activity in the United States measured by accelerometer'. *Medicine and Science in Sports and Exercise*, 40: 181–8.

Tudor-Locke, C., Henderson, K. A., Wilcox, S., Cooper, R. S., Durstine, J. L. and Ainsworth, B. E. (2003) 'In their own voices: Definitions and interpretations of physical activity'. *Women's Health Issues*, 13: 194–9.

U.S. Bureau of the Census. (2011) *The Black Population: 2010. US Department of Commerce* [Online]. Available: www.census.gov/prod/cen2010/briefs/c2010br-06.pdf (Accessed November 11, 2016).

U.S. Bureau of the Census. (2012) *Statistical Abstract of the United States: 2012 (131st Edition), Section 4: Education* [Online]. Available: http://census.gov/library/publications/2011/compendia/statab/131ed/education.html (Accessed November 11, 2016).

U.S. Department of Health and Human Services Office of Minority Mental Health. (2016) *Mental Health and African Americans* [Online]. Available: http://minorityhealth.hhs.gov/omh/browse.aspx?lvl=4&lvlid=24 (Accessed November 11, 2016).

Watson, K. B., Harris, C. D., Carlson, S. A., Dorn, J. M. and Fulton, J. E. (2016) 'Disparities in adolescents' residence in neighborhoods supportive of physical activity: United States, 2011–2012'. *MMWR Morbidity and Mortality Weekly Report*, 65: 598–601.

Whitt-Glover, M. C., Brand, D. J., Turner, M. E., Ward, S. A. and Jackson, E. M. (2009) 'Increasing physical activity among African-American women and girls'. *Current Sports Medicine Reports*, 8: 318–24.

Whitt-Glover, M. C., Goldmon, M. V., Karanja, N., Heil, D. P. and Gizlice, Z. (2012) 'Learning and Developing Individual Exercise Skills (L.A.D.I.E.S.) for a better life: A physical activity intervention for black women'. *Contemporary Clinical Trials*, 33: 1159–71.

Whitt-Glover, M. C., Ham, S. A. and Yancey, A. K. (2011) 'Instant Recess: A practical tool for increasing physical activity during the school day'. *Progress in Community Health Partnerships*, 5: 289–97.

Whitt-Glover, M. C., Keith, N. R., Ceaser, T. G., Virgil, K., Ledford, L. and Hasson, R. E. (2014) 'A systematic review of physical activity interventions among African American adults: Evidence from 2009 to 2013'. *Obesity Reviews*, 15 Suppl 4: 125–45.

Whitt-Glover, M. C. and Kumanyika, S. K. (2009) 'Systematic review of interventions to increase physical activity and physical fitness in African-Americans'. *American Journal of Health Promotion*, 23: S33–56.

Whitt-Glover, M. C., Porter, A. T. and Yancey, A. K. (2013) *Do physical activity breaks in classrooms work?* San Diego, CA: Active Living Research.

Whitt-Glover, M. C., Taylor, W. C., Heath, G. W. and Macera, C. A. (2007) 'Self-reported physical activity among blacks: Estimates from national surveys'. *American Journal of Preventive Medicine*, 33: 412–17.

Wilbur, J. (2003) 'Correlates of physical activity in urban Midwestern African-American women'. *American Journal of Preventive Medicine*, 25: 45–52.

Wilson, D. K., Lawman, H. G., Segal, M. and Chappell, S. (2011) 'Neighborhood and parental supports for physical activity in minority adolescents'. *American Journal of Preventive Medicine*, 41: 399–406.

Woods, C. D. (2011) *Evaluation of Instant Recess exercise breaks as a means for implementing LAUSD physical activity policy in elementary schools.* Doctor of Public Health Dissertation, University of California, Los Angeles.

Woolford, S. J., Woolford-Hunt, C. J., Sami, A., Blake, N. and Williams, D. R. (2016) 'No sweat: African American adolescent girls' opinions of hairstyle choices and physical activity'. *BMC Obesity*, 3: 31.

Yancey, A. K. (2010) *Instant Recess: Building a fit nation 10 minutes at a time*. Los Angeles, CA: University of California Press.

Yancey, A. K., Grant, D., Kurosky, S., Kravitz-Wirtz, N. and Mistry, R. (2011). Role modeling, risk, and resilience in California adolescents. *Journal of Adolescent Health*, 48: 36–43.

Yancey, A. K., McCarthy, W. J., Taylor, W. C., Merlo, A., Gewa, C., Weber, M. D. and Fielding, J. E. (2004) 'The Los Angeles lift off: A sociocultural environmental change intervention to integrate physical activity into the workplace'. *Preventive Medicine*, 38: 848–56.

Yancey, A. K., Winfield, D., Larsen, J., Anderson, M., Jackson, P., Overton, J., Wilson, S., Rossum, A. and Kumanyika, S. (2009) '"Live, learn and play": Building strategic alliances between professional sports and public health'. *Preventive Medicine*, 49: 322–5.

Young, D. R. and Voorhees, C. C. (2003) 'Personal, social, and environmental correlates of physical activity in urban African-American women'. *American Journal of Preventive Medicine*, 25: 38–44.

5

PHYSICAL ACTIVITY AMONG LATINOS

David X. Marquez, Susan Aguiñaga, Priscilla Vásquez, Isabela Gouveia Marques and Maricela Martinez

Understanding the Latino population

The Latino population is the fastest-growing minority group in the US, expected to reach 119 million by 2060 (Pew Hispanic Research Center 2014). Latinos are a heterogeneous group that vary in race, country of origin, immigration status, socio-economic characteristics, cultural values, beliefs, and practices. The term *Latino/ Hispanic* refers to immigrants from many different countries, and many times, unfortunately, does not consider the different subgroups. The three most common groups of Latinos in the United States are Mexican, Puerto Rican, and Cuban. However, it also comprises people coming from other countries from Central America, South America, and (sometimes) Spain (Rodriguez *et al.* 2014, Santiago-Rivera *et al.* 2001). More than half (55%) of the US Latino population live in three states, California, Texas, and Florida; and eight states have a Latino population of over 1 million (i.e., California, Texas, Florida, New York, Illinois, Arizona, New Jersey, and Colorado) (Brown and Lopez 2013).

The terms *Latino* and *Hispanic* have been used interchangeably in reports and in the literature; however, research has shown that the term *Latino* is often preferred instead of *Hispanic*. *Hispanic* was a term introduced in the 1970s by the Office of Management and Budget, serving as a label to characterize the group of people from Spanish origins without considering differences in culture, traditions, history, but focusing mainly on the Spanish language (Santiago-Rivera *et al.* 2001). The term is currently less preferred by the community itself given the imposition of the term on the group as well as implicitly referring to only European descent and negating Native indigenous roots (Santiago-Rivera *et al.* 2001). Instead, people often have a preference to be called by the country of origin (Pew Hispanic Center 2012) or the use of the term *Latino*. *Latino* is a gendered term whereby *Latino* refers to males and *Latina* to females and efforts to be more gender-inclusive have led to using *Latina/o* and other variations.

We will adopt the term *Latino* throughout this chapter, and the main idea is that either term should be interpreted as a heterogeneous group, especially considering health outcomes as they may vary broadly.

Demographic characteristics

According to the US Census (2015), the income of Latinos (about $40,000/year) is similar to that of Non-Latino Blacks, which is substantially lower than Non-Latino Whites (NLWs) (about $60,000/year). Regarding educational attainment, 65.3% of Latinos had a high school education or higher compared to 88.8% of NLWs, with lower educational attainment among foreign-born Latinos. Data also show that for the Latino population, 23.5% have no health insurance coverage compared to 10.4% for NLWs (Rodriguez *et al.* 2014, Santiago–Rivera *et al.* 2001).

Common cultural beliefs

As public health practitioners, an understanding of common cultural beliefs can assist in delivering culturally relevant information and may support efforts to develop culturally tailored interventions. Here we briefly describe some concepts that have characterized Latino culture. *Familismo* refers to the increased value given to family members as the main source of emotional and material support. *Personalismo* refers to an appropriate amount of time to institute a close and constant bond, also relating to the respect of older generations. *Machismo* refers to the patriarchal authority, and *Marianismo* represents "women values," as virtuous, but mainly as being available for the family needs, and prioritizing family duties over self-care. Spirituality also plays an important role in Latino culture, and an important aspect is the concept of *fatalismo*, where events are perceived as not preventable, something will happen if it is supposed to happen per "God's will" (Rodriguez *et al.* 2014). Another related and important component is language. Despite the fact that most Latin American countries predominantly speak Spanish (except for Brazil), there are differences in dialects and accents in addition to the presence of Native and indigenous languages. Health-related materials to be used in Spanish should be aware of these differences and adjust accordingly.

Historical background

Latin America has a history of several cultural influences starting with the colonization period. Racial and cultural mixing occurred especially after interracial marriage was legalized in the fifteenth century. Different groups were responsible for this heterogeneity, such as Spanish and Portuguese conquests. Thus, Latin American groups vary in geography, culture, and race (Rodriguez *et al.* 2014, Santiago–Rivera *et al.* 2001). The Latino population also varies in immigration status and reasons to immigrate to the US, and such factors have a great impact on health-related outcomes.

Mexicans are the largest and oldest Latino population in the US, since the fifteenth century (Rodriguez *et al.* 2014, Santiago-Rivera *et al.* 2001). Puerto Ricans, either born in the mainland, or in the US territory, are considered US citizens by birth, and thus do not face issues with the immigration process, like other Latino groups.

The first largest Cuban immigration occurred following the increased power of Fidel Castro, and was primarily composed of educated and wealthy Cubans (Rodriguez *et al.* 2014, Santiago-Rivera *et al.* 2001). The Dominican Republic comprises two-thirds of the island, and Haiti is located on the remaining area of the island. The Dominican community in the US is considerably recent (Rodriguez *et al.* 2014, Santiago-Rivera *et al.* 2001).

Central America is composed of people from countries such as Guatemala and El Salvador. Due to the geographical proximity to the US, this has allowed for the migration of individuals with low socioeconomic status (SES). Immigrants from South America usually have a higher socioeconomic profile, and probably due to the geographical distance, those of more disadvantaged social standing are unable to afford migration (Santiago-Rivera *et al.* 2001).

Health disparities and inequities among the Latino population

Approaches to address health inequities among Latinos are complex and should account for overarching and distinct characteristics from other underrepresented groups. The distinct characteristics have implications for how we can target this diverse population to alleviate the burden of chronic and infectious conditions across the lifespan.

Chronic diseases

Emerging research on chronic diseases affecting the Latino population demonstrates the importance of specifying Latino subgroups by country of origin, time living in the United States, and other characteristics in order to accurately depict the health status of the group (Castañeda *et al.* 2016, González *et al.* 2016, Penedo *et al.* 2015). Overall, social determinants of health play a major role in determining health outcomes for this population and should be considered as we frame our research and preventive efforts.

Cardiovascular and metabolic health

The Hispanic Community Health Study/Study of Latinos (HCHS/SOL) is a large US multicenter epidemiological study which includes adults aged 18–74 who are from Mexican, Puerto Rican, Cuban, Dominican, Central American, and South American backgrounds. Daviglus et al. report differences by Latino background and gender in the prevalence of major cardiovascular disease (CVD) risk factors including hypercholesterolemia, hypertension, obesity, diabetes, and smoking (Daviglus *et al.* 2014a). Findings demonstrate that a large proportion of the study sample had at least one CVD risk factor and the presence of three or more risk factors was highest among Puerto Ricans, those with less education, those living in the US for 10 years or more, those who were US-born, and lastly those who preferred the English language. Research with younger generations shows similar results, whereby Mexican American children have higher rates of diabetes and lower rates of ideal fasting glucose compared to their Black and Non-Latino White counterparts (Daviglus *et al.* 2014b). Metabolic health is determined by examining triglyceride levels, HDL cholesterol levels, blood pressure levels, fasting glucose levels, and examination of the metabolic syndrome includes abdominal obesity (Alberti *et al.* 2009). Examples of disparities in metabolic health include Latinos being 1.7 times as likely as Non-Latino Whites to be diagnosed with diabetes (OMH 2016a), and 77% of Mexican American women are overweight or obese, compared to only 64% of Non-Latina White women (OMH 2016b). Metabolic syndrome examined in the HCHS/SOL study observed a prevalence of 33.7% among men and 36.0% among women, with the highest among Puerto Ricans (Heiss *et al.* 2014).

Cognitive and mental health

The presence of a rapidly aging population, low educational levels, and high rates of diabetes among Latinos result in a higher risk for the development of dementia and warrants urgent attention. The Alzheimer's Association reported a projected six-fold increase of Latinos with Alzheimer's disease from fewer than 200,000 individuals in 2004 to 1.3 million by 2050 (Alzheimer's Association 2007). Physical inactivity has been identified as a modifiable risk factor for Alzheimer's disease. Approximately 21% (or >1.1 million) of cases are attributed to physical inactivity whereby a 10–25% reduction in this risk factor could prevent between 90,000–230,000 cases in the US. An increase in the levels of PA also has the potential to impact other risk factors such as diabetes, hypertension, and obesity (Barnes and Yaffe 2011).

An individual's mental health is complementary to cognitive health and includes an individual's emotional, psychological, and social well-being (CDC 2016). Recently 27% of Latinos reported high levels of depressive symptoms with the highest being among Puerto Ricans with 38% (Wassertheil-Smoller *et al.* 2014). Individuals 45–64 years old were 21% more likely to have symptoms of depression, women were twice as likely as men, and a higher number of cardiovascular disease risk factors resulted in a greater likelihood of reporting depressive symptoms.

The protective effects of engaging in regular leisure-time physical activity on cognitive health and emotional health exist. However, given the low levels of leisure-time physical activity among Latinos, this provides practitioners a unique challenge and opportunity to improve health outcomes among this population (Arredondo *et al.* 2012, Arredondo *et al.* 2016, Lautenschlager and Almeida 2006, Wilbur *et al.* 2012). Efforts in this area will both improve health and reduce the health inequities currently present in the US.

Mortality and the Hispanic Paradox

Given that the majority of Latinos have a lower SES in comparison to other groups, it would be expected for Latinos to have higher mortality rates in many of the leading causes of death. However, this has not been demonstrated in the large surveillance datasets. This epidemiological phenomenon is known as the Hispanic Paradox (Markides and Coreil 1986). Possible explanations have been described by Medina-Inojosa et al. such as the Salmon bias where Latinos who immigrate to the United States return to their country of origin once learning of terminal illness or death. The level of acculturation is another possible explanation whereby those who are the least acculturated retain their healthy behaviors from their country of origin. Another viable explanation would be the reliability of the data such that mortality data are not accurately captured for Latinos (Medina-Inojosa *et al.* 2014). As outlined in Chapter 2, often health outcomes are related to social, cultural, and environmental outcomes. Understanding this phenomenon can provide insight on how we can continue to support this group in maintaining the protective factors already in place while simultaneously alleviating the burden of chronic disease that disproportionately impact Latinos.

Physical activity among Latinos

Latinos are not less informed about the benefits of physical activity in comparison to their NLW counterparts. However, despite this knowledge, on average Latinos do not meet physical activity recommendations. From a social ecological perspective, Latinos of all ages, sexual orientation, and immigration status face complex barriers to engaging in PA. Common barriers to physical activity among Latinos are shown in Table 5.1.

Common barriers and facilitators to physical activity for Latinos

Starting at the individual level, self-efficacy, the confidence one has in his or her ability to successfully execute a specific task (Bandura 1997, Salinas *et al.* 2014), is among the strongest predictors of physical activity among Latinos (Marquez *et al.* 2009). Four sources impact levels of self-efficacy: mastery experiences, vicarious experiences, social persuasion, and interpretation of physiological and emotional states. Latinos may have a lack of mastery physical activity experiences, more specifically, a lack of history of engaging in traditional exercise (e.g., lifting weights, going to a gym) resulting in low self-efficacy. Latinos may also have a lack of vicarious experiences such as a lack of role models who are also physically active, thus resulting in low self-efficacy. Latinos may lack people encouraging them to become physically active. Feelings of embarrassment and stress levels due to financial constraints or neighborhood environment may impact Latinos' physiological and emotional state, also resulting in low self-efficacy.

Acculturation is another factor that may act as a barrier to physical activity. Acculturation (also refer to Chapter 3) is the degree to which individuals retain their

TABLE 5.1 Barriers and strategies to physical activity for Latinos

Barrier for PA	Barriers for PA for Latinos	Strategies to Overcome Barriers
Self-efficacy: mastery experiences	Lack of history of engaging in traditional exercise	Interventions can promote non-traditional types of exercise
Self-efficacy: vicarious experiences	Lack of role models who are also physically active	Use *promotoras*
Self-efficacy: social persuasion	Lack of people encouraging them to become physically active	Use *promotoras* and include family members
Self-efficacy: interpretation of physiological and emotional states	Unfamiliar with how exercise will make one feel, physically and emotionally	Education about the effects of exercise
	Acculturation	
	Language	Interventions could include materials and resources in Spanish and English
Time constraints	Latinos may work more than one job and may spend more time commuting	Include family members
Social support	Having no one to exercise with, lack social support to exercise	Use *promotoras* or community health workers to deliver the intervention; capitalize on strong social ties in Latino communities
Physical environment	Living in disadvantaged neighborhoods	Use strategies in existing resources, such as walking in a grocery store, shopping mall, etc.
Environmental issues	Disproportionate impact on Latinos and those living in low-income housing	Use multi-level interventions that focus on change at the family, community, and society level, in addition to the individual level

culture of origin while adopting certain aspects of the dominant culture in their new country of residence (Berry and Sabatier 2011). Acculturation may be very difficult to measure due to complex, dynamic, and multidimensional processes (Van Wieren *et al.* 2011). Some studies have shown that Latinos who are more accultur-ated to the English language and US culture and values participate in higher levels of physical activity (Crespo *et al.* 2001) (Martinez *et al.* 2012). Despite this evidence, acculturation should be interpreted with caution as ethnic culture is at times made culpable for physical activity differences. Examining the historical, political, and economic contexts of Latino subgroups is important to consider because physical activity levels may differ based on where Latinos come from and where they currently reside in the US.

Language is another complex individual-level factor that may act as a barrier to engaging in physical activity. Some studies have shown that language barriers may contribute to lack of access to physical activity information (Salinas *et al.* 2014). In more socially isolated Latino immigrant communities, language barriers may create and reinforce negative racial/ethnic perceptions, a lack of communication, and a limited access to broader social and economic networks and resources (Barrington *et al.* 2012).

Time constraints is another commonly cited barrier among Latinos. Although time is a common barrier among all groups, time may be especially pertinent among Latinos because they may work more than one job and may spend more time commuting; thus reducing leisure time that might otherwise be spent physically active.

The social environment is another aspect of the ecological model that impacts physical activity among Latinos. The social environment comprises the relationships, the culture, and the society with whom the individual interacts. Social support is an important predictor of physical activity in Latinos (Marquez and McAuley 2006) in which family, friends, and even broader social networks can play a role in encouraging or discouraging physical activity behaviors (Larson 2013). Studies have shown that Latinos may face social barriers such as having no one to exercise with (D'Alonzo and Fischetti 2008). Social support may be so salient for Latinos that one study found that Latinas who reported simply seeing people exercise in their neighborhood were more likely to exercise than those who did not (Wilbur *et al.* 2003).

The physical environment is the next layer of the social ecological model that impacts physical activity participation due to physical activity taking place in either the natural environment or the built environment. Latinos are more likely to live in disadvantaged neighborhoods in comparison to NLWs (Cubbin *et al.* 2000). Low SES neighborhoods have few physical activity resources (Estabrooks *et al.* 2003), and they may also be of lower quality (Lee *et al.* 2005). These neighborhoods may also have poorly maintained parks or uneven sidewalks, and fewer free activity resources than those in higher SES neighborhoods (Estabrooks *et al.* 2003). Furthermore, low SES neighborhoods may be less safe, thus Latinos of all ages may avoid spending time outdoors and ultimately reducing opportunities to engage in physical activities (Lee and Cubbin 2009). Environmental issues such as outdoor air pollution have a disproportionate impact on Latinos and those living in low-income housing. In an attempt to avoid these toxic environments, Latinos may not participate in outdoor physical activities. Many Latinos also live in three states that are being greatly impacted by climate change, such as California, Texas, and Florida (Environmental Defense Fund, 2016). The droughts in California, extreme heat in Texas, and flooding in Florida could substantially decrease Latinos' engagement in activity.

Policy level is the outermost layer of the social ecological model which refers to legislation and policy making actions that have the potential to impact physical activity. Macro-environmental-level policies can be used to increase physical activity participation; however, these may favor some groups more than others.

For example, dedicated bike lanes may be less likely to be implemented in low SES neighborhoods, which are the neighborhoods that might actually benefit the most. In fact, if activity policies could be implemented among the communities that need them the most, the positive effects could still trickle to more affluent communities who already have access to physical activity resources.

Unique influences among specific Latino groups

Men

Many Latino men engage in some type of manual labor work, and this can lead to perceptions of already being fit. Men who have more physically demanding occupations may not see a reason to be active during their leisure time. Currently there is not enough literature on the barriers faced by Latino men that prevents them from engaging in activity; however, following are some of the important lessons we have learned from our work across segments of the Latino population.

Women

Latina women present some well-established barriers to participating in physical activities. Regarding the *marianismo* value discussed earlier in this chapter, Latinas are culturally responsible for taking care of the family members, even at the risk of not taking care of themselves. This issue comes in situations with caregiving of partners/spouses, grandchildren, occupational roles, spousal and maternal roles, and lack of spousal/family support. It is expected that the women will take care of grandchildren, or a sick family member, or even long-term caregiving for some serious illnesses, for example. Most of the time, this extra task is of higher priority than other occupational tasks. Most women who work and have children spend more hours working and caring for children than do their male counterparts, leading to less time for recreational fitness pursuits (Lee and Cubbin 2009). Latinas, for example, have often cited a cultural norm of spending much of their time caring for others, particularly their children, and reported that the idea of "leisure time," when they could do something of their choosing, was foreign or frowned upon (Larsen *et al.* 2015). Also, Latinas have different cultural norms of body shape, they may want to be classified as "overweight" instead of "normal weight" due to the curvilinear shape being attributed to wealth and motherhood. In this aspect, exercising would conflict with cultural norms. Once again, this should be interpreted with caution, as this cultural norm may vary across different Latin American countries and individuals.

Youth

One of the common barriers for Latino children is the lack of physical environment and facilities that promote activity; although some strategies can assist in overcoming some of the lack of appropriate space and unfavorable weather conditions (Lindsay *et al.* 2015). One important component in childhood is the intensive amount of screen time used as leisure. Television, video games, online games and social media are being used as a tool to manipulate disruptive behavior in social environments (Lindsay *et al.* 2015). Other barriers are psychological control (verbal criticism and insults), physical and/or emotional abuse, lack of parental engagement, and parents being afraid of children getting hurt (O'Connor *et al.* 2013). Role modeling, parenting engagement in child activities, and creativity are essential strategies to decrease screen time and sedentary behavior in Latino youth.

Older adults

In general, older adults face many difficulties to engaging in physical activity relative to young adults. However, this is even more so among older Latinos. As discussed earlier, traditional exercise may not be part of the Latino culture, and older Latinos might not consider initiating an exercise program in a gym/fitness center. Age-related issues play an important role in preventing this population from being active. Poor health conditions such as hypertension, diabetes, and chronic pain that are very prevalent among Latinos may inhibit or even exclude participation in exercise programs, especially for those who do not have knowledge about the benefits of physical activity.

Physiological alterations like worsening balance and decreased strength can lead to older Latinos decreasing daily activities due to the fear of falling or getting hurt. Decreasing daily activities can lead to accelerated progress of diseases, as well as decreased mental health or even depression. From a social standpoint, lack of support from family members can be a great barrier. Older Latinos might not have social networks other than family, and overprotection of family members can prevent physical activity participation.

Caregiving is another major barrier. As previously discussed, it is expected that women have this role; however, men usually assume this responsibility if the affected one is the wife. Alzheimer's disease and related dementia are becoming increasingly common in the Latino community, and due to cultural values, Latinos often assume the role of caregiver instead of using services such as nursing homes. Latinos report the feeling of having failed the family member if one is not able to take care of the relative, especially when the parent is the one affected by the disease (Calderon and Tennstedt 1998).

Immigration status

Several social and environmental factors may contribute to low levels of physical activity among Latino immigrants. These include anti-immigrant sentiment and legislative initiatives, leading immigrants to voluntarily curb their public exposure and therefore limit options for physical activity. Perceived racism and discrimination may contribute to the fact that Latinos may be less inclined to go to gyms or exercise in parks (Salinas et al. 2014). Immigrant women have cited immigration status issues as a barrier to activity and were less likely to be physically active if they believed doing so risked deportation (Salinas et al. 2014). Another aspect of immigration status may be fear of engaging in certain activities due to increased risk of injury. For example, undocumented Latinos may have an insecurity of biking to work. Traffic accidents could lead to accidents, and in many cases, immigrants lack health insurance, consequently limiting any type of possibly dangerous activity. And as new technological devices are more readily available and accessible in the US, immigrants may start to adopt new habits that increase sedentary time.

Leisure-time activity is frequently modified in a new country. Family members and friends that used to accompany Latinos in those activities might not be present, and leisure activities themselves can also be different. The lack of social support and familiar places or events may create a snowball effect, leading the person to be isolated. In many Latin American countries, people engage in some type of PA, mainly transportation physical activity, such as walking and biking, and the weather more often than not allows people to engage in leisure-time physical activity. When moving to the United States, those aspects become more difficult to maintain.

Intervention strategies

Thus far we have learned that Latinos are a diverse group of people, yet share common values and behaviors. There is much morbidity and mortality among the Latino population, and some of that is the result of low levels of leisure-time physical activity. Given the barriers experienced by many Latinos, this is not surprising.

However, in order to overcome barriers, evidence-based, culturally appropriate strategies for promoting physical activity among Latinos are needed at both surface and deep levels. These include the following:

- Social support
- Modes of PA
- Community Health Workers
- Language
- Intergenerational
- Technology
- Faith-based

Social support

Latinos have been known to be very collectivist, meaning that they tend to be aware of the results of their actions on other Latinos, share resources with Latinos, feel interdependent with Latinos, and feel involved in the lives of Latinos (Triandis 1994). Latinos are very social, and spend a lot of time in groups. Thus, increasing social support for physical activity is one deep-level strategy that may be even more effective among Latinos than NLWs. Among Latina women, social support is the most commonly reported correlate of PA (Barrera *et al.* 2006, Eyler *et al.* 1999, Hovell *et al.* 1991, Keller and Fleury 2006, Marquez *et al.* 2004). Pregnant and post-partum Mexican-born Latinas saw social support as more essential to the maintenance of PA than women of other racial/ethnic groups (Evenson *et al.* 2003).

There has been much research done on different types of social support. Keller et al. used four different types of social support in order to increase activity among post-partum Latina women in their Madres para la Salud intervention (Keller *et al.* 2014). Details can be seen in Table 5.2.

TABLE 5.2 Social support

Social Support

Social Support Type	Provider of Support	Approach to Reach Goal	Support/Program Method
Emotional and Verbal Support	Promotoras and Family/Friends	Discussion leads to comfort amongst Latinos. Therefore it is safe to assume discussion is an adequate tool of encouragement.	Women shared ideas and experiences of ways to initiate and maintain walking, offer encouragement, and personalize strategies to maintain walking. Discussion of cultural concepts such as machismo and marianismo while participating in a walking group.
Instrumental (tangible) Support	Study staff, women from community	Reduce/eliminate barriers that prevent PA.	Use of pedometers for monitoring regular walking, maps showing safe walking routes, historic facts and local lore of interest around participants' neighborhoods, walking groups, stroller-loan program, child-care, and walking shoes.
Informational Support	Study staff, women from study	Latinos are likely to be family oriented, so explain the benefits of PA for family members.	Educational materials to promote walking, facilitate neighborhood safety, child-rearing tips such as infant sleep habits and breastfeeding, and avoiding musculoskeletal injury. Strategies for time management were key for the women's success PA.
Appraisal Support	Study staff, women from study	Use self-monitoring activities.	Self-evaluation included the use of accelerometers to provide study participants with precise information and feedback that the intensity and accumulation of activity they were participating in was adequate. Goal setting was done, and promotoras reviewed the participants' PA and goal attainment with them.

Modes of PA

Historically it was believed that people had to engage in high-intensity/vigorous exercise in order to achieve health benefits. Over time it has been established that it is not true. Latinos of all ages have been shown to participate in many different modes of physical activity (walking, biking, dancing, sports such as soccer), the most common of which are somewhat different than other ethnic/racial groups.

Among Latino youth, soccer is a very common way of engaging in physical activity. Arreola reported that, from a very young age, Latino children are encouraged to watch or play soccer, which may influence their preference for soccer (Arreola 2004). Olvera et al. assessed activity preferences in preadolescent Latino and NLW children and, as expected, a total of 44.9% of Latino children preferred soccer while only 31.2% of NLW children preferred soccer (Olvera *et al.* 2009).

Schober and colleagues capitalized on these preferences for soccer (Schober *et al.* 2015). A community–university partnership in Kansas City used a community-based participatory approach, *an orientation to research that focuses on relationships between academic and community partners, with principles of co-learning, mutual benefit, and long-term commitment that incorporates community theories, participation, and practices into the research efforts* (Wallerstein and Duran 2006). They developed an action plan for addressing chronic disease among Latinos, and a coalition voted to develop soccer tournaments to promote physical activity among overweight or obese Latino youth ages 6–15 (Schober *et al.* 2015). At the end of the program, both youth and parents were highly satisfied with the soccer program.

More recently the health impacts of Latin dance among Latinos has been examined. Dance has been an important form of leisure and socialization in Latin cultures for centuries (Delgado and Munoz 1997, Lewis 1994). In focus groups, older Latinos reported that dancing is a part of life in Latin culture, and dancing begins when Latinos are young. They liked that it is a social activity and thought that it could lead to as many, if not more, health benefits as other forms of physical activity. Currently trials are being conducted to examine if, and how, engaging in regular dance might influence the physical and cognitive health of Latinos (Marquez *et al.* 2014).

Community Health Workers

One common, more frequently seen, method of increasing physical activity among Latinos is the use of community health workers (CHWs), also referred to as lay health advisor, promotores (promoters), or promotoras (if workers are women). This is similar to the constituent-involving strategies outlined in Chapter 3. They are people who do not typically have formal education, but who are trained to promote health and advocate for change in their communities (Carrasquillo *et al.* 2013). CHWs are effective for several reasons, including their cultural competence, informal networks, social support they provide, and a positive source of social influence (Farrell *et al.* 2009). CHWs are mainly effective because of the cultural and linguistic connections they have with the communities they serve (Haughton *et al.* 2015), and have been called "the backbone of an intervention" because of the tools, knowledge, and support they provide to participants (Albarran *et al.* 2014). These individuals receive rigorous training before and during the intervention to ensure they are prepared to deliver the program (Haughton *et al.* 2015).

CHWs have been reported to be successful in their efforts to increase physical activity, and thus health. For example, Spinner and Alvarado trained promotoras to lead *Salud Para Su Corazon*, a culturally sensitive, community-based program to increase heart healthy knowledge and behaviors, including physical activity, among Latinos (Spinner and Alvarado 2012). Promotoras were trained with a 10-session manual to teach participants about heart disease risk factors and skills to achieve heart healthy behaviors. Results showed that among 435 Latinos, there were increases in PA outside of work (57%–78%) and heart health knowledge (49%–76%) after the program.

Language

Latinos in the US speak English only, Spanish only, English and Spanish, and indigenous languages. The more Latinos speak English, the more likely it is that there are programs they can participate in. Differences in activity and preferences in activity have been noted in English- and Spanish-speaking Latinos. Derose et al. found that English-speaking Latinos in Los Angeles were less likely than NLWs to report being physically active, exercising in the park, and exercising outside the park; and Spanish-speaking Latinos were equally likely as NLWs to report exercising in parks but less likely to report exercising outside the park and more likely to report using the parks for social interactions (Derose *et al.* 2015). It appears that urban parks are an important resource for activity and socialization particularly among Spanish-speaking Latinos.

Interventions that include materials and resources in Spanish and English are a surface-level strategy that can open up the possibility for many Latinos to participate. However, there are a number of Latinos who cannot read or write at a high level in Spanish or English. Thus, researchers such as Piziak (2014) created bilingual interactive video interventions to improve age-appropriate physical activity and improve nutritional intake in youth (Piziak 2014). There are audio-only exercises, and video and audio discs. Overall the program was well received and could provide a template for intervening not only with children, but with adults with limited literacy. Other research with older Latinos is solely intended for Spanish-speaking Latinos, involving a Spanish-language dance program with Spanish-speaking instructors and staff (Marquez *et al.* 2014).

Intergenerational

We have emphasized the importance of family in the physical activity, health, and lives of Latinos. Intervention strategies focused on families use deep structure approaches to enhance the effectiveness and acceptability of programs. Dolash and colleagues assessed factors associated with park use and PA among park users in predominantly Latino neighborhoods in San Antonio, Texas (Dolash *et al.* 2015). Adults reported coming to the park to play with their children, and they wanted to be healthy for their children. Interestingly, "children" included grand-children, nieces, nephews, and their own children. Latinos frequently went to the park with other family members, such as fiancé, sister, and/or husband. Thus, it was a family event.

Some researchers have tried to intervene with families, rather than individu-als. Arredondo noted that the physical activity rates among Latina girls are low, and thus examined the acceptability and feasibility of implementing a mother–daughter intervention targeting individual and family-level correlates of PA (Arredondo *et al.* 2014). Eleven mother–daughter dyads participated in an 8-week intervention promoting physical activity through a church. The intervention was informed by data from focus groups collected from eight mother-daughter dyads attending the same church. Mothers and daughters attended weekly 2.5 hour sessions on Saturday mornings. Each session began with a prayer, then mothers went to sessions co-led in Spanish by the study Principal Investigator and a promotora who was affili-ated with the church and employed by the study; and daughters went into sessions co-led in both Spanish and English by two youth leaders. Between the Saturday group sessions, mothers and daughters were encouraged to take walks together, which encouraged them to do activity together and to improve their communica-tion. Results of this pilot study suggested the feasibility of such an intervention, and increases in self-report physical activity, reductions in television watching, and improvements in parenting and mother–daughter communication were demon-strated (Arredondo *et al.* 2014).

Technology

PA interventions that incorporate or focus on technology use are becoming more prevalent given the advances in technology. Depending on the type of technology, such interventions might be more or less suited for Latinos. For example, data from the Pew Research Center show that there is a greater percentage of Latinos with cellphone and smartphones than NLWs. However, data also show that Latinos are less likely to have desktop computers in their homes (Lopez *et al.* 2013).

Technology has been used in some studies to help form an intervention among Latinos, often young Latinos. Morales-Campos and colleagues had innovative ideas by involving girls, parents, and the community in an intervention planning process in order to improve initiation and maintenance of physical activity in Latina adolescents (Morales-Campos *et al.* 2015). In short, the Partnership for Girls Project used a community-based participatory research approach to include different community stakeholders to design an intervention together that could be offered and sustained through a youth-serving community organization; and would include low-cost, mobile, and wireless technology to promote health and connect youth to community resources. They used a Participatory Photo Mapping (PPM) Method that uses participatory photography, photo elicitation interviews, and public participation geographic information systems to allow community-based research partnerships to produce shared practical knowledge about a topic of mutual interest (Dennis *et al.* 2009). Participating community residents took photos, discussed the meaning behind the photos with facilitators, and then produced a narrative. Using a portable GPS device, the qualitative narratives and photos of community residents were linked to a specific location on a map. Results of the intervention are pending, but this shows one way technology can be used as part of an intervention.

The use of technology is also increasing in Latino adults. Collins et al. conducted a two-part study among Latinos at risk for vascular disease in order to examine the prevalence of text messaging among Latinos in Kansas, and to report on a 6-week pilot study to determine the effect of text messaging on exercise behaviors (Collins *et al.* 2014). In the pilot, text messages were delivered once per day, 5 days per week, for 6 weeks. Results of the survey showed that 96% of participants owned a cellular telephone, 89% had texting capacity on their cellphones, and 89% received or sent text messages daily. The pilot study significantly increased exercise from about 56 minutes per week to over 200 minutes per week. Similar work is being conducted among Latina women (Marcus *et al.* 2015), but results have yet to be published.

Faith-based

One of the more common deep structure approaches to increasing the physical activity and health of Latinos is to intervene through churches and faith-based organizations. This has been successful among African Americans (Baruth and Wilcox 2013), but until recently was not done with Latinos. Churches provide social, emotional, and material support in addition to religious worship, and serve as focal points for social networking (Krause *et al.* 2001). Latinos and African Americans attend church more frequently and become more involved in faith-based services than their NLW counterparts (Newport 2010). Health can be seen as a dynamic process between faith and behavior, and participating in health behaviors can be viewed as an opportunity to honor God (Ellison and Levin 1998). A majority of Latinos are Catholic or Protestant and are associated with faith-based communities (Castro *et al.* 1995), so intervening through churches makes sense. Schwingel and Galvez reported that Latino priests, study participants, and promotoras found churches to be trustworthy and comfortable, natural and authentic, engaging and appealing, and holistic and spiritual; all positive traits that supported activity and positive lifestyle behaviors (Schwingel and Galvez 2016).

A small trial was conducted in Kansas, with two churches receiving an intervention, and one church was a comparison group (Bopp *et al.* 2011). The intervention was targeted to Latino church members, but the intervention was available to parishioners of any race/ethnicity in attempts to be more inclusive. Intervention materials were available in English and Spanish, were designed to be culturally relevant to Latinos, and incorporated the spiritual ideology of the Roman Catholic religion by using scriptures and Biblical references to reinforce health messages (Resnicow *et al.* 1999). Participants participated in an 8-week, team-based walking contest. It was found that 66% of intervention participants compared with 36% of comparison participants identified health reasons (e.g., diabetes, high blood pressure) for participating in physical activity, and 47% accurately described PA recommendations, compared with 16% of comparison participants (Bopp *et al.* 2011).

A previously mentioned intervention in San Diego that involved CHWs was faith-based. *Fe en Accion* (Faith in Action; Chapter 3) was a community-based, group-randomized trial to increase moderate-to-vigorous physical activity (MVPA) among churchgoing Latinas in San Diego, California (Arredondo *et al.* 2015, Haughton *et al.* 2015).

BOX 5.1 EVIDENCE FOR PRACTICE: FAITH IN ACTION

Multi-level physical activity interventions are unique in that they target physical activity from all angles. Churches are well-positioned settings for implementing such interventions. Faith in Action – Fe en Acción is a physical activity, multi-level intervention for Latina, churchgoing women in San Diego. Researchers partnered with churches throughout San Diego County and trained bilingual/bicultural promotoras (community health workers) from each church to deliver several components of the intervention. The promotoras led exercise classes at or near the church site (individual level), which were preceded by prayer, conducted motivational interviewing calls (interpersonal level), created promotional banners and posters to provide informational support (organizational level), and led environmental projects (environmental level). The promotoras were trained by Circulate San Diego, an organization that advocates for better transportation and more sustainable land use choices, on how to conduct walkability audits with the purpose of addressing the built environment and physical activity issues. After the training, the promotoras worked with church members to identify two projects, one at the church site and one in the community surrounding the church. The goals of both projects were to improve opportunities for physical activity and reduce environmental physical activity barriers. Some of the projects include increased lighting to enhance safety, trail restoration, traffic calming solutions, and sidewalk improvements. The project activities were open to all church members in participating sites. As a result of this multi-level physical activity intervention, thousands of parishioners have participated in Faith in Action's physical activity classes.

Implications for practice

Throughout this chapter we have tried to stress several things that we believe are extremely important when intervening to improve the physical activity and health of Latinos in the US. These include the fact that Latinos are a large and growing population. There is much variability among Latinos, including country of origin, language spoken, SES, and presence of one or more chronic diseases. There are many barriers to being physically active that go beyond excuses for not wanting to exercise. Culture is strong, and rooted in history. We recommend finding ways to work with Latino communities to overcome common barriers such as not speaking English, not having safe and available resources, traditional gender roles, physical activity preferences, and immigration status. Intervening using some of the strategies we have discussed, such as using social support, community health workers, intergenerational programs, and faith-based programs, can be useful, and addressing as many levels of the social ecological model as possible will have the best chances of success.

Summary points

- The Latino population is the fastest-growing minority group in the US, and Latinos are a heterogeneous group that vary in race, country of origin, immigration status, socioeconomic characteristics, cultural values, beliefs and practices.
- From a social ecological perspective, Latinos of all ages, sexual orientation, and immigration status face complex barriers to engaging in physical activity.
- Culturally appropriate strategies for promoting physical activity among Latinos are needed at both surface and deep levels, including focusing on the following: Social support; Modes of PA; Community Health Workers; Language; Intergenerational programs; Technology; Faith-based programs.

Critical thinking questions

1. How could immigration, and immigration history, impact engagement in regular physical activity?
2. How might cultural values and practices influence engagement in regular physical activity?
3. Which barriers do you see as the most powerful/influential in impeding Latinos from exercising on a regular basis?
4. Which intervention strategies do you think will be easiest to implement, and which do you think would have the most impact?

Acknowledgments

We would like to acknowledge the UIC Department of Kinesiology and Nutrition and the Training in CVD Epidemiology and Related Chronic Diseases in Minority Populations Program NIH/NHLBI T-32-HL-125–294–01A1 for funding support of the students.

References

Albarran, C. R., Heilemann, M. V. and Koniak-Griffin, D. (2014) 'Promotoras as facilitators of change: Latinas' perspectives after participating in a lifestyle behaviour intervention program'. *Journal of Advanced Nursing*, 70: 2303–2313.

Alberti, K. G. M. M., Eckel, R. H., Grundy, S. M., Zimmet, P. Z., Cleeman, J. I., Donato, K. A., Fruchart, J.-C., James, W. P. T., Loria, C. M. and Smith, S. C. (2009) 'Harmonizing the metabolic syndrome'. *Circulation*, 120: 1640.

Alzheimer's Association. (2007) Alzheimer's disease in Latinos expected to surge [Online]. Available https://www.alz.org/national/documents/release_111507_spanish.pdf (Accessed October 15 2016).

Arredondo, E. M., Haughton, J., Ayala, G. X., Slymen, D. J., Sallis, J. F., Burke, K., Holub, C., Chanson, D., Perez, L. G., Valdivia, R., Ryan, S. and Elder, J. (2015) 'Fe en Accion/Faith in Action: Design and implementation of a church-based randomized trial to promote physical activity and cancer screening among churchgoing Latinas'. *Contemporary Clinical Trials*, 45: 404–415.

Arredondo, E. M., Mendelson, T., Elder, J. P., Marshall, S. J., Flair, L. L. and Ayala, G. X. (2012) 'The relation of medical conditions to depressive symptoms among Latinos: Leisure time physical activity as a mediator'. *Journal of Health Psychology*, 17: 742–752.

Arredondo, E. M., Morello, M., Holub, C. and Haughton, J. (2014) 'Feasibility and preliminary findings of a church-based mother-daughter pilot study promoting physical activity among young Latinas'. *Family & Community Health*, 37: 6–18.

Arredondo, E. M., Sotres-Alvarez, D., Stoutenberg, M., Davis, S. M., Crespo, N. C., Carnethon, M. R., Castañeda, S. F., Isasi, C. R., Espinoza, R. A., Daviglus, M. L., Perez, L. G. and Evenson, K. R. (2016) 'Physical activity levels in U.S. Latino/Hispanic adults'. *American Journal of Preventive Medicine*, 50: 500–508.

Arreola, D. (2004) *Hispanic spaces, Latino places: Community and cultural diversity in contemporary America*, Austin, TX: University of Texas Press.

Bandura, A. (1997) *Self-efficacy: The exercise of control*, New York: Freeman.

Barnes, D. E. and Yaffe, K. (2011) 'The projected impact of risk factor reduction on Alzheimer's disease prevalence'. *Lancet Neurology*, 10: 819–828.

Barrera, M., Jr., Toobert, D. J., Angell, K. L., Glasgow, R. E. and Mackinnon, D. P. (2006) 'Social support and social-ecological resources as mediators of lifestyle intervention effects for type 2 diabetes'. *Journal of Health Psychology*, 11: 483–495.

Barrington, C., Messias, D. K. H. and Weber, L. (2012) 'Implications of racial and ethnic relations for health and well-being in new Latino communities: A case study of West Columbia, South Carolina'. *Latino Studies*, 10: 155–178.

Baruth, M. and Wilcox, S. (2013) 'Multiple behavior change among church members taking part in the Faith, Activity, and Nutrition program'. *Journal of Nutrition Education & Behavior*, 45: 428–434.

Berry, J. W. and Sabatier, C. (2011) 'Variations in the assessment of acculturation attitudes: Their relationships with psychological wellbeing'. *International Journal of Intercultural Relations*, 35: 658–669.

Bopp, M., Fallon, E. A. and Marquez, D. X. (2011) 'A faith-based physical activity intervention for Latinos: Outcomes and lessons'. *American Journal of Health Promotion*, 25: 168–171.

Brown, A. and Lopez, M. H. (2013) *Ranking Latino Populations in the States* [Online]. Available: www.pewhispanic.org/2013/08/29/ii-ranking-latino-populations-in-the-states/ (Accessed October 15 2016).

Calderon, V. and Tennstedt, S. L. (1998) 'Ethnic differences in the expression of caregiver burden: Results of a qualitative study'. *Journal of Gerontological Social Work*, 30: 159–178.

Carrasquillo, O., Patberg, E., Alonzo, Y., Li, H. and Kenya, S. (2013) 'Rationale and design of the Miami Healthy Heart Initiative: A randomized controlled study of a community health worker intervention among Latino patients with poorly controlled diabetes'. *International Journal of General Medicine*, 7: 115–126.

Castañeda, S. F., Buelna, C., Giacinto, R. E., Gallo, L. C., Sotres-Alvarez, D., Gonzalez, P., Fortmann, A. L., Wassertheil-Smoller, S., Gellman, M. D., Giachello, A. L. and Talavera, G. A. (2016) 'Cardiovascular disease risk factors and psychological distress among Hispanics/Latinos: The Hispanic Community Health Study/Study of Latinos (HCHS/SOL)'. *Preventive Medicine*, 87: 144–150.

Castro, F. G., Elder, J., Coe, K., Tafoya-Barraza, H. M., Moratto, S., Campbell, N. and Talavera, G. (1995) 'Mobilizing churches for health promotion in Latino communities: Companeros en la Salud'. *Journal of the National Cancer Institute Monographs*, 18: 127–135.

Centers for Disease Control and Prevention. (2016) *Mental Health Basics* [Online]. Available: www.cdc.gov/mentalhealth/basics.htm (Accessed April 15 2016).

Collins, T. C., Dong, F., Ablah, E., Parra-Medina, D., Cupertino, P., Rogers, N. and Ahlers-Schmidt, C. R. (2014) 'Text messaging to motivate exercise among Latino adults at risk for vascular disease: A pilot study, 2013'. *Preventing Chronic Disease*, 11: E192.

Crespo, C. J., Smit, E., Carter-Pokras, O. and Andersen, R. (2001) 'Acculturation and leisure-time physical inactivity in Mexican American adults: Results from NHANES III, 1988–1994'. *American Journal of Public Health*, 91: 1254–1257.

Cubbin, C., Hadden, W. C. and Winkleby, M. A. (2000) 'Neighborhood context and cardiovascular disease risk factors: The contribution of material deprivation'. *Ethnicity & Disease*, 11: 687–700.

D'Alonzo, K. T. and Fischetti, N. (2008) 'Cultural beliefs and attitudes of Black and Hispanic college-age women toward exercise'. *Journal of Transcultural Nursing*, 19: 175–183.

Daviglus, M. L., Pirzada, A. and Talavera, G. A. (2014a) 'Cardiovascular disease risk factors in the Hispanic/Latino population: Lessons from the Hispanic Community Health Study/Study of Latinos (HCHS/SOL)'. *Progress in Cardiovascular Diseases*, 57: 230–236.

Daviglus, M. L., Pirzada, A. and Van Horn, L. (2014b) 'Ethnic disparities in cardiovascular risk factors in children and adolescents'. *Current Cardiovascular Risk Reports*, 8: 1–9.

Delgado, C. F. and Munoz, J. E. (1997) *Everynight life: Culture and dance in Latino America*, Durham, NC: Duke University Press.

Dennis, S. F., Jr., Gaulocher, S., Carpiano, R. M. and Brown, D. (2009) 'Participatory Photo Mapping (PPM): Exploring an integrated method for health and place research with young people'. *Health & Place*, 15: 466–473.

Derose, K. P., Han, B., Williamson, S. and Cohen, D. A. (2015) 'Racial-ethnic variation in park use and physical activity in the City of Los Angeles'. *Journal of Urban Health*, 92: 1011–1023.

Dolash, K., He, M., Yin, Z. and Sosa, E. T. (2015) 'Factors that influence park use and physical activity in predominantly Hispanic and low-income neighborhoods'. *Journal of Physical Activity and Health*, 12: 462–469.

Ellison, C. G. and Levin, J. S. (1998) 'The religion-health connection: Evidence, theory, and future directions'. *Health Education and Behavior*, 25: 700–720.

Environmental Defense Fund. (2016) *Partnering for Latino Health and the Environment* [Online]. Available: www.edf.org/health/toxic-chemicals-and-latino-health (Accessed April 15 2016).

Estabrooks, P. A., Lee, R. E. and Gyurcsik, N. C. (2003) 'Resources for physical activity participation: Does availability and accessibility differ by neighborhood socioeconomic status?'. *Annals of Behavioral Medicine*, 25: 100–104.

Evenson, K. R., Sarmiento, O. L., Tawney, K. W., Macon, M. L. and Ammerman, A. S. (2003) 'Personal, social, and environmental correlates of physical activity in North Carolina Latina immigrants'. *American Journal of Preventive Medicine*, 25: 77–85.

Eyler, A. A., Brownson, R. C., Donatelle, R. J., King, A. C., Brown, D. and Sallis, J. F. (1999) 'Physical activity social support and middle- and older-aged minority women: Results from a US survey'. *Social Science Medicine*, 49: 781–789.

Farrell, M. A., Hayashi, T., Loo, R. K., Rocha, D. A., Sanders, C., Hernandez, M. and Will, J. C. (2009) 'Clinic-based nutrition and lifestyle counseling for Hispanic women delivered by community health workers: Design of the California WISEWOMAN study'. *Journal of Womens Health (Larchmt)*, 18: 733–739.

González, H. M., Tarraf, W., Rodríguez, C. J., Gallo, L. C., Sacco, R. L., Talavera, G. A., Heiss, G., Kizer, J. R., Hernandez, R., Davis, S., Schneiderman, N., Daviglus, M. L. and Kaplan, R. C. (2016) 'Cardiovascular health among diverse Hispanics/Latinos: Hispanic Community Health Study/Study of Latinos (HCHS/SOL) results'. *American Heart Journal*, 176: 134–144.

Haughton, J., Ayala, G. X., Burke, K. H., Elder, J. P., Montanez, J. and Arredondo, E. M. (2015) 'Community health workers promoting physical activity: Targeting multiple levels of the social ecological model'. *Journal of Ambulatory Care Management*, 38: 309–320.

Heiss, G., Snyder, M. L., Teng, Y., Schneiderman, N., Llabre, M. M., Cowie, C., Carnethon, M., Kaplan, R., Giachello, A., Gallo, L., Loehr, L. and Avilés-Santa, L. (2014) 'Prevalence of metabolic syndrome among Hispanics/Latinos of diverse background: The Hispanic Community Health Study/Study of Latinos'. *Diabetes Care*, 37: 2391.

Hovell, M., Sallis, J., Hofstetter, R., Barrington, E., Hackley, M., Elder, J., Castro, F. and Kilbourne, K. (1991) 'Identification of correlates of physical activity among Latino adults'. *Journal of Community Health*, 16: 23–36.

Keller, C., Ainsworth, B., Records, K., Todd, M., Belyea, M., Vega-Lopez, S., Permana, P., Coonrod, D. and Nagle-Williams, A. (2014) 'A comparison of a social support physical activity intervention in weight management among post-partum Latinas'. *BMC Public Health*, 14: 971.

Keller, C. and Fleury, J. (2006) 'Factors related to physical activity in Hispanic women'. *Journal of Cardiovascular Nursing*, 21: 142–145.

Krause, N., Ellison, C. G., Shaw, B. A., Marcum, J. P. and Boardman, J. D. (2001) 'Church-based social support and religious coping'. *Journal for the Scientific Study of Religion*, 40: 637–656.

Larsen, B. A., Noble, M. L., Murray, K. E. and Marcus, B. H. (2015) 'Physical activity in Latino men and women facilitators, barriers, and interventions'. *American Journal of Lifestyle Medicine*, 9: 4–30.

Larson, B. A., Pekmezi, D., Marquez, B., Benitez, T. J., and Marcus, B. (2013) 'Physical activity in Latinas: social and environmental influences'. *Women's Health*, 9(2): 201–210.

Lautenschlager, N. T. and Almeida, O. P. (2006) 'Physical activity and cognition in old age'. *Current Opinion in Psychiatry*, 19: 190–193.

Lee, R. E., Booth, K. M., Reese-Smith, J. Y., Regan, G. and Howard, H. H. (2005) 'The Physical Activity Resource Assessment (PARA) instrument: Evaluating features, amenities and incivilities of physical activity resources in urban neighborhoods'. *International Journal of Behavioral Nutrition and Physical Activity*, 2: 13.

Lee, R. E. and Cubbin, C. (2009) 'Striding toward social justice: The ecologic milieu of physical activity'. *Exercise and Sport Sciences Reviews*, 37: 10.

Lewis, D. (1994) 'Introduction: Dance in Hispanic cultures'. *Choreography and Dance*, 3: 1–5.

Lindsay, A. C., Salkeld, J. A., Greaney, M. L. and Sands, F. D. (2015) 'Latino family child-care providers' beliefs, attitudes, and practices related to promotion of healthy behaviors among preschool children: A qualitative study'. *Journal of Obesity*, 1–9.

Lopez, M. H., Gonzalez-Barrera, A. and Patten, E. (2013) Closing the digital divide: Latinos and technology adoption [Online]. Available http://www.pewhispanic.org/files/2013/03/Latinos_Social_Media_and_Mobile_Tech_03-2013_final.pdf (Accessed April 15 2016).

Marcus, B. H., Hartman, S. J., Pekmezi, D., Dunsiger, S. I., Linke, S., Marquez, B., Gans, K. M., Bock, B. C., Larsen, B. A. and Rojas, C. (2015) 'Using interactive Internet technology to promote physical activity in Latinas: Rationale, design, and baseline findings of Pasos Hacia La Salud'. *Contemporary Clinical Trials*, 44: 149–158.

Markides, K. S. and Coreil, J. (1986) 'The health of Hispanics in the southwestern United States: An epidemiologic paradox'. *Public Health Reports*, 101: 253–265.

Marquez, D. X., Bustamante, E. E., Blissmer, B. J. and Prohaska, T. R. (2009) 'Health promotion for successful aging'. *American Journal of Lifestyle Medicine*, 3: 12–19.

Marquez, D. X. and McAuley, E. (2006) 'Social cognitive correlates of leisure time physical activity among Latinos'. *Journal of Behavioral Medicine*, 29: 281–289.

Marquez, D. X., Mcauley, E. and Overman, N. (2004) 'Psychosocial correlates and outcomes of physical activity among Latinos: A review'. *Hispanic Journal of Behavioral Sciences*, 26: 195–229.

Marquez, D. X., Wilbur, J., Hughes, S. L., Berbaum, M. L., Wilson, R. S., Buchner, D. M. and Mcauley, E. (2014) 'B.A.I.L.A.: A Latin dance randomized controlled trial for older Spanish-speaking Latinos: Rationale, design, and methods'. *Contemporary Clinical Trials*, 38: 397–408.

Martinez, S. M., Ayala, G. X., Patrick, K., Arredondo, E. M., Roesch, S. and Elder, J. (2012) 'Associated pathways between neighborhood environment, community resource factors, and leisure-time physical activity among Mexican-American adults in San Diego, California'. *American Journal of Health Promotion*, 26: 281–288.

Medina-Inojosa, J., Jean, N., Cortes-Bergoderi, M. and Lopez-Jimenez, F. (2014) 'The Hispanic paradox in cardiovascular disease and total mortality'. *Progress in Cardiovascular Diseases*, 57: 286–292.

Morales-Campos, D. Y., Parra-Medina, D. and Esparza, L. A. (2015) 'Picture this!: Using Participatory Photo Mapping with Hispanic girls'. *Family & Community Health*, 38: 44–54.

Newport, F. (2010) 'Americans' church attendance inches up in 2010'. *Gallup*, June 25.

O'Connor, T. M., Cerin, E., Hughes, S. O., Robles, J., Thompson, D., Baranowski, T., Lee, R. E., Nicklas, T. and Shewchuk, R. M. (2013) 'What Hispanic parents do to encourage and discourage 3–5 year old children to be active: A qualitative study using nominal group'. *International Journal of Behavioral Nutrition and Physical Activity*, 10:93.

Office of Minority Health. (2016a) *US Dept of HHS, Office of Minority Health: Diabetes and Hispanic Americans* [Online]. Available: http://minorityhealth.hhs.gov/omh/browse.aspx?lvl=4&lvlID=63 (Accessed April 15 2016).

Office of Minority Health. (2016b) *US Dept of HHS, Office of Minority Health: Obesity and Hispanic Americans* [Online]. Available: http://minorityhealth.hhs.gov/omh/browse.aspx?lvl=4&lvlid=70 (Accessed April 15 2016).

Olvera, N., McCarley, K. E., Leung, P., Mcleod, J. and Rodriguez, A. X. (2009) 'Assessing physical activity preferences in Latino and white preadolescents'. *Pediatric Exercise Science*, 21: 400–412.

Penedo, F. J., Brintz, C. E., Llabre, M. M., Arguelles, W., Isasi, C. R., Arredondo, E. M., Navas-Nacher, E. L., Perreira, K. M., González, H. M., Rodriguez, C. J., Daviglus, M., Schneiderman, N. and Gallo, L. C. (2015) 'Family environment and the metabolic syndrome:

Results from the Hispanic Community Health Study/Study of Latinos (HCHS/SOL) Sociocultural Ancillary Study (SCAS)'. *Annals of Behavioral Medicine*, 49: 793–801.

Pew Hispanic Research Center. (2012) Report Looks at Hispanics and Their Views of Identity. The Hispanic Outlook in Higher Education: Paramus.

Pew Hispanic Research Center. (2014) With Few New Arrivals, Census Lower Hispanic Population Projections. The Hispanic Outlook in Higher Education: Paramus.

Piziak, V. (2014) 'The development of a bilingual interactive video to improve physical activity and healthful eating in a head start population'. *International Journal of Environmental Research in Public Health*, 11: 13065–13073.

Resnicow, K., Baranowski, T., Ahluwalia, J. S. and Braithwaite, R. L. (1999) 'Cultural sensitivity in public health: Defined and demystified'. *Ethnicity & Disease*, 9: 10–21.

Rodriguez, C. J., Allison, M., Daviglus, M. L., Isasi, C. R., Keller, C., Leira, E. C., Palaniappan, L., Piña, I. L., Ramirez, S. M., Rodriguez, B. and Sims, M. (2014) 'Status of cardiovascular disease and stroke in Hispanics/Latinos in the United States: A science advisory from the American Heart Association'. *Circulation*, 130: 593–625.

Salinas, J. J., Messias, D. K. H., Morales-Campos, D. and Parra-Medina, D. (2014) 'English language proficiency and physical activity among Mexican-origin women in South Texas and South Carolina'. *Journal of Health Care for the Poor and Underserved*, 25: 357.

Santiago-Rivera, A. L., Arredondo, P. and Gallardo-Cooper, M. (2001) *Counseling Latinos and la familia: A practical guide*. Thousand Oaks, CA: Sage Publications.

Schober, D. J., Zarate, J. and Fawcett, S. B. (2015) 'Developing an academic-community partnership to promote soccer-based physical activity among Latino youth'. *Progress in Community Health Partnerships*, 9: 397–404.

Schwingel, A. and Galvez, P. (2016) 'Divine interventions: Faith-based approaches to health promotion programs for Latinos'. *Journal of Religion & Health*, 55: 1891–1906.

Spinner, J. R. and Alvarado, M. (2012) 'Salud Para Su Carozon: A Latino promotora-led cardiovascular health education program'. *Family & Community Health*, 35: 111–119.

Triandis, H. C. (1994) 'Cultural differences in patterns of social behavior'. *Culture and Social Behavior*. New York: McGraw-Hill, Inc.

U.S. Census Bureau. (2015) *Income and Poverty in the United States: 2014* [Online]. Available: www.census.gov/content/dam/Census/library/publications/2015/demo/p60-252.pdf (Accessed March 27 2016).

Van Wieren, A. J., Roberts, M. B., Arellano, N., Feller, E. R. and Diaz, J. A. (2011) 'Acculturation and cardiovascular behaviors among Latinos in California by country/region of origin'. *Journal of Immigrant and Minority Health*, 13: 975–981.

Wallerstein, N. B. and Duran, B. (2006) 'Using community-based participatory research to address health disparities'. *Health Promotion Practice*, 7: 312–323.

Wassertheil-Smoller, S., Arredondo, E. M., Cai, J., Castenada, S., Choca, J. P., Gallo, L., Jung, M., Lavange, L. M., Lee-Rey, E. T., Mosley, T., Penedo, F. J., Santistaban, D. A. and Zee, P. C. (2014) 'Depression, anxiety, antidepressant use, and cardiovascular disease among Hispanic men and women of different national backgrounds: Results from the Hispanic Community Health Study/Study of Latinos (HCHS/SOL)'. *Annals of Epidemiology*, 24: 822–830.

Wilbur, J., Chandler, P. J., Dancy, B. and Lee, H. (2003) 'Correlates of physical activity in urban Midwestern Latinas'. *American Journal of Preventive Medicine*, 25: 69–76.

Wilbur, J., Marquez, D. X., Fogg, L., Wilson, R. S., Staffileno, B. A., Hoyem, R. L., Morris, M. C., Bustamante, E. E. and Manning, A. F. (2012) 'The relationship between physical activity and cognition in older Latinos'. *The Journals of Gerontology, Series B: Psychological Sciences and Social Sciences*, 67: 525–534.

6

PHYSICAL ACTIVITY AMONG ASIAN AMERICANS

Edith W. Chen, Grace J. Yoo, Elaine A. Musselman and Jane Jih

Understanding the Asian American population

In First Lady Michelle Obama's "Let's Move" campaign, which aimed at fighting childhood obesity through physical activity, African American and Latina/o youth were often prominently featured. Almost absent from these campaigns were Asian American children, furthering the idea in the popular imagination that Asian Americans are a healthy population. Often viewed as a model minority (Nguyen 2015), Asian Americans are rarely targeted as a group needing to increase physical activity. Yet Asian Americans have lower physical activity levels compared to other racial and ethnic groups (Afable-Munsuz et al. 2010, Bhattacharya Becerra et al. 2015, Kandula and Lauderdale 2005, Yu et al. 2015). Additionally, there is a misperception that thin Asian Americans are at a healthy weight and not at risk for chronic diseases. Although Asian Americans have a lower body mass index (BMI) than Whites and other racial/ethnic groups, they are more likely to develop diabetes, hypertension, and coronary heart disease at lower BMI (Aoki et al. 2014, Jih et al. 2014, Menke et al. 2015).

Demographic characteristics

Contrary to the stereotype of a monolithic racial group, Asian Americans are a diverse population representing over 50 different ethnic groups. In 2014, 20.3 million Asian Americans lived in the U.S. (US Census 2015a). California has the largest population of Asian Americans, with one third of Asian Americans calling California their home (Asian Americans Center for Advancing Justice 2013). The largest Asian American groups include Chinese Americans (4.4 million), Filipino Americans (3.8 million), Asian Indian Americans (3.8 million), Vietnamese Americans (2.0 million), Korean Americans (1.8 million), and Japanese Americans

(1.4 million) (U.S. Census Bureau 2015b). Asian American subgroups with fewer than 1 million include Pakistani Americans, Bangladeshi Americans, Cambodian Americans, Hmong Americans, Laotian Americans, Taiwanese Americans, and Thai Americans. Furthermore, Asian Americans range in immigration experiences from Japanese Americans, a predominantly American-born and well-established population, to Vietnamese and Cambodian Americans, who largely came to the U.S. involuntarily escaping from war and persecution in the 1970s and 1980s, with few material resources and less formal education. While many Asian Americans arrive to the U.S. with high levels of education and occupational skills, as the result of U.S. immigration policy that gives preferences to the skilled and educated elite, there is also a notable working-class segment that work in low-wage industries (Ray 2006, Pih et al. 2012).

Health disparities and inequities in the Asian American population

Despite the stereotype that these populations do not have health problems, there is an increasing incidence of chronic disease in these populations. Asian Americans have almost double the prevalence rates of diabetes as Whites (20.6% vs. 11.3%; Menke et al. 2015). Coronary heart disease is higher in Japanese Americans living in the U.S. compared with Japanese people living in Japan (Marmot et al. 1975). Second-generation Asian Americans are twice as likely to be obese as their immigrant parents (Harrison et al. 2005). The growing chronic disease health concerns among Asian Americans demonstrate the importance of understanding and promoting physical activity in Asian American communities. Physical activity has been shown to be important for overall health and wellness, and may lower the risk of diabetes, hypertension, cardiovascular disease, and some cancers (ODPHP 2016).

Physical activity among Asian Americans

As Asian Americans are a diverse group including differences in ethnic origin, socio-economic status, and immigration experiences (Chan 1991, Lowe 1991, Takaki 1998), this chapter attempts to summarize the commonalities as well as make distinctions between the groups relative to physical activity.

Unique influences among specific Asian American groups

Understanding the barriers and incentives to physical activity among Asian American populations requires examining their experiences from multiple levels. Using a social ecological approach (McLeroy et al. 1988, Sallis et al. 2008), this chapter examines the role of immigration and acculturation on physical activity and how it plays out at the intrapersonal and interpersonal levels by considering stages of life, ethnicities, socio-economic status, and gender. It also considers the community-level factors by examining the neighborhoods and built environments in which Asian Americans live. In addition, this chapter identifies culturally tailored interventions that have increased physical activity in specific subgroups of Asian Americans.

Asian American youth and younger adults

Younger Asian Americans have alarmingly low physical activity levels. For example, on average, younger Asian Americans (ages 18–44 years) in California have marked lower activity levels compared to other racial/ethnic groups (see Figure 6.1). Only 30% of Asian Americans in this age group engage in regular physical activity compared to Whites (41%), African Americans (46%), and Latina/os (41%) (UCLA Center for Policy Health Research 2016).

Perhaps Asian Americans are more likely to spend their leisure time in front of the screen instead of engaging in physical activity. In addition to watching television, Asian American children spend more time on the computer for recreational use such as social networking, watching videos, and playing video games than Whites, African Americans, and Latina/os (Allen et al. 2007, Babey et al. 2013, Rideout et al. 2011). Immigrant Asian parents may not always know what computer

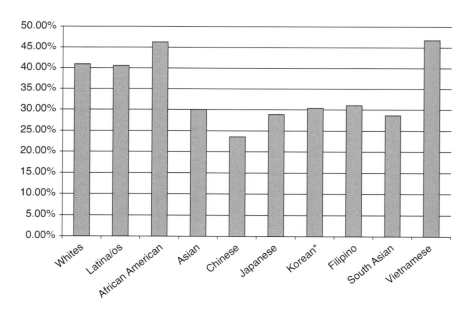

FIGURE 6.1 Regular physical activity for adults, ages 18–44, by race and Asian ethnicity in California

Source: California Health Interview Survey (2009).

Notes: Regular physical activity includes walking for transportation and leisure, vigorous physical activity, and moderate physical activity, and moderate leisure activity.

*Statistically unstable

activities their child is engaged in when they are not completing academic work and other scheduled activities (Babey et al. 2013). Acculturation has also been associated with lower frequency of physical activity for Asian American and Latina/o adolescents (Unger et al. 2004). For low-income Asian American families, parents may prefer their children to spend time indoors to playing outside where safety and air pollution may be an issue. Cambodian American youth in Long Beach, California, for example, are fearful of playing at the local park due to concerns about gang violence and personal safety according to Scott Chan, Program Director of Asian Pacific Islander Obesity Prevention Alliance (Chan 1991, personal communication).

Asian immigrant parents may emphasize academics due to a belief that education is one of the few pathways for social mobility (Sue and Okazaki 2009, Tran and Birman 2010). The emphasis on academic and intellectual activities may impede physical activity among young Asian American children and their families. Norms on how time should be spent and/or gendered ideas of physical activity impact how much time is spent on physical activity. For example, children of Asian immigrants may be encouraged to pursue intellectual activities, such as practicing a musical instrument, rather than engaging in physical activity (Im et al. 2012). Additionally, males in such households might be encouraged to participate in competitive sports and outdoor activities, while females may be expected to care for the family and home (Im et al. 2012).

Middle-aged adults and seniors

Generally, non-leisure-time physical activity such as activities that take place at the workplace are a major source of physical activity for many adult Asian immigrants (Afable-Munsuz et al. 2010, Coronado et al. 2011, Kandula and Lauderdale 2005). This is especially true for immigrants who are not engaged in office-based or white-collar professions. Immigrants who are engaged in small family businesses such as restaurants, donut shops, mom and pop grocery stores, and dry cleaners may meet much of the daily physical activity requirement running their businesses. In a study of Korean immigrant dry cleaner married couples, most worked over 60 hours a week with little time for leisure activities (Ju et al. 2011). The daily task of running their business and taking care of their household comprised the bulk of their lifestyle physical activity. Vietnamese and Cambodian Americans, on the other hand, are much more likely to be engaged in physically demanding work as employees in blue-collar, manual services, farming and military positions (Asian American Legal Center and Asian American Justice Center 2011, Chen and Arguelles 2012, Coronado et al. 2011, Kandula and Lauderdale 2005, Le 2016). Filipinos also have one of the higher occupational physical activity levels among Asian Americans (Afable-Munsuz et al. 2010, Kandula and Lauderdale 2005), perhaps due to their concentration in the health professions in physically active roles as nurses and health care workers and in military service (Espiritu 1995, Tung 2000).

For Asian American adults, occupational physical activity tends to decline with greater socio-economic status and greater assimilation into American society

(Kandula and Lauderdale 2005, Taylor et al. 2007). The concentration of Asian Americans in engineering, high-tech, research, and other desk jobs may be a reason why many Asian Americans' overall physical activity levels are low. While representing about 6% of the nation's population, Asian Americans make up between 29–50% of the San Francisco Bay and Silicon Valley area's high-tech jobs (Cameron 2015, Nakaso 2012). Many of these workers are immigrants from China and India, which may explain why the 18- to 44-year-olds of this group have some of the lower physical activity scores (see Figure 6.1). Similarly, second-generation Asian Americans have lower occupational physical activity compared to their immigrant counterparts, which may reflect their greater assimilation to white-collar and professional positions. However, leisure-time physical activity tends to increase with greater assimilation (Afable-Munsuz et al. 2010, Kandula and Lauderdale 2005).

Dedicated time devoted to physical activity for the sake of enjoyment may be seen as a luxury, rather than essential for health and well-being among some Asian

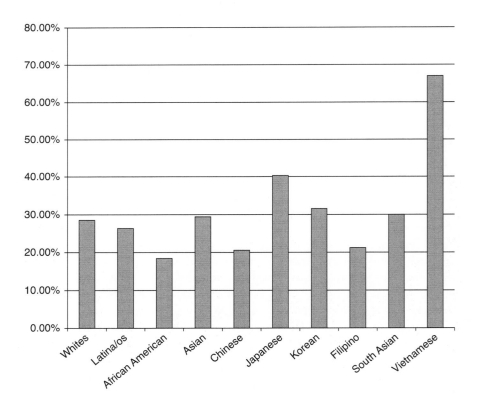

FIGURE 6.2 Regular physical activity for Californian adults, ages 65–85, by race and Asian ethnicity

Source: California Health Interview Survey, 2009.

Note: Regular physical activity includes walking for transportation and leisure, vigorous physical activity, and moderate physical activity, and moderate leisure activity.

American groups (Kandula and Lauderdale 2005, Lawton et al. 2006). During their initial years in the U.S., Asian Americans immigrants are often busy establishing themselves, surviving, and providing for their families (de Castro et al. 2008). It may be not until later, after having established their careers and their children are grown, that Asian Americans make time for physical activity as increased physical activity (Im et al. 2012, Kandula and Lauderdale 2005, Kao et al. 2016, Taylor et al. 2007). Older Asian American adults, in particular, may have more time to engage in leisurely physical activity (Kandula and Lauderdale 2005, Li and Wen 2013) as well as see the importance of exercise in addressing and preventing chronic health conditions (Fitzpatrick et al. 2012, Kao et al. 2016).

There is wide variation in the level of physical activity among the different Asian American ethnicities, with Chinese and Korean immigrants the least likely to engage in leisure-time physical activity (Kandula and Lauderdale 2005, Kao et al. 2016, Li and Wen 2013). South Asian Indians – most who are professional migrants with higher levels of education – may have more leisure time for physical activity, more so than their Korean American counterparts (Daniel et al. 2013). Japanese Americans, who are primarily American-born and the most established Asian American group, have leisure-time physical activity similar to Whites (Li and Wen 2013). Second-generation Asian Americans generally are more likely to engage in leisure-time physical activity than their immigrant peers, which furthers the idea that dedicated time for exercise and sports may be a reflection of assimilation to U.S. society and the reduced stress of having to adapt to a new country (Kandula and Lauderdale 2005, Kao et al. 2016, Yu et al. 2015).

Asian American females

In addition to preventing chronic diseases, being physically active is important for increasing bone density and preventing osteoporotic fractures for Asian American women (Crespo et al. 2011, US Department of Health and Human Services 2015). Asian American females are particularly at risk for not meeting the recommended physical activity levels that maintain health and well-being, having the lowest physical activity levels of all racial/ethnic and gender groups (Babakus and Thompson 2012, Im et al. 2012, 2013, Kandula and Lauderdale 2005, UCLA Center for Policy Health Research 2016).

Going to the gym and dedicating time specifically for physical activity may seem like a foreign concept for some Asian immigrant women (Babakus and Thompson 2012, Im et al. 2012, Lawton et al. 2006, Sriskantharajah and Kai 2007). Prior to immigration, physical activities may have been more incorporated into their daily lives such as walking and bicycling to shop for groceries, visiting friends, and going to work (Im et al. 2012). Additionally, some middle-aged Asian immigrant women believe that daily household activities constitute sufficient physical activity (Im et al. 2012). In a study of South Asian women in the United Kingdom, meaningful physical activity revolved around caring and nurturing for family members, or those activities that contribute to the household income (Lawton et al. 2006).

As children and adolescents, Asian American females may not have been encouraged to participate in sports and other forms of physical activity due to the perception of their bodies being weak and small (Dave et al. 2015, Im et al. 2012). As mothers, some Asian American women feel compelled to sacrifice their own needs for exercise to care for the children, family, and attending to household activities (Dave et al. 2015, Im et al. 2012). Employment and number of children has an inverse association with exercise among mid-life Asian American women (Lee and Im 2010). As immigrants trying to establish themselves in their new adopted country, recreational exercise unrelated to their duties as mothers, daughters, and wives may be seen as selfish (Lawton et al. 2006). Interestingly, Asian American men usually report higher leisurely physical activity (Im et al. 2012, Ju et al. 2011). Even when they make plans for exercise, Asian American women will compromise their own schedules for family and social events more so than their male counterparts (Im et al. 2012).

As their children grow up and become more independent, Asian American women may have more time to dedicate themselves to their own needs (Im et al. 2012). Cultural and religious taboos about exposing their bodies to members of the opposite sex and the lack of availability of single-sex facilities with same-sex instructors may impede some South Asian women from engaging in physical activities (Babakus and Thompson 2012, Dave et al. 2015, Lawton et al. 2006). The longer Asian American immigrant women stay in the U.S., the more likely they are to be physically inactive (Kandula and Lauderdale 2005).

Neighborhood and built environment

Community-level factors such as the characteristics of the built environment are also important in understanding the physical activity of Asian Americans. Characteristics of built environment include the walking distance to stores or recreational

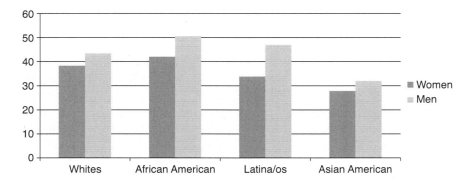

FIGURE 6.3 Regular physical activity for Californian adults, ages 18–44, by race and gender

Source: California Health Interview Survey 2009.

Note: Regular physical activity includes walking for transportation and leisure, vigorous physical activity, and moderate physical activity, and moderate leisure activity.

facilities, existence and condition of sidewalks in the neighborhood, street connectedness, traffic speed, and the availability of nearby parks. Asian and Latina/o immigrant enclaves may have worse walkability, worse neighborhood safety, and fewer recreational exercise facilities than neighborhoods with less immigrants (Osypuk et al. 2009). Depending on the neighborhood context prior to immigration, physical activity may have been more integrated in the daily lives of Asian immigrants in their home countries. Walking and bicycling – common means of getting to work and accomplishing daily tasks – have given way to the American style of transportation, driving regardless of distance to these destinations (Im et al. 2012). Kandula and Lauderdale (2005) have suggested that Asian Americans may be more likely to participate in non-leisure-time physical activity, such as bicycling or walking to work, rather than traditional leisure-time physical activities. Moreover, Asian Americans are more likely to participate in leisure-time physical activities if they live in neighborhoods that are near parks, playgrounds, and open spaces (Li and Wen 2013, Taylor et al. 2012). Older Vietnamese Americans in California, one of the poorer Asian American groups, are also the least likely to report living nearby a park (Yu et al. 2015). In short, improving the walkability, safety, and access to recreational facilities may be especially important in increasing the overall physical activity in Asian immigrant populations (Bhattacharya Becerra et al. 2015, Bungum et al. 2012, Kelley et al. 2016).

Social cohesion, how connected residents of a neighborhood feel, is a key environmental factor impacting physical activity levels. Residents of neighborhoods with high social cohesion collaborate to reduce violence and provide an environment more conducive to being physically active (Sampson et al. 1997). Ironically, Asian immigrant enclaves may have the worst social cohesion/trust according to a study on Chinese Americans living in Los Angeles and Chicago (Osypuk et al. 2009). Furthermore, older Asian American adults in California reported living in neighborhoods with less social cohesion compared to their White counterparts (Li et al. 2015). However, there is considerable variation among the Asian American subgroups, with Vietnamese Americans reporting the lowest social cohesion levels. On the other hand, Japanese Americans, the most residentially and culturally assimilated of all the Asian American groups (Logan and Zhang 2013), also reported the highest neighborhood social cohesion (Li et al. 2015). When parks are nearby and environments are socially cohesive, older Asian Americans are more likely to walk on a regular basis (Li et al. 2015).

Asian Americans live in a variety of neighborhoods from typical American suburbs, ethnic enclaves, and urban centers (Li 2009, Logan and Zhang 2013, Skop and Li 2005, Zhou et al. 2008), and their perception of neighborhood safety reflects the types of neighborhoods in which they reside. Poorer and working-class Asian American communities, such as Chinese American youth and immigrants in Chinatowns; Cambodian Americans in Long Beach, California; and Vietnamese Americans in the Tenderloin area of San Francisco, may be more particularly vulnerable to crime such as burglary and physical safety (Adebiyi et al. 2013, Mai and Chen 2013, Opatrny 1996), posing an environmental barrier to physical activity.

In a study on Asian American adults living in California, Filipino Americans and Vietnamese Americans were the most likely to report neighborhood safety as a significant barrier to physical activity (Bhattacharya Becerra et al. 2015). Asian American preschoolers who live in neighborhoods that the mothers perceive as unsafe spend more time watching television than preschoolers in perceived safe neighborhoods (Datar et al. 2013).

Neighborhood safety may be especially important for Asian American older adults (Choi et al. 2016, Li et al. 2015), as they generally walk considerably more for transportation and leisure than their White counterparts (Li et al. 2015). For many Asian American older adults, walking may be one of the more economically viable forms of transportation and recreation as they are generally poorer with less education than their White counterparts (Li et al. 2015). Moreover, when living in a multi-generational home, older Asian immigrants may be responsible for the majority of grocery shopping and childcare responsibilities including walking the children to school (Li et al. 2015).

Intervention strategies

Culturally competent approaches

Asian Americans may encounter adaptation challenges such as limited English proficiency (LEP), discrimination experiences, limited social networks, and cultural and racial/ethnic differences that may pose barriers to leisure physical activity (Fitzpatrick et al. 2012, Islam et al. 2013, Kim et al. 2014). For those with LEP, even if they are interested in going to an exercise class, it could be difficult for them to know where and when there is the opportunity to engage in physical activities outside their home. Examples of institutional-level strategies include local parks and recreational facilities offering culturally specific physical activities, such as Tai Chi and yoga to Chinese and South Asian immigrants, respectively. These activities may be of greater interest to these immigrant populations than facilities offering aerobic exercise classes (Daniel et al. 2013, Lin et al. 2007). Many Asian Americans believe incorporating physical activity into their daily routine is important for remaining healthy and happy (Belza et al. 2004, Coronado et al. 2011, Taylor et al. 2008).

Culturally tailored interventions that increase education and awareness on the importance of physical activity are particularly needed especially among older Asian Americans who often are LEP and who have low levels of health literacy (Bender et al. 2014). Several culturally tailored interventions have been created by researchers to increase physical activity in Asian American populations. To increase nutrition and physical activity among older LEP Chinese immigrants, one study utilized culturally tailored Chinese-language health educator presentations and in-language presentation print materials compared to in-language presentation print materials only in a randomized control trial (RCT) study (Jih et al. 2016a). As outlined in Chapter 3, constituent-involving and linguistic strategies are intrapersonal or surface-level approaches to tailoring. The written and lecture-based curriculum to promote physical activity was designed to be simple and engaging with culturally appropriate mnemonic techniques to help participants remember the basic recommendations regarding optimal aerobic physical activity level based on the 2008 Physical Activity Guidelines (U.S. Department of Health and Human Services 2008). For example, the health educators used simple hand gestures with a Chinese poem as a learning aid to help participants recall the recommended number of minutes of aerobic moderate physical activity. Knowledge of recommended level of physical activity modestly increased for both groups, but the greatest increase was with the group of participants that received the presentations with print materials. In terms of reported levels of physical activity, both the group that received print materials alone and the group that received Chinese-language health educator lectures with print materials had increases in self-reported physical activity behaviors.

Community health workers

Community participatory methods, including the active engagement of community organizations and training community members to implement health interventions to promote physical activity, have been an effective, tailored way of increasing physical activity in immigrant and minority communities. Filipino Americans have among the highest rates of obesity, type 2 diabetes, and cardiovascular disease including hypertension among Asian Americans with physical activity as a modifiable risk factor (Barnes et al. 2008, Holland et al. 2011, Jih et al. 2014, Karter et al. 2013). A nutrition and physical activity intervention called *Siglang Buhay* (meaning "active life" in Tagalog) conducted among Filipino Americans in social clubs in San Diego, California, was a multi-level approach using both interpersonal and community-level strategies (Dirige et al. 2013). Committee members at each social club were trained to deliver a nutrition and physical activity intervention or cancer education. In the nutrition and physical activity intervention, the committee led exercise activities including group aerobic classes, dancing, kickboxing, basketball tournaments, and gardening. Each committee also facilitated policy changes within each organization such as creating a regular walking club. After 18 months of follow-up, the participants receiving the nutrition and physical activity intervention had significant increases in physical activity meeting recommended guidelines.

Community members trained to conduct health interventions, also known as community or lay health workers (a constituent-involving strategy), have also been found effective in promoting physical activity among other Asian American subgroups including Vietnamese Americans. An intervention with lay health workers (LHW) was conducted to increase fruit and vegetable intake and physical activity among Vietnamese Americans living in the San Francisco Bay Area (Jih et al. 2016b). LHWs were recruited through Vietnamese community-based organizations and led group sessions using flip charts in Vietnamese to promote healthy eating and physical activity. The intervention LHWs led 2 group sessions on healthy nutrition and physical activity and the comparison LHWs led 2 group sessions on colorectal cancer screening. For the participants that received the LHW nutrition and physical activity intervention, knowledge of physical activity recommendations increased by almost 60% and self-reported physical activity meeting recommendations increased by 25%.

BOX 6.1   EVIDENCE-BASED PRACTICE: ASIAN AND PACIFIC ISLANDER OBESITY PREVENTION ALLIANCE TACKLES OBESITY BY IMPROVING NEIGHBORHOODS

Scott Chan, Program Director

Increasing physical activity in Asian Americans can serve a greater purpose. The Asian and Pacific Islander Obesity Prevention Alliance (APIOPA) is a community-based organization that combats the growing levels of obesity, diabetes, and heart disease in Asian and Pacific Islander communities through environmental changes. It is not enough to simply ask community members to change health behaviors, but instead we must engage the community to advocate for healthier neighborhoods to live in.

Specific to physical activity, APIOPA organized the "Bike to China" program in 2013 targeted to Asian American high school youth living in Los Angeles Chinatown. Bike to China was a program in which a class of 15 high school students was challenged to bike the equivalent distance of Chinatown to China (5,000 miles). Over the summer, APIOPA organized rides once a week and if the class attended a majority of sessions and biked all 5,000 miles, every participant would be given a bicycle to keep. Each ride APIOPA organized focused on larger issues impacting Chinatown. From gentrification to environmental justice, APIOPA coordinated rides throughout Los Angeles County and invited community leaders from each area to share with the youth more about how they are fighting similar issues in urban planning. The program culminated with the youth not only riding 5,000 miles and keeping their bikes, but they also organized their own bike tour of Chinatown for Assembly member Jimmy Gomez, in which they educated their elected official on key issues impacting Chinatown, and what they believe are the necessary solutions to improve their community.

Mode of physical activity

Understanding the meaning of physical activity and motivating types of physical activity among the diverse Asian American subgroups is particularly important in the design and implementation of community and institutional-level interventions, particularly as they may reinforce socio-cultural factors to engage in physical activity. This can allow for deep structure strategies in designing interventions. Institutional-based strategies include making available activities with other co-ethnics, which also enables Asian Americans to maintain friendships (Belza et al. 2004, Taylor et al. 2008) and a sense of belonging to their respective cultures (Im et al. 2012, Kim et al. 2014). Asian immigrant women who would like to participate in exercise classes often prefer classes with other co-ethnics, eliminating language barriers experienced in classes with women of other cultures (Dave et al. 2015, Im et al. 2012, Ju et al. 2011).

The Bollywood dance style, popularized by India's film industry, is modeled after traditional Indian dance forms and can be aerobically intense. A study of a culturally relevant Bollywood dance exercise intervention, which included a 1-hour class meeting twice per week over an 8-week period, for South Asian women with diabetes was effective in improving glycemic control and in weight loss (Natesan et al. 2015).

Technology-based

While many physical activity promotion interventions among Asian American groups have focused on self-reported levels of physical activity, there have been emerging pilot studies using mobile technologies, such as mobile phone applications and wearable activity trackers. In a feasibility study testing an in-language iPhone application to promote physical activity among adult Chinese, Filipino, and Vietnamese speakers, the participants had minimal problems with wearing a Fitbit pedometer to provide an objective measure of number of steps walked each day (Yu et al. 2015). In this feasibility study that focuses on intrapersonal-level strategies, wearing the pedometer and using the application increased physical activity by an average of > 2,000 steps daily after 5 weeks with walking as the most commonly reported mode of physical activity.

Healthcare settings

Physical inactivity and the associated chronic conditions among youth including Asian Americans remains a significant public health priority. In a feasibility study of immigrant Chinese youth aged 7–12 and a parent conducted in partnership with a community-based center and integrated with primary care provided by a pediatrician, Chinese children participated in an 8-week, 1.5-hour educational play-based activities curriculum focused on nutrition and physical activity (Chen et al. 2013). During each session, youth engaged in 1 hour of exercise such as basketball, dodgeball, and badminton. Each child also received physical activity education materials and a pedometer to motivate them toward 10,000 steps/day. Parents attended a 1-hour workshop in Chinese and English to reinforce the principles being taught to their children, blending both Chinese and Western perspectives in nutrition and physical activity. This study used interpersonal as well as community approaches to tailor the intervention through both surface- and deep-level approaches to tailoring. At the end of the study, immigrant Chinese American children receiving the intervention had improvements in BMI and blood pressure.

Implications for practice

Gaps in evidence-based, culturally appropriate strategies for promoting physical activity among Asian Americans remain and is a fertile area for further research and community-engaged efforts. Conventional approaches with cultural tailoring and in-language such as print materials and/or discussion or lecture-based interventions may promote physical activity. However, further research is needed to explore the effect of alternative educational methods that can influence behaviors, such as LHWs that provide social support and mobile technologies that provide regular reminders and feedback among the heterogeneous Asian American subgroups to prevent and manage chronic diseases and its risk factors related to physical inactivity. Additionally, increased attention to the low levels of physical activity among Asian Americans must also be addressed at the policy level. Due to the misperception that Asian Americans are "skinny" and therefore healthy, funding, research, and programs dedicated to Asian American populations have been limited.

Summary points

This chapter examines various factors that influence physical activity among Asian Americans including acculturation and social and community context. Asian Americans are a diverse, growing population that is often invisible at policy making and national programs to increase physical activity. Because Asian Americans face significant risk for chronic diseases, it is vital to understand the barriers, challenges, and strategies to increase physical activity in this growing population. Key findings of this chapter include:

- The meaning and experiences of physical activity among Asian Americans differs across stages of life, ethnicities, socio-economic status, gender, and immigration experiences.
- Built environment can impact levels of physical activity.
- Among younger Asian Americans, physical inactivity and the associated chronic conditions remains a significant public health priority.
- For older Asian immigrants, culturally competent interventions to promote physical activity are particularly needed because of LEP and low levels of health literacy.
- Designing and implementing physical activity interventions should take into account the meaning and motivations behind physical activity in ethnic minority communities.

Critical thinking questions

1   How does the built environment shape and influence physical activity among individuals in your neighborhood?
2   How does the immigrant experience shape physical activity levels of Asian Americans? How might it vary by gender? Explain why there are variations between the different Asian American ethnic groups.

3　What messages regarding physical activity were you given while growing up?
4　How might the physical activity concerns be different for younger American-born Asian Americans versus Asian American older adults who may have more limited English-speaking abilities? How would you propose to increase physical activity across the different age groups and levels of English abilities?

Acknowledgment

Research for this chapter was supported by a National Institute of Health Building Infrastructure Leading to Diversity grant #8RL5GM118975, and California State University, College of Humanities Faculty Fellowship.

References

Adebiyi, A., Cheng, A., Kim, J., Kim, T., Men, A., Ly, M., Pech, C., Luna, B., Sestich, M., Sithounnolat, D. and Tse, L. (2013). *The State of Cambodia Town*. Asian Pacific Policy and Planning Council (A3PCON), the UCLA Asian American Studies Center (AASC), and the UCLA Department of Urban Planning.

Afable-Munsuz, A., Ponce, N.A., Rodriguez, M. and Perez-Stable, E.J. (2010). 'Immigrant generation and physical activity among Mexican, Chinese & Filipino adults in the US.' *Social Science & Medicine*, 70: 1997–2005.

Allen, M., Elliott, M., Morales, L., Diamant, A., Hambarsoomian, K., et al. (2007). 'Adolescent participation in preventive health behaviors, physical activity, and nutrition: Differences across immigrant generations for Asians and Latinos compared with whites.' *American Journal of Public Health*, 97: 337–343.

Aoki, Y., Yoon, S.S., Chong, Y. and Carroll, M.D. (2014). 'Hypertension, abnormal cholesterol, and high body mass index among non-Hispanic Asian adults: United States, 2011–2012.' *NCHS Data Brief*, 140: 1–8.

Asian American Center for Advancing Justice (2013). *A Community of Contrasts: Asian Americans, Native Hawaiians and Pacific Islanders in California*. Los Angeles and San Francisco, CA: Asian American Center for Advancing Justice.

Asian American Legal Center and Asian American Justice Center (2011). *A Community of Contrasts: Asian Americans in the United States*. Los Angeles and Washington, DC: Asian American Center for Advancing Justice.

Babakus, W.S. and Thompson, J.L. (2012). 'Physical activity among South Asian women: A systematic, mixed-methods review.' *International Journal of Behavioral Nutrition and Physical Activity*, 9: 1–18.

Babey, S.H., Hastert, T.A. and Wolstein, J. (2013). 'Adolescent sedentary behaviors: Correlates differ for television viewing and computer use.' *Journal of Adolescent Health*, 52: 70–76.

Barnes, P.M., Adams, P.F. and Powell-Griner, E. (2008). 'Health characteristics of the Asian adult population: United States, 2004–2006.' US Department of Health & Human Services, Centers for Disease Control and Prevention, National Center for Health Statistics.

Becerra, M.B., Herring, P., Marshak, H.H. and Banta, J.E. (2015). 'Social determinants of physical activity among adult Asian-Americans: Results from a population-based survey in California.' *Journal of Immigrant and Minority Health*, 17: 1061–1069.

Belza, B., Walwick, J., Shiu-Thornton, S., Schwartz, S., Taylor, M. and LoGerfo, J. (2004). 'Older adult perspectives on physical activity and exercise: Voices from multiple cultures.' *Preventing Chronic Disease*, 1: A09.

Bender, M.S., Choi, J., Won, G.Y. and Fukuoka, Y. (2014). 'Randomized controlled trial lifestyle interventions for Asian Americans: A systematic review.' *Preventive Medicine*, 67: 171–181.

Bhattacharya Becerra, M., Herring, P., Marshak, H. and Banta, J. (2015). 'Social determinants of physical activity among adult Asian Americans: Results from a population-based survey in California.' *Journal of Immigrant and Minority Health*, 17: 1061–1069.

Bungum, T. J., Landers, M., Azzarelli, M. and Moonie, S. (2012). 'Perceived environmental physical activity correlates among Asian Pacific Islander Americans.' *Journal of Physical Activity and Health*, 9: 1098.

Cameron, D. (2015). 'Tech's diversity problem: It's not just a pipeline issue.' *Washington Post.* July 13, 2015.

Chan, S. (1991). *Asian Americans: An Interpretive History*. New York, NY: Twayne Publishers.

Chen, E. and Arguelles, D. (2012). 'Bamboo Ceilings, the Working Poor, and the Unemployed: The Mixed Economic Realities of Asian Americans and Pacific Islanders.' *In:* Shrake, E. and Chen, E. W. (eds.) *Asian Pacific Americans: Past, Present, and Future.* Dubuque: Kendall-Hunt Publishers.

Chen, J.L., Kwan, M., Mac, A., Chin, N.C. and Liu, K. (2013). 'iStart smart: A primary-care based and community partnered childhood obesity management program for Chinese-American children: Feasibility study.' *Journal of Immigrant and Minority Health*, 15: 1125–1128.

Choi, S.E., Kwon, I., Chang, E., Araiza, D., Thorpe, C.L. and Sarkisian, C.A. (2016). 'Developing a culturally tailored stroke prevention walking programme for Korean immigrant seniors: A focus group study.' *International Journal of Older People Nursing.* 11(4): 255–265.

Coronado, G., Sos, C., Talbot, J., Do, H. and Taylor, V. (2011). 'To be healthy and to live long, we have to exercise: Psychosocial factors related to physical activity among Cambodian Americans.' *Journal of Community Health*, 36: 381–388.

Crespo, N.C., Yoo, E. J. and Hawkins, S.A. (2011). 'Anthropometric and lifestyle associations of bone mass in healthy pre-menopausal Mexican and Asian American women.' *Journal of Immigrant & Minority Health*, 13: 74–80.

Daniel, M., Wilbur, J., Marquez, D. and Farran, C. (2013). 'Lifestyle physical activity behavior among South Asian Indian immigrants.' *Journal of Immigrant and Minority Health*, 15: 1082–1089.

Datar, A., Nicosia, N. and Shier, V. (2013). 'Parent perceptions of neighborhood safety and children's physical activity, sedentary behavior, and obesity: Evidence from a national longitudinal study.' *American Journal of Epidemiology*, 177: 1065–1073.

Dave, S.S., Craft, L.L., Mehta, P., Naval, S., Kumar, S. and Kandula, N.R. (2015). 'Life stage influences on US South Asian women's physical activity.' *American Journal of Health Promotion*, 29(3): e100–e108.

De Castro, A.B., Gee, G.C. and Takeuchi, D.T. (2008). 'Job-related stress and chronic health conditions among Filipino immigrants.' *Journal of Immigrant and Minority Health*, 10: 551–558.

Dirige, O.V., Carlson, J.A., Alcaraz, J., Moy, K.L., Rock, C.L., Oades, R. and Sallis, J.F. (2013). 'Siglang Buhay: Nutrition and physical activity promotion in Filipino-Americans through community organizations.' *Journal of Public Health Management and Practice*, 19: 162–168.

Espiritu, Y. (1995). *Filipino American Lives*. Philadelphia: Temple University Press.

Fitzpatrick, A.L., Steinman, L.E., Tu, S.P., Ly, K.A., Ton, T.G., Yip, M.P. and Sin, M.K. (2012). 'Using photovoice to understand cardiovascular health awareness in Asian elders.' *Health Promotion Practice*, 13: 48–54.

Harrison, G.G., Kagawa-Singer, M., Foerster, S.B., Lee, H., Pham Kim, L., Nguyen, T.U., Fernandez-Ami, A., Quinn, V. and Bal, D.G. (2005). 'Seizing the moment.' *Cancer*, 104: 2962–2968.

Holland, A.T., Wong, E.C., Lauderdale, D.S. and Palaniappan, L.P. (2011). 'Spectrum of cardiovascular diseases in Asian-American racial/ethnic subgroups.' *Annals of Epidemiology*, 21: 608–614.

Im, E.O., Ko, Y., Hwang, H., Chee, W., Stuifbergen, A., Lee, H. and Chee, E. (2012). 'Asian American midlife women's attitudes toward physical activity.' *Journal of Obstetric, Gynecologic, & Neonatal Nursing*, 41: 650–658.

Im, E., Ko, Y., Hwang, H., Chee, W., Stuifbergen, A., et al. (2013). Racial/ethnic differences in midlife women's attitudes toward physical activity. *Journal of Midwifery & Women's Health*, 58(4): 440–450.

Islam, N.S., Zanowiak, J.M., Wyatt, L.C., Chun, K., Lee, L., Kwon, S.C. and Trinh-Shevrin, C. (2013). 'A randomized-controlled, pilot intervention on diabetes prevention and healthy lifestyles in the New York City Korean community.' *Journal of Community Health*, 38: 1030–1041.

Jih, J., Le, G., Woo, K., Tsoh, J.Y., Stewart, S., Gildengorin, G., Burke, A., Wong, C., Chan, E., Fung, L.C. and Yu, F. (2016a). 'Educational interventions to promote healthy nutrition and physical activity among older Chinese Americans: A cluster-randomized trial.' *American Journal of Public Health*, 106: 1092–1098.

Jih, J., Mukherjea, A., Vittinghoff, E., Nguyen, T.T., Tsoh, J.Y., Fukuoka, Y., Bender, M.S., Tseng, W. and Kanaya, A.M. (2014). 'Using appropriate body mass index cut points for overweight and obesity among Asian Americans.' *Preventive Medicine*, 65: 1–6.

Jih, J., Stewart, S., Luong, T.N., Nguyen, T.T., McPhee, S. and Nguyen, B.H. (2016b). 'A Cluster Randomized Controlled Trial of a Lay Health Worker Intervention to Increase Healthy Eating and Physical Activity among Vietnamese Americans.' *In preparation*.

Ju, S., Wilbur, J., Lee, E. and Miller, A. (2011). 'Lifestyle physical activity behavior of Korean American dry cleaner couples.' *Public Health Nursing*, 28: 503–514.

Kandula, N.R. and Lauderdale, D.S. (2005). 'Leisure time, non-leisure time, and occupational physical activity in Asian Americans.' *Annals of Epidemiology*, 15: 257–265.

Kao, D., Gulati, A.C. and Lee, R.E. (2016). 'Physical activity among Asian American adults in Houston, Texas: Data from the Health of Houston Survey 2010.' *Journal of Immigrant and Minority Health*, 18: 1470–1481.

Karter, A.J., Schillinger, D., Adams, A.S., Moffett, H.H., Liu, J., Adler, N.E. and Kanaya, A.M. (2013). 'Elevated rates of diabetes in Pacific Islanders and Asian subgroups: The Diabetes Study of Northern California (DISTANCE).' *Diabetes Care*, 36: 574–579.

Kelley, E., Kandula, N., Kanaya, A. and Yen, I. (2016). 'Neighborhood walkability and walking for transport among South Asians in the MASALA study.' *Journal of Physical Activity & Health*, 13(5): 514.

Kim, J., Heo, J. and Kim, J. (2014). 'The benefits of in-group contact through physical activity involvement for health and well-being among Korean immigrants.' *International Journal of Qualitative Studies on Health and Well-Being*, 9: 1–11.

Lawton, J., Ahmad, N., Hanna, L., Douglas, M. and Hallowell, N. (2006). ' "I can't do any serious exercise": Barriers to physical activity amongst people of Pakistani and Indian origin with Type 2 diabetes.' *Health Education Research*, 21: 43–54.

Le, C.N. (2016). 'Employment & Occupational Patterns.' *Asian-Nation: The Landscape of Asian America* [Online]. Available: www.asian-nation.org/employment.shtml (Accessed May 24 2016).

Lee, S.H. and Im, E.O. (2010). 'Ethnic differences in exercise and leisure time physical activity among midlife women.' *Journal of Advanced Nursing*, 66: 814–827.

Li, K. and Wen, M. (2013). Racial and ethnic disparities in leisure-time physical activity in California: Patterns and mechanisms. *Race and Social Problems*, 5: 147–156.

Li, W. (2009). *Ethnoburb: The New Ethnic Community in Urban America*. Honolulu: University of Hawai'i Press.

Li, Y., Kao, D. and Dinh, T. (2015). 'Correlates of neighborhood environment with walking among older Asian Americans.' *Journal of Aging and Health*, 27: 17–34.

Lin, Y., Huang, L., Young, H. and Chen, Y. (2007). 'Beliefs about physical activity: Focus group results of Chinese community elderly in Seattle and Taipei.' *Geriatric Nursing*, 28: 236–244.

Logan, J.R. and Zhang, W. (2013). 'Separate and equal: Asian Nationalities in the U.S. US2010 Project Report.' Brown University: Advisory Board of the US2010 Project.

Lowe, L. (1991). 'Heterogeneity, hybridity, multiplicity: Marking Asian American differences.' *Diaspora: A Journal of Transnational Studies*, 1: 24–44.

Mai, R. and Chen, B. (2013). 'The State of Chinatown Los Angeles.' Asian Pacific Policy and Planning Council (A3PCON), the UCLA Asian American Studies Center (AASC), and the UCLA Department of Urban Planning.

Marmot, M., Syme, S.L., Kagan, A., Kato, H., Cohen, J. and Belsky, J. (1975). 'Epidemiologic studies of coronary heart disease and stroke in Japanese men living in Japan, Hawaii and California: Prevalence of coronary and hypertensive heart disease and associated risk factors.' *American Journal of Epidemiology*, 102: 514–524.

McLeroy, K.R., Bibeau, D., Steckler, A. and Glanz, K. (1988). 'An ecological perspective on health promotion programs.' *Health Education Quarterly*, 15: 351–377.

Menke, A., Casagrande, S., Geiss, L. and Cowie, C.C. (2015). 'Prevalence of and trends in diabetes among adults in the United States, 1988–2012.' *JAMA*, 314(10): 1021–1029.

Nakaso, D. (2012). 'Asian workers now dominate Silicon Valley tech jobs.' *The Mercury News*, November 30.

Natesan, A., Nimbal, V.C., Ivey, S.L., Wang, E.J., Madsen, K.A. and Palaniappan, L.P. (2015). 'Engaging South Asian women with type 2 diabetes in a culturally relevant exercise intervention: A randomized controlled trial.' *BMJ Open Diabetes Research & Care*, 3: e000126.

Nguyen, T.T. (2015). 'Not your model minority: The reality of the Asian American and Pacific islander community [Online].' Available: www.huffingtonpost.com/dr-tung-thanh-nguyen/not-your-model-minority-t_b_8513548.html (Accessed November 9 2015).

Office of Disease Prevention and Health Promotion (ODPHP) (2016). 'Physical activity has many health benefits [Online].' Available: http://health.gov/paguidelines/guidelines/chapter2.aspx (Accessed June 9 2016).

Opatrny, D. (1996). 'Immigrants brave risks to settle in Tenderloin families flourish despite high crime.' Second Edition. *San Francisco Examiner*. <http://www.sfgate.com/news/article/Immigrants-brave-risks-to-settle-in-Tenderloin-3160388.php> Accessed March 27th, 2017.

Osypuk, T.L., Roux, A.V.D., Hadley, C. and Kandula, N.R. (2009). 'Are immigrant enclaves healthy places to live? The Multi-ethnic study of atherosclerosis.' *Social Science & Medicine*, 69: 110–120.

Pih, K., Hirose, A. and Mao, K. (2012). 'The invisible unattended: Low-wage Chinese immigrant workers, health care, and social capital in Southern California's San Gabriel Valley.' *Sociological Inquiry*, 82: 236–256.

Ray, M. (2006). 'Undocumented Asian American workers and state wage laws in the aftermath of Hoffman plastic compounds.' *Asian American Law Journal*, 13: 91–233.

Rideout, V., Lauricella, A. and Wartella, E. (2011). *Children, Media, and Race: Media Use among White, Black, Hispanic, and Asian American Children*. Evanston, IL: Center on Media and Human Development, School of Communication, Northwestern University.

Sallis, J.F., Owen, N. and Fisher, E.B. (2008). 'Ecological Models of Health Behavior.' *In*: Glanz, K., Rimer, B.K. and Viswanath, K. (eds.) *Health Behavior and Health Education: Theory, Research and Practice*. 4th ed. San Francisco: Jossey-Bass.

Sampson, R.J., Raudenbush, S.W. and Earls, F. (1997). 'Neighborhoods and violent crime: A multilevel study of collective efficacy.' *Science*, 27: 918–924.

Skop, E. and Li, W. (2005). 'Asians in America's suburbs: Patterns and consequences of settlement.' *Geographical Review*, 95: 167–188.

Sriskantharajah, J. and Kai, J. (2007). 'Promoting physical activity among south Asian women with coronary heart disease and diabetes: What might help?' *Family Practice*, 24: 71–76.

Sue, S. and Okazaki, S. (2009). 'Asian-American educational achievements: A phenomenon in search of an explanation.' *Asian American Journal of Psychology*, S(1): 45–55.

Takaki, R. (1998). *Strangers from a Different Shore: A History of Asian Americans*. Boston: Little, Brown.

Taylor, V.M., Cripe, S.M., Acorda, E., Teh, C., Coronado, G., Do, H., Woodall, T. and Hislop, G. (2008). 'Development of an ESL curriculum to educate Chinese immigrants about physical activity.' *Journal of Immigrant & Minority Health*, 10: 379–387.

Taylor, V.M., Liu, Q., Yasui, Y., Talbot, J., Sos, C., Coronado, G. and Bastani, R. (2012). 'Physical activity among Cambodian Americans: An exploratory study.' *Journal of Community Health*, 37: 1040–1048.

Taylor, V.M., Yasui, Y., Tu, S.P., Neuhouser, M.L., Li, L., Woodall, E., Acorda, E., Cripe, S.M. and Hislop, T.G. (2007). 'Heart disease prevention among Chinese immigrants.' *Journal of Community Health*, 32: 299–310.

Tran, N. and Birman, D. (2010). 'Questioning the model minority: Studies of Asian American academic performance.' *Asian American Journal of Psychology*, 1: 106–118.

Tung, C. (2000). 'The cost of caring: The social reproductive labor of Filipina live-in home health caregivers.' *Frontiers: A Journal of Women Studies*, 21: 61–82.

UCLA Center for Policy Health Research. (2016). 'AskCHIS 2009–2010 [Online].' Available at http://ask.chis.ucla.edu. (Exported February 22 2016).

Unger, J.B., Reynolds, K., Shakib, S., Spruijt-Metz, D., Sun, P. and Johnson, C.A. (2004). 'Acculturation, physical activity, and fast-food consumption among Asian-American and Hispanic adolescents'. *Journal of Community Health*, 29: 467–481.

U.S. Census Bureau, Population Division. (2015a). 'Annual estimates of the resident population by sex, race alone or in combination, and Hispanic origin for the United States, states, and counties: April 1, 2010 to July 1, 2014 [Online].' Available at http://factfinder.census.gov/faces/tableservices/jsf/pages/productview.xhtml?src=bkmk (Accessed June 2 2016).

U.S. Census Bureau, Population Division. (2015b). 'Annual estimates of the resident population by sex, race alone or in combination, and Hispanic origin for the United States, states, and counties: April 1, 2010 to July 1, 2014 [Online].' Available at http://factfinder.census.gov/faces/tableservices/jsf/pages/productview.xhtml?src=bkmk (Accessed June 2 2016).

U.S. Department of Health and Human Services, Office of Disease Prevention and Health Promotion, U.S. Department of Health and Human Services and Office of Disease Prevention and Health Promotion. (2008). *Physical Activity Guidelines for Americans*. Washington, DC: U.S. Department of Health and Human Services.

U.S. Department of Health and Human Services, Office on Women's Health. (2015). 'Minority women's health: Osteoporosis [online].' Available at http://womenshealth.gov/minority-health/asian-americans/osteoporosis.html (Accessed June 3 2016).

Yu, F., Jih, J., Tsoh, J., Gildengorin, G., Wong, C., Lam, H., Fukuoka, Y. and Ngueyn, T. (2015). 'A community-based feasibility study of an in-language mobile phone application to promote physical activity among Asian Americans.' *2015 American Public Health Association Annual Meeting*. Chicago, IL.

Zhou, M., Tseng, Y. and Kim, R.Y. (2008). 'Rethinking residential Assimilation: The case of a Chinese ethnoburb in the San Gabriel Valley, California.' *Amerasia Journal*, 34: 55.

7

PHYSICAL ACTIVITY AMONG NATIVE AMERICANS

Heather J. A. Foulds

Understanding the Native American population

Indigenous peoples of continental North America include Native Americans of the United States: American Indians and Alaskan Natives, and Canadian First Nations, Métis and Inuit peoples. These peoples descend from two distinct lineages: American Indian/First Nations and Métis, and Native Alaskan/Inuit, arriving in North America from separate migrations (Schurr 2004, Dulik *et al.* 2012). Native American populations have inhabited North America for more than 15,000 years (Dickason 1992). From populations upwards of 18 million people prior to the arrival of Europeans to North America, Native Americans now represent 1.7% of the United States population (5.2 million) and 4.3% of the Canadian population (1.4 million) (Norris *et al.* 2012, Statistics Canada 2013).

Native American peoples have survived devastating experiences of infectious diseases, colonialist policies, relocations and reservations, and boarding and residential schools (Braveheart 1998, Milloy 1999, Muckle 2007, British Columbia Provincial Health Officer 2009, Coates 2016). Diseases including smallpox, tuberculosis, scarlet fever, influenza and measles brought by fur traders, gold rushes and settlers decimated populations. The advent of reservations limited access to traditional territory, leading to breakdowns in traditional social relations, and limiting resources and traditional subsistence methods. Further, many Native American tribes in the United States were relocated to reservations away from their traditional territories. Forced attendance at boarding schools in the United States and residential schools in Canada has also had a well-documented negative impact on Native American populations. These experiences have been directly linked to increased prevalence of disease, poorer health and quality of life and intergenerational post-traumatic stress response and disproportionately high stress loads (Duran and Duran 1995, Whitbeck *et al.* 2004, Barton *et al.* 2005, Mitchell and Maracle 2005, Muckle 2007,

Craib *et al.* 2009). Diagnosed chronic conditions are more frequent among Native American adults who attended residential schools (76.1% vs. 59.1%) (First Nations Information Governance Centre 2012).

Health disparities and inequities among Native Americans

Many chronic conditions and health risks are higher among Native American populations (Peschken and Esdaile 1999, Story *et al.* 1999, Janz *et al.* 2009, Oster and Toth 2009, Reading and Wien 2009, Tjepkema *et al.* 2009, Garner *et al.* 2010, Wilson and Macdonald 2010, Foulds *et al.* 2011b, Frieden *et al.* 2011, Public Health Agency of Canada 2011, Foulds *et al.* 2013a, Krieger 2014, Kelley *et al.* 2015). Obesity, diabetes, cardiovascular disease, asthma, arthritis and many other conditions have become widespread health issues for Native Americans. Further, Native American populations currently experience social challenges including reduced education, income, employment, food security and safe housing. Data from NHANES, BRFSS and California Health Interview Study in the United States and Canadian Aboriginal Peoples Surveys, Canadian Community Health Surveys, National Household Survey and smaller research studies where necessary highlight many health disparities among Native American adults (Table 7.1).

Chronic disease

Many chronic conditions are experienced at much higher rates among Native Americans (Ferucci *et al.* 2008, Barnes *et al.* 2010, Public Health Agency of Canada 2011, Rotenberg 2016). Throughout North America, rates of diabetes are roughly three times higher among Native Americans and obesity more than 50% greater. Heart disease and asthma are also more prevalent among Native Americans. In Canada, cancer and arthritis are more frequent among Native Americans.

Determinants of health

Determinants of health among Native American populations present a significant health challenge and potential area for improving outcomes (Kirmayer *et al.* 2007, Barnes *et al.* 2010, Dogra *et al.* 2010, Foulds *et al.* 2016b, Rotenberg 2016). Behaviors such as smoking and sedentary behavior are 50–80% more prevalent among Native Americans. Physical inactivity is also more prevalent among Native Americans. Suicide among Native American populations is a significant concern, where rates reach double that of the general population.

Social determinants of health present a significant challenge for Native American populations and contribute to the increased health challenges (Kirmayer *et al.* 2007, Barnes *et al.* 2010, Garner *et al.* 2010, Jernigan *et al.* 2013, Krieger 2014, Kelly-Scott and Smith 2015, Foulds *et al.* 2016b, Rotenberg 2016). Food insecurity

TABLE 7.1 The prevalence of health disparities among Native American populations

	Canada		United States	
	Native American (%)	General Population (%)	Native American (%)	White (%)
Heart disease	7.1[†]	5.0[†]	14.7[§]	12.2[§]
Diabetes	16.2[ε]	5.0[ε]	17.5[§]	6.6[§]
Cancer	4.0[†]	2.0[†]	7.0[§]	8.4[§]
Asthma	12.7[†]	7.0[†]	14.2[§]	11.6[§]
Obesity	31.0[‡]	17.0[‡]	39.4[§]	24.3[§]
Arthritis	22.3[†]	16.0[†]	22.5[δ]	21.5[δ]
Suicide	0.024[φ]	0.012[φ]	0.019[φ]	0.011[φ]
Smoking	29.0[‡]	16.0[‡]	32.7[§]	22.5[§]
Physical inactivity	56.8[α]	54.1[α]	43.8[§]	34.6[§]
2 or more hours television viewing[θ]	32.1[χ]	23.7[χ]	39.8[χ]	23.1[χ]
Unemployment	13.0[‡]	7.8[‡]	14.6[β]	7.2[β]
Food insecurity	20.0[‡]	8.0[‡]	38.7[γ]	15.0[γ]
Less than high school education	29.9[†]	16.0[†]	21.1[§]	10.7[§]
Poverty	23.9[†]	12.4[†]	24.4[§]	8.7[§]
No regular physician	20.0[‡]	15.0[‡]	16.0[§]	15.1[§]

† Garner et al. (2010);
‡ Rotenberg (2016);
§ Barnes et al. (2010);
ε Public Health Agency of Canada (2011);
β Krieger (2014);
α Dogra (2010);
γ Jernigan et al. (2013);
δ Ferucci et al. (2008);
φ Kirmayer et al. (2007);
χ Foulds et al. (2016b);
θ only includes children/youth

is 150% more prevalent among Native Americans and unemployment is close to double. Poverty and lower levels of education affect 2–3 times as many Native Americans. Native Americans also experience lower access to regular physicians. Health disparities among Native American populations have been linked to social determinants of health as outlined in Chapter 1. Reduced education and income levels have been associated with poorer health outcomes (Wilson and Macdonald 2010). Historical trauma including family residential school experiences and losses of culture contribute to health disparities among Native Americans (Craib *et al.* 2009, Greenwood and De Leeuw 2012, Foulds *et al.* 2016a, Hackett *et al.* 2016).

Addressing health disparities among this population requires strategies which consider the historical experiences among Native Americans and utilize wholistic and inclusive methods.

Physical activity among Native Americans

Physical activity levels among Native Americans

In past, Native American peoples were traditionally a very healthy people, with skeletal evidence demonstrating greater health than peoples elsewhere in the world (Steckel *et al.* 2002; Dapice 2006). Among the Aboriginal Sport Circle, sport and recreation are considered "powerful medicine that can prevent many of the social ills facing Aboriginal peoples, and foster community healing" (Aboriginal Sport Circle 2016). Traditional Native American culture included lifestyles of hunting, gathering, fishing and farming (Fredericks 1999). Similar to experiences of other cultures, Native Americans have experienced decreases in physical activity and physical fitness and changes in lifestyles with the introduction of a Western lifestyle (Rode and Shephard 1994). Physical activity levels among Native American populations are often found to be higher than other North American groups (Foulds *et al.* 2013b). However, physical activity levels still lag behind recommendations and may contribute to health risks (Young and Katzmarzyk 2007, Foulds *et al.* 2013b).

Historical physical activity

Many traditional activities common among Native American populations require extensive physical fitness (Miller 1996, Fisher 2002, Kirby *et al.* 2007, Forsyth 2012, Bruner and Chad 2013). Traditional survival required cutting and hauling wood, fishing, hunting, carrying water and other survival activities. Pow wow dancing, canoeing, lacrosse (Figure 7.1A), snowshoeing (Figure 7.1B) and many other games and sports derive from traditional Native American activities. From 1880–1951 in Canada and 1889–1934 in the United States, legislation outlawed traditional dancing, including Pow wows and Sun Dances (Mathias and Yabsley 1991, Kracht 1994). These limits to traditional activities may have reduced physical activities among this population by preventing common recreational physical activities.

Native American students attending residential and boarding schools commonly participated in sports such as hockey, basketball, skating, football and softball (Miller 1996, Waldrum *et al.* 2006). However, traditional Native American sports such as lacrosse were not played at these schools, despite reduced expenses and easier access to facilities. Sports teams from residential schools often played in leagues with non–Native American teams from nearby communities, where Native American residential school teams often won handedly. For many Native American children attending residential schools, participation in sports was a coping mechanism for dealing with the trauma and difficulties of these institutions, particularly when sports and recreational activities were played outdoors. Participation in sports

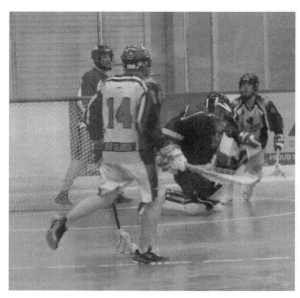

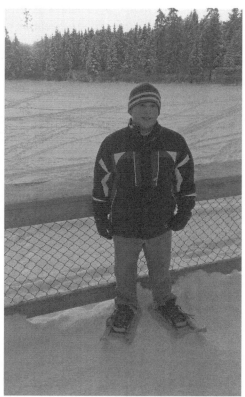

FIGURES 7.1A AND 7.1B Sports and activities such as lacrosse (A) and snowshoeing (B) are derived from traditional Native American games and activities

among residential school students was often hampered by insufficient funds. Funding to purchase sporting equipment and travel to games was difficult to obtain. This financial limitation was more often experienced by female students. While equipment for boys' participation in sports was often scrounged up, equipment for female students was much less common. Experiences of sports and recreation, and gender biases therein, may still influence physical activity participation among residential school survivors and their families.

Modern physical activity

Physical activity levels among many Native American populations may differ from that of other North American populations (Dogra *et al.* 2010, Holm *et al.* 2010, Foulds *et al.* 2013b). The prevalence of Native Americans meeting physical activity guidelines is similar to that of the general population, based on self-reports. In the United States, 49.7% of Native Americans meet recommended moderate or vigorous activity guidelines, compared to 49.1% of the overall United States population. In Canada, 22.7% of Native Americans are considered active and 20.5% moderately active, compared to 21.3% and 24.6% of the general population, respectively. Based on objectively measured physical activity levels, Native American populations are generally found to be moderately active (5,000–9,999 steps/day) or physically inactive (< 5,000 steps/day), with women more likely than men to be physically inactive.

Native American children engage in physical activity an average of 4 times per week, performing an average of 5 hours per week of activity (Paradis *et al.* 2005, Jollie-Trottier *et al.* 2009). Among Native American children in Canada, 65% participate in sports at least once per week (Findlay and Kohen 2007). Physical inactivity is identified among high levels of Native American children and youth, including 51.9% of female children and 29.9% of male children (Foulds *et al.* 2013b). Screen time use is also high among Native American children and youth, averaging 3.65 ± 1.26 hours per day, greater than averages among White children and youth (Foulds *et al.* 2016b). Outdoor play is greatest among preschool-aged Native American children and declines with age (Adams and Prince 2010). Physical activity among Native American adults is similar to that of children/youth, with 22.1% achieving physical activity below recommendations and 47.9% considered inactive (Foulds *et al.* 2013b). In Canada, 56% of First Nations participate in sports, games or recreational activities (Kirby *et al.* 2007). Native American adults report physical activity 3.6 times per week, with elders reporting 1.2 times per week (Ruthig and Allery 2008, Coble *et al.* 2009). Screen time behavior is also high among Native American adults, including 3.61 ± 2.95 hours per day (Foulds *et al.* 2016b).

Across Native American groups, physical activity levels vary (Findlay and Kohen 2007, Young and Katzmarzyk 2007, Duncan *et al.* 2009, Redwood *et al.* 2009, Findlay 2011). In the United States, physical inactivity is more common among Alaskan Natives (53.4%) compared to American Indians (46.5%). Conversely, American Indians are more likely to be physically active (27.5% vs. 24.2%) or moderately active (25.9% vs. 22.4%) than Alaskan Natives. American Indians living in the Northern Plains are more physically active than those in the Southwest (50% vs. 44%). Within Canada, Métis populations achieve the greatest proportions of adults achieving physical activity recommendations, followed by First Nations and then Inuit. Similarly, physical inactivity was lowest among Métis and highest among Inuit. First Nations people residing off-reserve demonstrate greater prevalence of the population meeting physical activity guidelines, compared to those residing on-reserve. Among Native American children and youth, those who participate in sports are more likely to reside off-reserve, come from two-parent households, be male, and have more educated parents. Further, Inuit and Métis children and youth are more likely to participate in sports at least once per week.

Over time, physical inactivity has increased among Native American adults, with greater levels of physical inactivity and lower levels of insufficient physical activity identified from the 1990s to the 2000s, suggesting a shift toward less active lifestyles (Foulds *et al.* 2013b). Native American adults who engage in more traditional life-styles and experience lower levels of psychosocial stress are generally more physically active, highlighting the importance of traditional culture for increasing physical activity (Bersamin *et al.* 2014). Similarly, psychosocial stress and colonial experiences such as residential schools have also been linked to other health risks including diabetes, metabolic syndrome quality of life (Barton *et al.* 2005, Craib *et al.* 2009).

While physical activity levels may be similar or greater among Native American adults compared to non–Native Americans, sedentary behavior is also greater among Native American adults (Kriska *et al.* 2006, Withrow *et al.* 2014, Foulds *et al.* 2016b). Native American populations generally report greater physical activity during occupational and/or household activities and lower physical activity during leisure time compared to other ethnicities (Brownson *et al.* 2000, Dogra *et al.* 2010, Bruner and Chad 2013, Bruce *et al.* 2014). Native Americans report higher levels of walking (70.8% vs. 68.3%) and commuting (60.5% vs. 53.15) activity, and lower exercise (31.0% vs. 36.6%), sports (25.0% vs. 28.8%) and recreation (51.7% vs. 60.0%) activity compared to the White population (Dogra *et al.* 2010). These behavior patterns of higher occupational physical activity and lower leisure-time physical activity are common among lower socioeconomic populations, such as Native American populations (Wilson and Macdonald 2010, Frieden *et al.* 2011, Beenackers *et al.* 2012).

Common barriers and facilitators to physical activity for Native Americans

Few studies have evaluated barriers and facilitators to physical activity among Native American populations (Kirby *et al.* 2007, Coble *et al.* 2009, Mason and Koehli 2012, Jahns *et al.* 2014). Many barriers and facilitators relate to social and geographical position and resources, which may be common to many Native Americans. However, as Native American peoples live in many different communities, environments and represent a variety of distinct cultures, barriers and facilitators may differ across individuals and communities. Barriers to physical activity among this population span from intrapersonal and interpersonal to institutional, community and policy factors, as outlined in the social ecological model in Chapter 1.

Intrapersonal factors

Interpersonal factors to physical activity for Native Americans include both psychological and physical factors. Psychological factors can include challenges such as a lack of willpower, shy personalities, fear of injury and perceived intimidation of gym or exercise environments. Positive beliefs about the physical and mental benefits of physical activity, including living longer, improved appearance and disease prevention are important psychological facilitators. Physical barriers to physical activity among Native American peoples include higher rates of disability, infectious disease and chronic disease than other populations. Personal use of drugs or alcohol and personal challenges with mental health can also be barriers to physical activity for some Native American people.

Interpersonal factors

Native American individuals identify barriers to physical activity including obligations and demands of time from jobs, family and other responsibilities. Native American individuals generally have more children than other ethnicities and many grandparents are raising grandchildren. Native American children are more likely to live in single-parent households and live in poverty. Consequently, responsibilities and time commitments within the home environment can be significant barriers to physical activity of caregivers. Many Native Americans report experiencing racism or racial discrimination in their daily lives. Experiences of discrimination or racially based assumptions within sports and exercise environments can deter Native Americans from participating. Facilitators to physical activity among Native Americans include community-based programs where members of all ages are included. When children are included and welcomed to physical activity programs, families and caregivers are better able to participate. Conducting these programs within Native American communities provides a safe opportunity for exercise and sports participation where individuals are more welcomed and encouraged.

Institutional factors

Many exercise facilities in Native American communities are unsafe or in poor condition. These facilities may be in need of repair and upkeep; they may have uneven surfaces covered with broken glass making it difficult to participate in sporting activities. Additionally, many Native American sporting programs and tournaments exist including national and international events such as the North American Indigenous Games. These tournaments provide opportunities and encouragement for youth and adults to participate in sporting activities at a high level, within, supported and coached by individuals of the local or regional Native American community. Conversely, these opportunities are available for more elite or higher-skilled individuals, while excluding those who are outside the target age ranges or not as skilled. Additional community-level programming open to members of all ages and skill levels is needed to encourage activity across all members of the community.

Community factors

A lack of physical infrastructure for structured physical activity presents a barrier to active lifestyles among this population. Many communities or neighborhoods have limited infrastructure for exercise and sports. Some communities lack even school gymnasiums or community halls. Within Native American communities, barriers to physical activity include challenges of safety. While urban and rural communities may present different types of threats, individual safety while exercising outdoors can be challenging in either setting, ranging from challenges of wild animals, violence and lack of lighting to sidewalks and roadways in need of repair. Conversely, some communities report aesthetically pleasing environments as facilitators to physical activity. Facilitators to physical activity include programs conducted within communities by community members. Providing opportunities to be physically active within Native American communities enhances participation and programs conducted in groups increase feelings of safety. Many evening and weekend programs in Native American communities are conducted in school gymnasiums or community halls, providing a community-based location familiar to most community members where physical activity opportunities can be provided. The companionship gained from participating in group activities and sports further facilitates physical activity among this population. Traditional cultural activities, such as pow wows, fishing, hunting and trapping present important facilitators for physical activity. Culturally based activities facilitate physical activity within the wholistic realms and beliefs common to many Native American communities.

Policy factors

Due to a combination of historical and political factors, Native American children are vastly overrepresented in foster care. Despite policies and legislations aiming to keep Native American children within their own culture, historically high numbers of Native American children continue to be apprehended, commonly for (perceived) neglect. This removal of children from their familial homes, and placement in often temporary homes presents a significant barrier to participation in sports activities for children and youth. Placement of children within their familial home with support and education for primary caregivers, or placement of children in homes within their community can facilitate continuation of participation in sports and activities within home communities.

Policies and resources for schools and school infrastructure in Native American communities often differs from that of local state or provincial funding and policies.

These differences often present barriers to building and maintaining infrastructure such as school and community gymnasiums. Such differences can present barriers to physical activity when isolated communities do not have gymnasiums or community halls, particularly among winter months when weather can limit outdoor activities. While governments may offer income tax deductions for physical activity expenses, the lower income of many Native American families precludes the ability to invest in organized or pay-per-use physical activity opportunities.

Unique influences among specific Native American groups

Some barriers and facilitators to physical activity are experienced more readily by specific groups of Native Americans. Enhancing physical activity among Native Americans may require consideration of specific needs and challenges unique to the specific group (Abonyi 2001, Coble and Rhodes 2006, Findlay and Kohen 2007, Kirby et al. 2007, Garner et al. 2010, Mason and Koehli 2012, Jahns et al. 2014).

Youth

Native American children who participate in sports are more likely to come from more affluent families, have parents with a higher degree of education, live in two-parent households and have fewer siblings. These parents may be better able to transport, observe and encourage their children in sports due to increased financial security and time available. Physical activity promotion should address the family and community as a whole, encouraging and promoting physical activity among all sectors of the community. Native Americans who know others who are physically active or have active neighbors are more likely to be physically active themselves, further highlighting the community involvement in promoting physical activity.

Living on reservation

Youth on-reserve report lower levels of sports participation than those residing off-reserve. For many Native American youth, participation in sporting activities is limited by the travel distances; sport activities are often conducted in neighboring towns, or bus transportation home from school is not available following after-school sports. Reservations provide additional barriers to physical activity including risking attacks from wild dogs or other wild animals.

Rural and remote communities

Native American peoples are more likely to reside in rural and remote communities. Rural communities limit the availability of structured physical activity opportunities due to a lack of facilities and infrastructure. One challenge of physical activity in rural and remote areas is the transient nature of many physical activity instructors. When Western methods of physical activity, such as aerobics, are introduced to Native American communities, individuals from outside the community often deliver the programs. Sustainability of these programs is lost when these individuals move on and leave the community. Many Native American peoples also reside in northern locations where weather may limit the ability to participate in outdoor physical activities during some months of the year. Participation in sports among Native American youth appears not to vary by urban/rural or northern location.

Socioeconomic status

The lower socioeconomic status of many Native Americans limits the ability to participate in physical activities requiring membership, registration or drop-in fees, such as access to gyms, purchase of sporting equipment or rental of equipment or facilities. Native American adults of lower socioeconomic status may be limited in their ability to participate in traditional physical activities such as hunting or fishing due to a lack of funds. Costs for fuel and other equipment to go hunting or fishing may cost more than purchasing the meat frozen. These losses of traditional activities are even greater among females, where traditional activities such as berry picking and gathering may no longer be available.

Intervention strategies

Many physical activity interventions have been pursued among this population. Most interventions use a multimodal approach including promotion of physical activity and other health behaviors. Many interventions also include a cross-generational model where children and adults are involved in the program, hitting on deep structure strategies for cultural tailoring.

Approaches for promoting physical activity

Physical activity programs among this population are most successful when undertaken at a community level (Heath *et al.* 1991, Narayan *et al.* 1998, First Nations Centre 2007, Kirby *et al.* 2007, Foulds *et al.* 2011a, Bersamin *et al.* 2014). Deep structure strategies involving the community in development, design and implementation of a program reflect cultural process and respect the autonomy and authority of local Native American communities. Community-level interventions considering local patterns of stress and enculturation are most likely to be effective in improving physical activity patterns.

Those promoting physical activity for Native American populations should consider three strategies: incorporate traditional activities to reconnect to land and culture (deep structure strategies), decrease financial barriers to physical activity and utilize opportunities appealing to both men and women. Peripheral and linguistic strategies including promotion of traditional activities, use of traditional language or words and images of active Native American people can enhance this promotion in a good way. Physical activity is often conducted as part of healthy lifestyle promotion including healthy eating and smoking cessation. Many successful strategies include local leaders or champions (constituent-involving strategies), with community members in leadership roles and demonstrating positive lifestyles. These champions conduct education and physical activity sessions among their peers and/or community members.

School-based approaches

All interventions to date among Native American children and youth have been conducted in the school setting. School-based physical activity interventions have been implemented in several communities, including the Kahnawake Schools Diabetes Prevention Project, Kitigan Zibi school program and Zhiiwapenewin Akino'maagewin: Teaching to Prevent Diabetes in Canada and the Cherokee Choices, Pathways and Zuni high school diabetes prevention program interventions in the United States (Scott and Myers 1988, Macaulay *et al.* 1997, Cook and Hurley 1998, Caballero *et al.* 2003, Ritenbaugh *et al.* 2003, Bachar *et al.* 2006, Ho *et al.* 2008). Among adults, physical activity interventions have included individual, group fitness and community-level programs primarily including aerobic activities. Most interventions include durations or follow-ups of only a few months; however, school-based interventions have evaluated physical activity and other health behaviors and risk factors over several years.

School-based interventions have included a multimodal approach: increased school time physical activity and educational components around healthy eating and lifestyle habits aimed at both children in classrooms and parents and other adults in the community. Successful school-based programs included deep structure strategies involving the community in designing the project and in some cases including traditional games and sports. These community-designed wholistic programs brought together physical activity with healthy eating and other health behaviors. These successful community-based programs incorporated the whole cross-generational community in education and physical activity promotion activities. Surface-level strategies including linguistic strategies (e.g. names of programs), constituent-involving strategies (e.g. community leaders or mentors) and peripheral strategies (e.g. traditional foods, locally developed promotional materials) have also been incorporated. The Pathways intervention used the Sports, Play and Active Recreation for Kids program with the American Indian Games module to increase physical activity among intervention schools. The Zuni high school diabetes prevention program included educational components to improve health behaviors and provided a drop-in fitness center for youth and partnered on activities such as aerobics, basketball, hiking, rock climbing, running, mountain biking and dances. The Kahnawake Schools Diabetes Prevention Program included community collaborations such as walking clubs, line-dancing clubs, figure skating and development of walking and cycling infrastructure. Cherokee Choices included several components of health promotion and education, including promotion of physical activity within the school setting. Challenges of these programs have included limited long-term success. Successful school-based interventions may require greater increases in physical activity components, greater involvement of families and communities and longer-term interventions to make sustainable life-long changes in physical activity behaviors. Despite a lack of changes in obesity with school-based physical activity interventions, improvements in health behaviors and physiology may be experienced.

Community-based approaches

Physical activity interventions among Native American adults have utilized a variety of approaches including structured physical activity training programs, community-based exercise training sessions, drop-in unstructured physical activity and online or pedometer monitoring of physical activity (Reitman *et al.* 1984, Heath *et al.* 1991, Narayan *et al.* 1998, Dyck *et al.* 1999, Heffernan *et al.* 1999, Kochevar *et al.* 2001, Wing *et al.* 2004, Foulds *et al.* 2011a). Adult interventions successful in improving health have included community-based group exercise sessions culturally tailored for Native American populations. These interventions incorporate deep structure strategies of wholistic approaches combining healthy eating and smoking cessation education with physical activity, are designed and promoted by local communities and may include traditional physical activities, sports and games. These programs often utilized group training sessions led by community leaders or volunteers trained in delivering the program; these are constituent-involving strategies that help with tailoring the program to the population. Interventions to date have largely focused on aerobic exercise, through walking, running, aerobics classes and access to gym facilities. Most of these programs offered group physical activity sessions or access to facilities where multiple individuals could be training together, further tailoring these programs by including multigeneration activities to welcome all members of the community.

Health-focused strategies

Over the short term, health benefits of physical activity programs among this population have included improved lipoprotein cholesterol levels, blood pressure, body weight and waist circumference, and physical strength and fitness (Heath *et al.* 1991, Kochevar *et al.* 2001, Ritenbaugh *et al.* 2003, Wing *et al.* 2004, Foulds *et al.* 2011a). Reductions in body weight and waist circumference, along with improvements in blood glucose, cholesterol and insulin levels, may contribute to reduced risks of diabetes and heart disease when engaging in a regular physical activity program. The medicine wheel, a common model to health approach among many Native American populations, highlights the interconnected nature of the four realms, where physical activity, sport and recreation can be healing tools for mental, emotional and spiritual well-being (Lavallee and Levesque 2013). Native American cultures often reflect a wholistic approach to health, believing the realms of physical, mental, spiritual and emotional health are interconnected. The interconnectedness of this model allows for physical realm activities such as physical activity to bring balance with mental, emotional and spiritual realms.

Among children and youth some beneficial changes in health-related knowledge and fat intake were observed after several years of follow-up, though long-term physiological changes are less consistently observed (Caballero *et al.* 2003, Ritenbaugh *et al.* 2003, Paradis *et al.* 2005, Ho *et al.* 2008). After 3 years of a youth fitness center and activities, diabetes risk factors including insulin levels are more similar to non–Native American youth, highlighting a benefit of physical activity promotion and availability among this population. However, after as many as 8 years, many school-based interventions do not observe differences in body size or obesity. Native American youth experience positive self-esteem and decreased smoking when participating in sports (Findlay and Kohen 2007).

Of the interventions to date, the most successful for improving physical activity and health risk factors and maintaining participation are culturally tailored community or group-based interventions. These programs are developed in conjunction with local community members and community members are involved in the distribution and delivery of programs. Physical activity can lead to improvements in both physical and mental health.

BOX 7.1   EVIDENCE-BASED PRACTICE: ABORIGINAL RUNWALK PROGRAM

Susan Nguyen, Manager, SportMed Aboriginal RunWalk

Improving health and healthy living among Native American populations requires a wholistic approach incorporating physical activity and exercise with healthy behaviors in a cross-generational community-based approach. The Aboriginal RunWalk Program is an ongoing province-wide community-based exercise training program which improves health and fitness of Native American communities. This program, which began in 2007, reduces risks of heart disease and diabetes while improving obesity, cholesterol levels and blood pressure through community engagement and a culturally tailored program.

In partnership with the Aboriginal Sport, Recreation and Physical Activity Partners Council (ASRPAPC), SportMedBC coordinates annual 13- to 21-week outdoor walk-and-run programs within Native American communities around the province of British Columbia. These programs are intended to support Native American participants of all ages and levels of fitness in training for and completing 5- or 10-km walk or run events. Community leaders plan, conduct and oversee exercise training programs within their communities designed to meet the unique needs of each community. Leader Training Sessions offered by ASRPAPC in partnership with SportMedBC provide community leaders with training and education including wholistic topics across nutrition, physical literacy, sport injury, mental health and a variety of exercise modes. Each community conducts its own training program, determining the length of program, timing of the year, program intensities and run/walk distances appropriate to its specific participants. This program also promotes healthy living, healthy eating, including a Native American–specific food guide and recipes, and reduced tobacco misuse to all participants. Community leaders are provided with weekly training, coaching and educational support in motivating and inspiring their participants. Within each community, cultural events including a 5- to 10-km walk/run event are coordinated to celebrate the achievements of this program.

Implications for practice

When conducting physical activity training, or physical education classes among this population, attempts should be made to ground programs in traditional culture. Inclusion of traditional activities, sports or games can encourage cultural significance and enhance participation. The use of activities on the land can also engage connection to the land within the physical activity experience.

Making low-cost programs available using community centers or existing infrastructure that minimizes costs to parents reduces barriers for low-income families (Findlay and Kohen 2007). Partnerships with community schools to use gymnasiums could be one such possibility (Findlay and Kohen 2007). Encouragement and engagement of Native American coaches can also improve connections and participation of Native American youth in sports (Findlay and Kohen 2007). Cultural training among non–Native American coaches, such as the Aboriginal Coaching Modules offered by the Coaching Association of Canada, can provide additional understanding and cultural awareness to better facilitate and encourage participation of Native American youth in sports (Coaching Association of Canada 2016).

Summary points

- Native American traditional culture includes activities requiring physical fitness and strength.
- Increased physical activity among Native American populations is associated with greater involvement in culture and traditional activities.
- Regular physical activity can improve physiological measures among Native American adults.
- Physical activity can contribute to improved mental health and resilience among Native Americans.
- Financial and environmental barriers can limit participation of Native Americans in physical activities.
- Community involvement in development and delivery of physical activity promotion and training programs increases success and reach of the program.

Critical thinking questions

1   What sports or recreational activities could be engaged in on the land among rural Native American communities: in the winter? In the summer? In northern communities? In southern desert communities?

2   How can a recreational program involve all members of a community? How can you incorporate young children, elders who may have mobility issues and individuals who may have limited or no experience with sports and recreation?

3   When designing a physical activity program to be offered in a Native American community, what components could be similar between various nations, such as the Pima in Arizona and the Tlingit in Alaska and the Yukon? What would be different?

References

Abonyi, S. (2001). 'Sickness and symptom: Perspectives of diabetes among the Mushkegowuk Cree.' Ph.D., Hamilton, Ontario, Canada: McMaster University.

Aboriginal Sport Circle. (2016). 'Aboriginal Sport Circle [Online].' Akwasasne, ON. Available: www.aboriginalsportcircle.ca/main/about.html (Accessed May 25 2016).

Adams, A. and Prince, R. (2010). 'Correlates of physical activity in young American Indian children: Lessons learned from the Wisconsin Nutrition and Growth Study.' *Journal of Public Health Management & Practice*, 16: 394–400.

Bachar, J. J., Lefler, L. J., Reed, L., McCoy, T., Bailey, R. and Bell, R. (2006). 'Cherokee Choices: A diabetes prevention program for American Indians.' *Preventing Chronic Disease*, 3: A103.

Barnes, P. M., Adams, P. F. and Powell-Griner, E. (2010). *Health Characteristics of the American Indian or Alaska Native Adult Population: United States, 2004–2008*. Hyattsville, MD: National Center for Health Statistics.

Barton, S. S., Thommasen, H. V., Tallio, B., Zhang, W. and Michalos, A. C. (2005). 'Health and quality of life of Aboriginal residential school survivors, Bella Coola Valley, 2001.' *Social Indicators Research*, 73: 295–312.

Beenackers, M. A., Kamphuis, C. B., Giskes, K., Brug, J., Kunst, A. E., Burdorf, A. and Van Lenthe, F. J. (2012). 'Socioeconomic inequalities in occupational, leisure-time, and transport related physical activity among European adults: A systematic review.' *International Journal of Behavioral Nutrition and Physical Activity*, 9: 116.

Bersamin, A., Wolsko, C., Luick, B. R., Boyer, B. B., Lardon, C., Hopkins, S. E., Stern, J. S. and Zidenberg-Cherr, S. (2014). 'Enculturation, perceived stress, and physical activity: Implications for metabolic risk among the Yup'ik – the center for Alaska native health research study.' *Ethnicity & Health*, 19: 255–69.

Braveheart, M. Y. H. (1998). 'The return to the sacred path: Healing the historical traum and historical unresolved grief response among the Lakota through a psychoeducation group intervention.' *Smith College Studies in Social Work*, 68: 287–305.

British Columbia Provincial Health Officer. (2009). *Pathways to Health and Healing: 2nd Report on the Health and Well-Being of Aboriginal People in British Columbia. Provincial Health Officer's Annual Report 2007*. Office of the Provincal Health Officer. Victoria, BC: British Columbia Ministry of Healthy Living and Sport.

Brownson, R. C., Eyler, A. A., King, A. C., Brown, D. R., Shyu, Y. L. and Sallis, J. F. (2000). 'Patterns and correlates of physical activity among US women 40 years and older.' *American Journal of Public Health*, 90: 264–70.

Bruce, S. G., Riediger, N. D. and Lix, L. M. (2014). 'Chronic disease and chronic disease risk factors among First Nations, Inuit and Metis populations of northern Canada.' *Chronic Disease and Injuries in Canada*, 34: 210–7.

Bruner, B. and Chad, K. (2013). 'Physical activity attitudes, beliefs, and practices among women in a Woodland Cree community.' *Journal of Physical Activity and Health*, 10: 1119–27.

Caballero, B., Clay, T., Davis, S. M., Ethelbah, B., Rock, B. H., Lohman, T., Norman, J., Story, M., Stone, E. J., Stephenson, L. and Stevens, J. (2003). 'Pathways: A school-based, randomized controlled trial for the prevention of obesity in American Indian schoolchildren.' *American Journal of Clinical Nutrition*, 78: 1030–8.

Coaching Association of Canada. (2016). 'Aboriginal Coaching Modules [Online].' Ottawa, ON: Coaching Association of Canada. Available: www.coach.ca/aboriginal-coaching-modules-p158240 (Accessed May 26 2016).

Coates, J. (2016). 'The Wiley-Blackwell Encyclopedia of Race, Ethnicity and Nationalism.' *In*: Stone, J., Rutledge, D. M., Smith, A. D., Rizova, P. S. and Hou, X. (eds.) *Encyclopedia of Race, Ethnicity and Nationalism*. Chicester, United Kingdom: Wiley-Blackwell.

Coble, J. D. and Rhodes, R. E. (2006). 'Physical activity and Native Americans: A review.' *American Journal of Preventive Medicine*, 31: 36–46.

Coble, J. D., Rhodes, R. E. and Higgins, J. W. (2009). 'Physical activity behaviors and motivations in an adult First Nation population: A pilot study.' *Ethnicity & Disease*, 19: 42–8.

Cook, V. V. and Hurley, J. S. (1998). 'Prevention of type 2 diabetes in childhood.' *Clinical Pediatrics*, 37: 123–9.

Craib, K. J., Spittal, P. M., Patel, S. H., Christian, W. M., Moniruzzaman, A., Pearce, M. E., Demerais, L., Sherlock, C. and Schechter, M. T. (2009). 'Prevalence and incidence of hepatitis C virus infection among Aboriginal young people who use drugs: Results from the Cedar Project.' *Open Medicine*, 3: e220–7.

Dapice, A. N. (2006). 'The medicine wheel.' *Journal of Transcultural Nursing*, 17: 251–60.

Dickason, O. P. (1992). *Canada's First Nations: A History of Founding Peoples from Earliest Times*. Toronto, ON: University of Oklahoma Press.

Dogra, S., Meisner, B. A. and Ardern, C. I. (2010). 'Variation in mode of physical activity by ethnicity and time since immigration: A cross-sectional analysis.' *International Journal of Behavioral Nutrition and Physical Activity*, 7: 75.

Dulik, M. C., Owings, A. C., Gaieski, J. B., Vilar, M. G., Andre, A., Lennie, C., Mackenzie, M. A., Kritsch, I., Snowshoe, S., Wright, R., Martin, J., Gibson, N., Andrews, T. D. and Schurr, T. G. (2012). 'Y-chromosome analysis reveals genetic divergence and new founding native lineages in Athapaskan- and Eskimoan-speaking populations.' *Proceedings of the National Academy of Sciences U S A*, 109: 8471–6.

Duncan, G. E., Goldberg, J., Buchwald, D., Wen, Y. and Henderson, J. A. (2009). 'Epidemiology of physical activity in American Indians in the education and research towards health cohort.' *American Journal of Preventive Medicine*, 37: 488–94.

Duran, E. and Duran, B. (1995). *Native American Postcolonial Psychology*. New York, NY: State University of New York Press.

Dyck, R. F., Sheppard, M. S., Klomp, H., Tan, L. and Chad, K. (1999). 'Using exercise to prevent gestational diabetes among Aboriginal women: Hypothesis and results of a pilot/feasibility project in Saskatchewan.' *Canadian Journal of Diabetes Care*, 23: 32–38.

Ferucci, E. D., Schumacher, M. C., Lanier, A. P., Murtaugh, M. A., Edwards, S., Helzer, L. J., Tom-Orme, L. and Slattery, M. L. (2008). 'Arthritis prevalence and associations in American Indian and Alaska Native people.' *Arthritis and Rheumatism*, 59: 1128–36.

Findlay, L. C. (2011). *Physical Activity among First Nations People off Reserve, Métis and Inuit*. Ottawa, Ontario: Statistics Canada.

Findlay, L. C. and Kohen, D. E. (2007). 'Aboriginal children's sport participation in Canada.' *Pimatisiwin: A Journal of Aboriginal and Indigenous Community Health*, 5: 185–206.

First Nations Centre. (2007). 'OCAP: Ownership, control, access and possession.' First National Information Governance Committee. National Aboriginal Health Organization. Ottawa: Assembly of First Nations.

First Nations Information Governance Centre. (2012). 'First Nations regional health survey 2008/10: National report on adults, youth and children living in First Nations communities.' First Nations Information Governance Centre. Ottawa: First Nations Information Governance Centre.

Fisher, D. M. (2002). *Lacrosse: A History of the Game*. Baltimore, MD: John Hopkins University Press.

Forsyth, J. (2012). 'Bodies of meaning: Sports and games at Canadian residential schools.' *In*: Forsyth, J. and Giles, A. R. (eds.) *Aboriginal Peoples and Sport in Canada: Historical Foundations and Contemporary Issues*. Vancouver, BC: UBC Press.

Foulds, H. J., Bredin, S. S. and Warburton, D. E. (2011a). 'The effectiveness of community based physical activity interventions with Aboriginal peoples.' *Preventive Medicine*, 53: 411–6.

Foulds, H. J., Bredin, S. S. and Warburton, D. E. (2011b). 'The prevalence of overweight and obesity in British Columbian Aboriginal adults.' *Obesity Reviews*, 12: e4–e11.

Foulds, H. J., Bredin, S. S. and Warburton, D. E. (2016a). 'The vascular health status of a population of adult Canadian indigenous peoples from British Columbia.' *Journal of Human Hypertension*, 30: 278–84.

Foulds, H. J., Rodgers, C. D., Duncan, V. and Ferguson, L. J. (2016b). 'A systematic review and meta-analysis of screen time behaviour among North American indigenous populations.' *Obesity Reviews*, 17: 455–66.

Foulds, H. J., Shubair, M. M. and Warburton, D. E. (2013a). 'A review of the cardiometabolic risk experience among Canadian Metis populations.' *Canadian Journal of Cardiology*, 29: 1006–13.

Foulds, H. J., Warburton, D. E. and Bredin, S. S. (2013b). 'A systematic review of physical activity levels in Native American populations in Canada and the United States in the last 50 years.' *Obesity Reviews*, 14: 593–603.

Fredericks, J. I. (1999). 'America's first Nations: The origins, history and future of American Indian sovereignty.' *Journal of Law and Policy*, 7: 347–410.

Frieden, T. R. and Centers for Disease Control and Prevention. (2011). 'Forward: CDC Health Disparities and Inequalities Report: United States, 2011.' *MMWR Surveillance Summary*, 60(Suppl.): 1–2.

Garner, R., Carriere, G. and Sanmartin, C. (2010). 'The health of Inuit, Metis and First Nations adults living off-reserve in Canada: The impact of socio-economic status on inequalities in health.' Health Research Working Paper Series. Ottawa: Statistics Canada.

Greenwood, M. L. and De Leeuw, S. N. (2012). 'Social determinants of health and the future well-being of Aboriginal children in Canada.' *Paediatric and Child Health*, 17: 381–4.

Hackett, C., Feeny, D. and Tompa, E. (2016). 'Canada's residential school system: Measuring the intergenerational impact of familial attendance on health and mental health outcomes.' *Journal of Epidemiology and Community Health*, 70: 1096–1105.

Heath, G. W., Wilson, R. H., Smith, J. and Leonard, B. E. (1991). 'Community-based exercise and weight control: Diabetes risk reduction and glycemic control in Zuni Indians.' *American Journal of Clinical Nutrition*, 53: 1642S–6S.

Heffernan, C., Herbert, C., Grams, G. D., Grzybowski, S., Wilson, M. A., Calam, B. and Brown, D. (1999). 'The Haida Gwaii Diabetes Project: Planned response activity outcomes.' *Health and Social Care in the Community*, 7: 379–86.

Ho, L. S., Gittelsohn, J., Rimal, R., Treuth, M. S., Sharma, S., Rosecrans, A. and Harris, S. B. (2008). 'An integrated multi-institutional diabetes prevention program improves knowledge and healthy food acquisition in northwestern Ontario First Nations.' *Health Education & Behavior*, 35: 561–73.

Holm, J. E., Vogeltanz-Holm, N., Poltavski, D. and Mcdonald, L. (2010). 'Assessing health status, behavioral risks, and health disparities in American Indians living on the northern plains of the U.S.' *Public Health Reports*, 125: 68–78.

Jahns, L., Mcdonald, L. R., Wadsworth, A., Morin, C. and Liu, Y. (2014). 'Barriers and facilitators to being physically active on a rural U.S. Northern Plains American Indian reservation.' *International Journal of Environmental Research in Public Health*, 11: 12053–63.

Janz, T., Seto, J. and Turner, A. (2009). 'Aboriginal peoples survey, 2006: An overview of the health of the Métis population.' Social and Aboriginal Statistics Division. Ottawa: Statistics Canada.

Jernigan, V. B., Garroutte, E., Krantz, E. M. and Buchwald, D. (2013). 'Food insecurity and obesity among American Indians and Alaska Natives and Whites in California.' *Journal of Hunger and Environmental Nutrition*, 8: 458–71.

Jollie-Trottier, T., Holm, J. E. and Mcdonald, J. D. (2009). 'Correlates of overweight and obesity in American Indian children.' *Journal of Pediatric Psychology*, 34: 245–53.

Kelley, A., Giroux, J., Schulz, M., Aronson, B., Wallace, D., Bell, R. and Morrison, S. (2015). 'American-Indian diabetes mortality in the Great Plains Region 2002–2010.' *BMJ Open Diabetes Research and Care*, 3: e000070.

Kelly-Scott, K. and Smith, K. (2015). 'Aboriginal peoples: Fact sheet for Canada.' *In*: Statistics Canada (ed.). Ottawa, ON: Minister of Industry.

Kirby, A. M., Levesque, L. and Wabano, V. (2007). 'A qualitative investigation of physical activity challenges and opportunities in a Northern-Rural Aboriginal community: Voices from within.' *Pimatisiwin: A Journal of Aboriginal and Indigenous Community Health*, 5: 5–24.

Kirmayer, L. J., Brass, G. M., Holton, T., Paul, K., Simpson, C. and Tait, C. (2007). 'Suicide among Aboriginal people in Canada.' *In*: The Aborginal Health Foundation (ed.). Ottawa, ON, Canada: Aboriginal Healing Foundation.

Kochevar, A. J., Smith, K. L. and Bernard, M. A. (2001). 'Effects of a community-based intervention to increase activity in American Indian elders.' *Journal of the Oklahoma State Medical Association*, 94: 455–60.

Kracht, B. R. (1994). 'Kiowa Powwows: Continuity in ritual practice.' *American Indian Quarterly*, 18: 321–48.

Krieger, N. (2014). 'Discrimination and health inequalities.' *International Journal of Health Services*, 44: 643–710.

Kriska, A. M., Edelstein, S. L., Hamman, R. F., Otto, A., Bray, G. A., Mayer-Davis, E. J., Wing, R. R., Horton, E. S., Haffner, S. M. and Regensteiner, J. G. (2006). 'Physical activity in individuals at risk for diabetes: Diabetes prevention program.' *Medicine and Science in Sports and Exercise*, 38: 826–32.

Lavallee, L. and Levesque, L. (2013). 'Two-eyed seeing: Physical activity, sport, and recreation promotion in indigenous communities.' *In*: Forsyth, J. and Giles, A. R. (eds.) *Aboriginal Peoples and Sport in Canada: Historical Foundations and Contemporary Issues*. Vancouver, BC: UBC Press.

Macaulay, A. C., Paradis, G., Potvin, L., Cross, E. J., Saad-Haddad, C., McComber, A., Desrosiers, S., Kirby, R., Montour, L. T., Lamping, D. L., Leduc, N. and Rivard, M. (1997). 'The Kahnawake Schools Diabetes Prevention Project: Intervention, evaluation, and baseline results of a diabetes primary prevention program with a native community in Canada.' *Preventive Medicine*, 26: 779–90.

Mason, C. and Koehli, J. (2012). 'Barriers to physical activity for Aboriginal youth: Implications for community health, policy, and culture.' *Pimatisiwin: A Journal of Aboriginal and Indigenous Community Health*, 10: 97–108.

Mathias, C. J. and Yabsley, G. R. (1991). 'Conspiracy of legislation: The suppression of Indian rights in Canada.' *BC Studies*, 89: 34–47.

Miller, J. R. (1996). *Shingwauk's Vision: A History of Native Residential Schools.* Toronto, ON: University of Toronto Press.

Milloy, J. S. (1999). *A National Crime: The Canadian Government and the Residential School System, 1879–1986.* Winnipeg: University of Manitoba Press.

Mitchell, T. L. and Maracle, D. T. (2005). 'Healing the generations: Post-traumatic stress and the health status of Aboriginal populations in Canada.' *Journal of Aboriginal Health*, 2: 14–25.

Muckle, R. J. (2007). *The First Nations of British Columbia.* Vancouver, BC: UBC Press.

Narayan, K. M., Hoskin, M., Kozak, D., Kriska, A. M., Hanson, R. L., Pettitt, D. J., Nagi, D. K., Bennett, P. H. and Knowler, W. C. (1998). 'Randomized clinical trial of lifestyle interventions in Pima Indians: A pilot study.' *Diabetic Medication*, 15: 66–72.

Norris, T., Vines, P. L. and Hoeffel, E. M. (2012). 'The American Indian and Alaska Native Population: 2010.' Suitland, Maryland, USA: U.S. Department of Commerce, U.S. Census Bureau.

Oster, R. T. and Toth, E. L. (2009). 'Differences in the prevalence of diabetes risk-factors among First Nation, Metis and non-Aboriginal adults attending screening clinics in rural Alberta, Canada.' *Rural and Remote Health*, 9: 1170.

Paradis, G., Levesque, L., Macaulay, A. C., Cargo, M., McComber, A., Kirby, R., Receveur, O., Kishchuk, N. and Potvin, L. (2005). 'Impact of a diabetes prevention program on body size, physical activity, and diet among Kanien'keha:ka (Mohawk) children 6 to 11 years old: 8-year results from the Kahnawake Schools Diabetes Prevention Project.' *Pediatrics*, 115: 333–9.

Peschken, C. A. and Esdaile, J. M. (1999). 'Rheumatic diseases in North America's indigenous peoples.' *Seminars in Arthritis and Rheumatism*, 28: 368–91.

Public Health Agency of Canada. (2011). 'Diabetes in Canada: Facts and figures from a public health perspective.' Chronic Disease Surveillance and Monitoring Division. Ottawa: Public Health Agency of Canada.

Reading, C. L. and Wien, F. (2009). *Health Inequalities and Social Determinants of Aboriginal Peoples' Health.* Prince George, BC, Canada: National Collaborating Centre for Aboriginal Health.

Redwood, D., Schumacher, M. C., Lanier, A. P., Ferucci, E. D., Asay, E., Helzer, L. J., Tom-Orme, L., Edwards, S. L., Murtaugh, M. A. and Slattery, M. L. (2009). 'Physical activity patterns of American Indian and Alaskan Native people living in Alaska and the Southwestern United States.' *American Journal of Health Promotion*, 23: 388–95.

Reitman, J. S., Vasquez, B., Klimes, I. and Nagulesparan, M. (1984). 'Improvement of glucose homeostasis after exercise training in non-insulin-dependent diabetes.' *Diabetes Care*, 7: 434–41.

Ritenbaugh, C., Teufel-Shone, N. I., Aickin, M. G., Joe, J. R., Poirier, S., Dillingham, D. C., Johnson, D., Henning, S., Cole, S. M. and Cockerham, D. (2003). 'A lifestyle intervention improves plasma insulin levels among Native American high school youth.' *Preventive Medicine*, 36: 309–19.

Rode, A. and Shephard, R. J. (1994). 'Physiological consequences of acculturation: A 20-year study of fitness in an Inuit community.' *European Journal of Applied Physiology and Occupational Physiology*, 69: 516–24.

Rotenberg, C. (2016). 'Social determinants of health for the off-reserve First Nations population, 15 years of age and older, 2012.' *In:* Statistics Canada (ed.). Ottawa, ON: Minister of Industry.

Ruthig, J. C. and Allery, A. (2008). 'Native American elders' health congruence: The role of gender and corresponding functional well-being, hospital admissions, and social engagement.' *Journal of Health Psychology*, 13: 1072–81.

Schurr, T. G. (2004). 'The peopling of the new world.' *Annual Reviews in Anthropology*, 33: 551–83.

Scott, K. A. and Myers, A. M. (1988). 'Impact of fitness training on native adolescents' self-evaluations and substance use.' *Canadian Journal of Public Health*, 79: 424–9.

Statistics Canada. (2013). 'Aboriginal peoples in Canada: First Nations people, Métis and Inuit.' Statistics Canada. Ottawa, ON: Statistics Canada.

Steckel, R. H., Rose, J. C., Larsen, C. S. and Walker, P. L. (2002). 'Skeletal health in the Western Hemisphere from 4000 BC to the present.' *Evolutionary Anthropology*, 11: 142–55.

Story, M., Evans, M., Fabsitz, R. R., Clay, T. E., Holy Rock, B. and Broussard, B. (1999). 'The epidemic of obesity in American Indian communities and the need for childhood obesity-prevention programs.' *American Journal of Clinical Nutrition*, 69: 747S–54S.

Tjepkema, M., Wilkins, R., Senecal, S., Guimond, E. and Penney, C. (2009). 'Mortality of Metis and registered Indian adults in Canada: An 11-year follow-up study.' *Health Reports*, 20: 31–51.

Waldrum, J. B., Herring, D. A. and Young, T. K. (2006). *Aboriginal Health in Canada: Historical, Cultural, and Epidimiological Perspectives.* Toronto, Ontario: University of Toronto Press Incorporated.

Whitbeck, L. B., Adams, G. W., Hoyt, D. R. and Chen, X. (2004). 'Conceptualizing and measuring historical trauma among American Indian people.' *American Journal of Community Psychology*, 33: 119–30.

Wilson, D. and Macdonald, D. (2010). 'The income gap between Aboriginal peoples and the rest of Canada.' Ottawa, Ontario, Canada: Canadian Centre for Policy Alternatives.

Wing, R. R., Hamman, R. F., Bray, G. A., Delahanty, L., Edelstein, S. L., Hill, J. O., Horton, E. S., Hoskin, M. A., Kriska, A., Lachin, J., Mayer-Davis, E. J., Pi-Sunyer, X., Regensteiner, J. G., Venditti, B. and Wylie-Rosett, J. (2004). 'Achieving weight and activity goals among diabetes prevention program lifestyle participants.' *Obesity Research*, 12: 1426–34.

Withrow, D. R., Amartey, A. and Marrett, L. D. (2014). 'Cancer risk factors and screening in the off-reserve First Nations, Metis and non-Aboriginal populations of Ontario.' *Chronic Diseases and Injuries in Canada*, 34: 103–12.

Young, T. K. and Katzmarzyk, P. T. (2007). 'Physical activity of Aboriginal people in Canada.' *Canadian Journal of Public Health*, 98(Suppl 2): S148–60.

8

PHYSICAL ACTIVITY AMONG NATIVE HAWAIIANS AND PACIFIC ISLANDERS

*Cheryl L. Albright, Marjorie M. Mau,
Lehua B. Choy and Tricia Mabellos*

Understanding the Native Hawaiian and Pacific Islander population

Native Hawaiians, the indigenous people of the State of Hawai'i are culturally, ancestrally and linguistically linked with other indigenous populations throughout the Pacific region such as Samoans, Tahitians, Cook Islanders, Micronesians, Melanesians and New Zealand Maoris (Kim *et al.* 2012). Figure 8.1 shows their geographic locations across the South Pacific. Since 1998, the U.S. Office of Management and Budget (OMB) has categorized Native Hawaiians and other Pacific Islanders (NHPIs) as a separate racial group that defines this group as the *"original peoples of Hawai'i (Native Hawaiians), Guam (Chamorros), Samoa (Samoans), or other Pacific Islands"* (Hixson *et al.* 2012). For purposes of this chapter, NHPIs will refer to the OMB 1998 definition of this racial category.

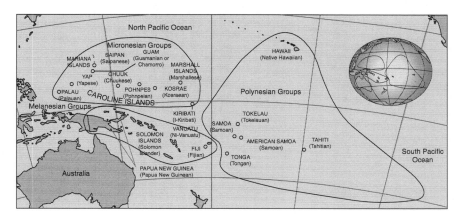

FIGURE 8.1 Geographic regions in the South Pacific for Native Hawaiians and Pacific Islanders
Source: Adapted from Hixson *et al.* (2012).

Demographic characteristics

The NHPI population in the U.S. is one of the fastest-growing racial groups with a 35% increase resulting in 1.22 million NHPIs counted in the 2010 U.S. Census (Hixson *et al.* 2012). NHPIs in the U.S. are also one of the most racially diverse groups with 56% of its members ethnically identifying with more than one race and/or NHPI sub-group (Hixson *et al.* 2012). New survey methods and data analyses first used in the Census 2010 provided detailed information on people who reported more than one race/ethnicity, and thus, the health information and social characteristics of NHPI could be described in more detail and with increased accuracy. Thus, when feasible, this chapter will report as much racial/ethnic detail available on each NHPI subgroup as possible (i.e. NHPI subgroups of Tongans, Marshallese, Fijians as well as the numerically larger groups of Native Hawaiians, Samoans and Chamorros).

According to the Census 2010, the Native Hawaiian population comprises the largest proportion of NHPIs at 527,077 (45%) followed by Samoans 184,440 (16%) and Chamorro 147,798 (13%) (Hixson *et al.* 2012). Nearly 20% of all NHPIs self-identified as "Other Pacific Islander" while Tongan, Marshallese, Fijiian and Other Micronesian groups each comprise 5% or less of the overall total. Within the 50 states, over half of all NHPIs (52%) live in just two states, Hawai'i (*n* = 356,000) and California (*n* = 286,000). Significant number of NHPIs also reside in Washington (70,000), Texas (48,000), Florida (40,000), Utah (37,000), New York (36,000), Nevada (33,000), Oregon (26,000) and Arizona (25,000). Thus, more

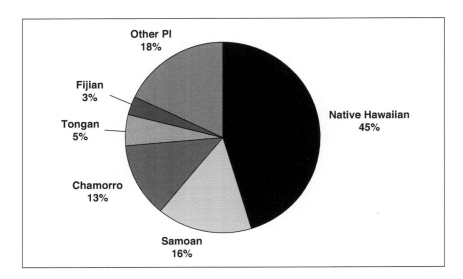

FIGURE 8.2 Native Hawaiian, Other Pacific Islander percentages of Hawai'i population
Source: Hixson *et al.* (2012).

than three-fourths of the entire NHPI population (78%) lives in just 10 states with the vast majority residing in the Western regions of the U.S. (Hixson *et al.* 2012).

Because of the numerically small number of NHPIs that comprise the overall U.S. population (0.4%), many national data reports often omit NHPIs or aggregate NHPIs with Asian American populations. At least one recent study has confirmed that aggregation of Asian Americans and NHPIs results in the masking of important health risk factors in both sub-populations and should be avoided. This is particularly important when the intent is to examine physical activity levels and its effect on health and wellness (Bitton *et al.* 2010). Thus, when disaggregated national data was not available, other reliable data sources from state or local sources were utilized and presented in this chapter. The State of Hawai'i has historically (since the late 1800s) collected extensive multi-ethnic and racial data with granularity from its diverse resident population and thus Hawai'i State-level data is presented when appropriate and available.

Health disparities and inequities among the NHPI population

Cardiovascular and metabolic health

Physical activity and chronic diseases measured by two major studies, the Molokai Heart Study and the Native Hawaiian Health Research Project (NHHRP) have largely focused only on the NH population. Both large studies started in the late 1980s to early 1990s and over the last 20+ years have provided much-needed descriptive data on the occurrence of diabetes mellitus (DM) and heart disease (HD) risk factors in adult NHs. Standardized data from both studies include lifestyle behaviors such as dietary intake and physical activity as well as information on social factors, body weight measurements, race/ethnicity, age and sex. It is well known that the prevalence of DM, pre-diabetes and obesity are increased among NHPIs and that a weight loss of 5–7% is clinically meaningful for multiple chronic diseases (i.e. diabetes, obesity, etc.) (Aluli *et al.* 2009, Grandinetti *et al.* 1998, Knowler *et al.* 2002).

In NH adults > 30 years old the frequency of DM is 22% with another 15% at high risk for DM based on standardized research glucose tolerance testing (i.e. 2 hr OGTT) (Grandinetti *et al.* 1998). Similar DM frequencies of 22.6% and 25.1% among 862 NH women and men, respectively, were also found in another NH population–based sample living in Hawai'i (Aluli *et al.* 2009). Moreover, Maskarinec et al. found NHs and Asians had higher rates of DM compared with Whites at all levels of BMI (Maskarinec *et al.* 2009). Thus, there are consistent findings that show NHPIs and Asians are at greater risk for developing DM even at the same BMI level as Whites (Shai *et al.* 2006).

Grandinetti et al. examined cross-sectional data on 1,440 multi-ethnic adults and found that physical activity was significantly associated with insulin resistance (an indicator that the body is not handling blood glucose (or sugar) efficiently) across all ethnic/racial groups (NH, Japanese, Filipino, White and mixed ethnicities) in Hawai'i. This study found that increased resting heart rate and low levels of physical activity were each independently associated with insulin resistance, which is a key factor related to the development of the metabolic syndrome. Metabolic syndrome is increased among NH adults and is defined as a clustering of CVD risk factors and insulin resistance that had been previously described in NHs by Mau et al. (Grandinetti *et al.* 1998, Mau *et al.* 1997). Thus, physical activity among NH adults is associated with insulin resistance, which in turn is associated with the development of DM, pre-DM and the metabolic syndrome.

Among other Pacific Islander populations few studies are available that have examined physical activity and its association with health disparities such as obesity, pre-DM, DM and metabolic syndrome. A pilot study of college-aged Samoan women (*n* = 48) investigated factors associated with percent body fat and found that sedentary behavior (little-to-no physical activity) was associated with a higher percentage of body fat and percent of Samoan ancestry was also associated with higher percent body fat. This pilot study supports the idea that Samoan women in particular tend to be sedentary and that this is strongly correlated with modifiable factors such as physical activity (Black *et al.* 2011).

Few studies are available on Chamorros; however, a national survey (i.e. Behavioral Risk Factor Surveillance System (BRFSS)) conducted in 2006 found that physical *in*activity was more common in Chamorros compared with the U.S. general population and they were also more likely to report high levels of cholesterol and diabetes. This study provided preliminary data on the public health burden of heart disease risk factors and suggests potential areas of improvements such as increasing physical activity as well as improved dietary changes may be warranted (Chiem *et al.* 2006).

Despite the overwhelming literature on the association of obesogenic lifestyles (sedentarism and physical inactivity and a high-fat, high-caloric dietary intake) being linked to overweight/obesity, pre-DM, DM and metabolic syndrome, most epidemiological studies have *not* found a consistent relationship with physical activity levels **alone** with BMI and/or DM. This is also a consistent finding among NHPIs (Grandinetti *et al.* 2015). One explanation for the lack of association between physical activity and obesity may relate to the cross-sectional nature of the data itself as individuals with high BMI may be reporting high levels of physical activity because they are trying to lose weight. Or other studies have suggested that physical activity levels were found to only weakly be associated with the incidence of Type 2 DM in individuals who are at high genetic risk such as NHPIs (Klimentidis *et al.* 2014). Alternatively, the lack of association between physical activity and BMI may reflect a NHPI-specific threshold that requires a higher dose of physical activity to have a beneficial impact on BMI or excess weight–associated diseases such as DM, pre-DM and metabolic syndrome.

Cancer

Physical inactivity has been associated with 1 in 10 deaths in the U.S., including cancer deaths (Danaei *et al.* 2009). Complex data analyses that combined data from several large population-based studies have found an association between physical activity and eight different forms of cancer including head/neck, colon, lymphoma, lung, prostate, kidney, breast and thyroid (Behrens and Leitzmann 2013, Boyle *et al.* 2012, Latino-Martel *et al.* 2016, Liu *et al.* 2011, Nicolotti *et al.* 2011, Schmid *et al.* 2013, Sun *et al.* 2012, Vermaete *et al.* 2013, Wu *et al.* 2013). Low levels of physical activity have been strongly associated with an increased risk for colon cancer and a moderately higher risk for postmenopausal breast cancer (Latino-Martel *et al.* 2016). Depending on the intensity level of physical activity, being more active was associated with a slight reduction in the risk of lung cancer (Sun *et al.* 2012). The link between physical activity and other cancers has been mixed and was thus described as "inconclusive" (Latino-Martel *et al.* 2016). In summary, an active life-style can reduce risk of some forms of cancer, particularly colon cancer.

New cancer diagnoses and cancer deaths for all race/ethnic groups including Asian and Pacific Islander (API) populations are tracked and compared using national cancer registries and state-specific vital records (i.e. death certificate data) (Miller *et al.* 2008). Analyses of this data have shown Native Hawaiian women had higher rates across *all* newly diagnosed cancers compared to White women (NHPI = 488.5 per 100,000; White = 448.5 per 100,000 (Miller *et al.* 2008). In particular, breast and lung cancer rates were higher in Native Hawaiian and Samoan women. Similar rates for both new cancer diagnoses and deaths were the highest in Native Hawaiian men, specifically prostate, lung and colorectal cancer, with high rates of prostate, lung, liver and stomach among Samoan men. Additional recent national data has shown NH and Samoan women's cancer rates for breast cancer were as high as Whites and higher than Asian Americans (Torre *et al.* 2016). Lung cancer rates were the highest for Samoan men with Hawaiian and Whites having comparable rates but these were also higher than most Asian American subgroups (Torre *et al.* 2016). Thus, NHPI men and women have significantly higher risks of being diagnosed with cancer and dying of cancer compared to Whites or Asian Americans.

To investigate health behaviors of children who had survived cancer, a study was conducted in Hawai'i to investigate physical activity levels in a sample of NHPI adolescent and young adult survivors of childhood cancers who were 13–24 years of age (*n* = 64), and 63% were leukemia/lymphoma survivors. The survivors' physical activity levels were compared to levels of physical activity reported by similarly aged persons without a history of cancer from Hawai'i and from across the U.S. (Wada *et al.* 2013). Although many of the young Hawai'i cancer survivors met age-specific physical activity recommendations, 44% of those less than 18 years old and 29% of those older than 18 years still failed to meet national guidelines, and these rates were significantly different from the rates of comparably aged people without a history of cancer. Low levels of physical activity place these young, ethnic minority cancer survivors at higher risk for secondary cancers and other chronic diseases.

Physical activity among NHPI

As noted in Chapter 1, physical activity levels assessed as part of the BRFSS report the proportion of adults that are meeting physical activity recommendations (i.e. 150 minutes of moderate-to-vigorous physical activity a week) both nationally and by state. According to the BRFSS in 2011, more than 50% of NHPI adults reported meeting these physical activity recommendations. The percentage for NHPIs was similar to Whites and was higher compared to all other racial/ethnic groups. Figure 8.3 shows the percent meeting physical activity recommendation by race/ethnicity and sex (Centers for Disease Control and Prevention *et al.* 2015).

The State of Hawai'i also collects racial/ethnic–specific physical activity data and has reported that NHs have the second-highest proportion of individuals who meet the recommended physical activity levels. Additionally, in surveys collected from

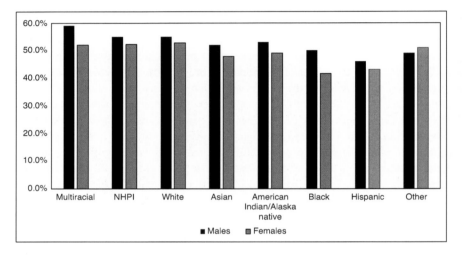

FIGURE 8.3 BRFSS 2011 data – percent meeting national guidelines for physical activity by race and sex

Source: Centers for Disease Control and Prevention *et al.* (2015).

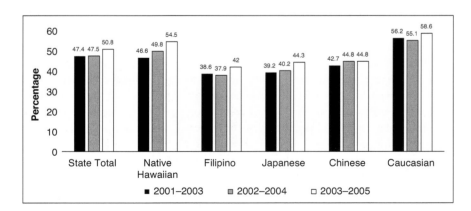

FIGURE 8.4 Percent meeting recommended physical activity levels by race in Hawai'i

Source: Hawai'i Health Data Warehouse (2009).

2001 to 2005, the race/ethnicity with the greatest increase in the number of people meeting the recommended levels (8% increase) from 2001 to 2005 was NH, and this increase was higher than all other ethnicities and races (Hawai'i Health Data Warehouse 2009).

Native Hawaiians and Other Pacific Islanders living in Hawai'i

In addition to Hawai'i data collected as part of the BRFSS or other population-based surveys, a number of research studies have surveyed large numbers of people living in Hawai'i or in other states in order to describe health behaviors, including the physical activity levels of NHPI and other race/ethnic groups. Although there were differences across these studies in how they reported various intensity levels of physical activity or types of physical activities included (e.g. including occupational, household/gardening or only leisure-time activities), they provide important comparisons between NHPI and other races/ethnicities. One large multi-ethnic study included 215,000 males and females between the ages of 45 and 75 living in Hawai'i or Southern California who were White, African American, Hispanic, Japanese American, or NH. Among the 13,971 NHs, 47% of NH men and 23% of NH women were doing strenuous or vigorous physical activity per week and these rates for strenuous physical activity were equal to Whites but higher than the other race/ethnic groups (Kolonel *et al.* 2000). A follow-up survey of this same sample's physical activity levels reported 11–14 years later found again more NHs (men and women) reported doing more vigorous work for > 4 hours a week (29.6% and 10.4%, respectively) than their respective genders across all other race/ethnic groups. Rates for moderate physical activity did not vary across different races of men; however, more White women (22.9%) reported +11 hours a week of moderate activity compared to Native Hawaiian (16.8%) or Japanese women (15.8%) (Kim *et al.* 2012, Steinbrecher *et al.* 2012).

A different population-based study surveyed 3,588 adults between 18 and 54 years of age who lived in Hawai'i and 16.4% of its sample was NH ($n = 590$). (Zou *et al.* 2012). There were significant differences between race/ethnic groups for the number of persons who met the national physical activity guidelines with a higher percentage (52.8%) of Whites and NH meeting the guidelines, compared to other race/ethnic groups (i.e. 45% of Chinese, 43.7% of Filipinos and 37.8% of Japanese). Factors that were significantly associated with meeting the physical activity guidelines were male gender, age (younger), Native Hawaiian race, having a normal or overweight BMI, having a job with mostly walking or heavy labor, being in excellent health, having a high self-efficacy for physical activity, spending less time sitting and walking a dog more frequently (Zou *et al.* 2012). Thus, studies with large samples of ethnic minorities found NHs had high levels of physical activity that was often equal to or greater than the rates for other race/ethnic groups. Since NHPI are underrepresented in the physical activity literature, it is important to also review the results of smaller-scale research studies. However, due to their small sample sizes their results may not be as representative or applicable as the data from larger samples. A survey of 381 adults in Hawai'i (mean age 46.5 ± 17.13) with 23% (n = 86) NHPI found that although Whites had the highest average minutes per week of physical activity, the levels for NHPI were the second highest with all other races (e.g. Asians) being lower (Geller *et al.* 2015). For example, NHPI reported 19 minutes/week of moderate physical activity with Whites reporting 22 minutes/week, with NHPI reporting 23 minutes/week of strenuous physical activity and Whites 25 minutes/week.

In contrast, a small survey conducted in Southern California (n = 100, aged 40–59) was unique because of the variety of NHPI that were included, such as 57% Samoans, 11% Guamanian/Chamorros, 6% Tongans, 3% Marshallese and 24% NHPI (many of whom reported having more than one race) (Moy *et al.* 2010a, Moy *et al.* 2010b). The majority of the sample (80%) was classified as having low levels of physical activity (i.e. those not meeting national guidelines); however, there were significant differences by gender, with women being significantly more active across all levels of physical activity intensity (p < 0.05). Almost all (93%) of NHPI men were classified as having low levels of physical activity, while 7.1% were moderately active and none reported vigorous activities. But, 64% of females had low-intensity, 32% moderate and 4.5% high physical activity levels. Moy *et al.* (2010b) also investigated the factors associated with physical activity in NHPI (Moy *et al.* 2010b). They found that after adjusting for gender and education, the only significant predictor of physical activity was servings of fruit and vegetables per day.

Tongans

A study of Tongans living in Utah included 21 women and 9 men with a mean age = 40 ± 15 measured physical activity levels using accelerometers (Behrens *et al.* 2011). The percent who met national guidelines was 11% for men (n = 1) and zero for women. Minutes of moderate to vigorous physical activity a day was 9 minutes/day for men and 4 minutes/day for women. Although this study had a small sample size (n = 30), it is noteworthy because it used objective measures of physical activity with a Pacific Island population that is very rarely included in research on physical activity.

In summary, national and Hawai'i-specific survey data that included large sample sizes found NHPIs had moderate to vigorous intensity levels that are equal to or higher than other races/ethnicities and about half meet the national physical activity recommendations. Thus, these findings were consistent across several studies with large sample sizes. However, studies with smaller but demographically unique sub-samples of NHPI found lower levels of physical activity across the different NHPI samples, with one small objectively measured physical activity (accelerometer) study finding extremely low levels of moderate to vigorous intensity activity in one NPHI subsample. Nonetheless, much of the population-based data for NHPI adults show high levels of physical activity comparable to Whites and higher than other ethnic minorities.

NHPI youth

Limited data, besides that from the Youth Risk Behavioral Survey (YRBS), are available on the physical activity levels of NHPI youth. In Hawai'i, YRBS physical activity data from 2015 are available from students attending public middle and high schools. Overall, 19.9% of middle school students and 16.4% of high school students met the guideline for being physically active for > 60 minutes on 7 of the past 7 days and doing muscle-strengthening activities on > 3 days of the past 7 days. Among Native Hawaiians, 23% of middle school students and 22% of high school students met guidelines, while for Other Pacific Islander students 23% of middle school students and 15% of high school students met the guideline. Except for Other Pacific Islander high school students, the physical activity rates for NHPI youth tended to be slightly higher than the overall state rate (Hawai'i Health Data Warehouse 2016).

Common barriers and facilitators to physical activity for NHPI

Community-level supports for physical activity, such as well-maintained parks and sidewalks on neighborhood streets, are not always available to NHPI populations. Later in this chapter, we discuss strategies to create more supportive community environments for NHPI.

Environment and community influences

Research findings are mixed for how community design and availability of physical activity resources/facilities in a neighborhood impact the physical activity levels of NHPI. In a study of adults living in Hawai'i, Geller and colleagues (2015) found no differences by ethnicity (among Caucasians, Asian Americans, Native Hawaiians and Other Pacific Islanders and Other/Mixed) in nearness of physical activity resources (e.g. swimming pools, parks and fitness centers) to their homes (Geller *et al.* 2015). However, the quality of the physical activity resources may differ. One study conducted on the island of O'ahu in Hawai'i found that a community with high percentage of Native Hawaiian residents had physical activity resources (e.g. playgrounds and walking/running trails) that were in poorer condition than two other communities with a lower percentage of Native Hawaiian residents (Mau *et al.* 2008). Yet, the observed utilization of the physical activity resources was high in all three communities.

Similarly, in another study focused on just public parks in Honolulu, Hawaii, researchers found that parks in low-income neighborhoods with slightly higher proportions of Pacific Islander populations tended to have more incivilities (e.g. litter, graffiti, dog refuse) than parks in higher-income neighborhoods (Jokura *et al.* 2010). Despite these incivilities, the parks in lower-income neighborhoods had a higher proportion of physically active users and fewer sedentary users (Chung-Do *et al.* 2011). A limitation was that the researchers were unable to classify individual park users by ethnicity. Taken together, these studies suggest that the availability of environmental resources supports physical activity in Native Hawaiian and Pacific Islander communities, even though efforts may be needed to improve the condition of the environmental resources.

In one of the few studies to examine the association between the built or physical environment and physical activity levels in NHPI, Moy and colleagues (2010b) assessed adults' perceptions of what resources for physical activity were available in their neighborhood and how their environment presented barriers to physical activity, in a convenience sample of 100 NHPI adults living in California (Moy *et al.* 2010b). As previously described, overall physical activity levels were low, with only 20% of the sample meeting physical activity guidelines. Most participants reported having destinations and transit stops within walking distance of their homes, but perceived that traffic volume and crime were barriers to walking in their neighborhoods. The majority also reported a lack of well-maintained sidewalks (55%) or bike paths (63%) and did not see their neighbors being physically active in the neighborhood (56%). A more supportive neighborhood environment was positively associated with the participant's physical activity level, but other lifestyle variables appeared to be more strongly related to physical activity. In another study, neighborhood environmental influences (e.g. living within walking distance to a grocery store, presence of sidewalks and presence of recreational facilities) were found to be correlated with physical activity levels of Asian American and Pacific Islander adults residing in Las Vegas, Nevada (Bungum *et al.* 2012). Although a methodological strength of this study was the use of random digit dialing techniques to generate the sample, the final sample comprised predominately Asian Americans. Native Hawaiians, Chamorro and Samoan participants represented less than 10% of the total sample. This study illustrates the lack of empirical data on physical activity correlates specific to NHPI.

Intervention strategies

Traditional, indigenous activities are often overlooked as methods to initiate and maintain physical activity. NHPIs participate in a number of activities that they inherently understand to be physical in nature, but some have not been quantitatively studied to determine the energy expenditure required to complete the task for an extended period of time. Without scientific evidence, these cultural activities such as canoe paddling, fishing, surfing, working in a traditional taro patch and dancing are not considered exercise. While other non-traditional forms of exercise have been evaluated (e.g. Tai Chi, yoga and gardening), there is little research associated with the NHPI cultural physical activities with one exception – hula dancing.

Hula: the traditional dance of Native Hawaiians

Hula is the traditional dance of Native Hawaiians, the indigenous people of the Hawaiian Islands (Kaeepler 1993). It has had a wide range of appeal to all people and cultures in Hawai'i, as well as worldwide. In Hawai'i, there are more than 100 *Hula Hālau* (hula schools), with almost every ethnicity represented among the students (Look *et al.* 2012). People across the state have learned to enjoy and appreciate this dance from the indigenous population.

Hula is rooted in the traditional Hawaiian values such as spirituality, religion and health and is an example of a sociocultural element that could be included as a part of deep structure strategies for cultural tailoring (Barrere 1980, Emerson 1909). Today, hula is divided into two main forms: (1) *kāhiko* and (2) *'auana*. *Kāhiko* is the traditional form of hula and is typically accompanied with a traditional Native Hawaiian instrument, such as an *ipu* or *ipu heke* (gourd instrument) or a *pahu* (drum) and chanting in Native Hawaiian language. *'Auana* is the modern form of hula, which is accompanied by stringed instruments (guitar, ukulele, bass) and singing in English and/or Native Hawaiian language. In both forms of hula, it is expected that the dancer have an understanding of not only the literal translation of the words, but also of the hidden, poetic meaning of the words and song. It is through this complete understanding that an appropriate performance of hula can take place. The movements of hula, both hands and feet, enhance the performance of a song by giving the audience a visual tool to bring the story to life (Kaeepler 1993, Kanaka'ole 1997). The surface or literal meaning in both traditional and modern song will often utilize components of the natural world found in Hawai'i as a way to spiritually connect the song back to the islands and people through nature or the land (Emerson 1915, Kanahele 1993, Pukui and Korn 1973). This connection back to the land can be important for improving the psychological well-being of people, as it deepens their spiritual connection to their culture. Hula has the ability not only to improve physical fitness, mobility, flexibility, but psychological well-being through stress and anxiety reduction as well.

Practitioners of hula know that while the dance is beautiful and appears effortless, there is a tangible physical aspect to properly perform and execute a dance. In order for hula to be utilized in a more formal capacity for health programs or interventions, it needs to be measured and tested as an activity that meets the level of exertion that would satisfy the definitions for moderate and/or vigorous physical activity (Haskell *et al.* 2007). In addition, this would allow health professionals like physicians and trainers to encourage their patients to engage in more hula dancing to increase their total physical activity time during the week. Dancers could take additional classes or dance on their own at home. This activity could maintain its cultural components, while providing the benefits of a more traditional exercise regimen if dancers keep in mind that they need to achieve a certain level of physical exertion. One study determined the physical exertion required of low- and high-intensity hula dancing (Usagawa *et al.* 2014). The primary goal of this small study was to determine the metabolic equivalent (MET) levels for the two different forms of hula, *'auana* and *kāhiko*, as a way to compare hula to other forms of activities with established MET values (Ainsworth *et al.* 2011, Ainsworth *et al.* 1993, Ainsworth *et al.* 2000). For moderate physical activity, the CDC recommends MET values of 3.0–5.9 METs, and for vigorous physical activity the CDC recommends MET values of 6.0 and higher (Haskell *et al.* 2007, Pate *et al.* 1995). It was found that when hula was stratified into low- and high-intensity dancing, '*auana* hula reached 5.7 METs or moderate physical activity and *kāhiko* hula reached 7.7 METs or vigorous physical activity (Usagawa *et al.* 2014). The results of this study provided quantifiable evidence that hula could be used in a comprehensive health intervention that focused on physical as well as psychological well-being that was culturally tailored at both surface and deep levels.

A five-year project called the "Hula Enabling Lifestyles Adaptation (HELA)" evaluated the use of hula as the physical activity for a cardiac rehabilitation program. Participants that had recently experienced a cardiac event (myocardial infarction, heart surgery or heart failure) were recruited for the study. The intervention was 12 weeks in duration, three times a week for one hour, and was held at Queen's Medical Center in Honolulu, Hawai'i. Classes were conducted by a *Kumu hula* (hula teacher and expert) and registered nurses to ensure the safety of participants that attended each class. The results from the intervention group were compared to a control group that did not participate in the hula class.

The HELA study was designed as a culturally appropriate approach, with principles of community-based participatory research employed in the design and implementation of the program. Demonstrating deep structure by validating the appropriateness of the study, multiple kumu hula were interviewed and agreed upon. All agreed hula would be appropriate for a health intervention, if implemented correctly by maintaining the culturally integrity of the dance (Look *et al.* 2012). A community partner, Hālau Mōhala 'Ilima (a school of traditional NH dance, language and culture), participated in the design and delivery of the intervention with their kumu hula teaching each of the study's groups. The results of the study did not show significant differences between the control group and intervention group; however, improvement in peak oxygen consumption or VO_2max occurred in 68% of intervention participants compared to 56% of control participants. In addition, 83% of intervention participants walked farther during the 6-minute walk test compared to 60% of the control participants at 3 months post-intervention.

BOX 8.1   EVIDENCE FOR PRACTICE: A PHYSICAL ACTIVITY INTERVENTION IN HAWAI'I USING HULA DANCING

In an effort to disseminate the intervention from HELA (tested in a clinical setting) to the community, a pilot study was conducted. *Ola Hou i ka Hula* (translation: "Return to Health with Hula") was a randomized controlled trial conducted at two community organizations that serve NHPI adults. The sites were Kula no na Po'e Hawai'i (a community non-profit organization serving three NH communities in Honolulu) and Kokua Kalihi Valley Comprehensive Family Services (a federally qualified community health center).

Ola Hou i ka Hula tested whether an intervention with hula as the main form of physical activity could reduce blood pressure in 55 NHPI adults with known hypertension. Participants attended hula classes for one hour, twice a week, for 12 weeks and received three hours of heart health education. The primary outcome was changes in systolic and diastolic blood pressure readings at the end of 12 weeks. Results showed a significant reduction in systolic blood pressure in the intervention group when compared to the control group; however, there was no change in diastolic blood pressure (Kaholokula *et al.* 2015). The results of this study suggested that a culturally relevant intervention using hula dancing as the primary physical activity could effectively reduce systolic blood pressure in NHPI adults with hypertension.

The PILI 'Ohana Program was a culturally adapted intervention of the Diabetes Prevention Program lifestyle program designed for NHs, Chuukese and Other Pacific Islanders and delivered using community-based participatory research approaches (Mau *et al.* 2010). As previously noted, rates of diabetes in this population are greater than many other population groups. The intervention was tested in a 9-month randomized control trial of 100 NHPIs. The authors found that weight loss in the first 3 months of the trial and a lower dietary fat intake at baseline were significant predictors of weight loss (defined as greater than 3% of their baseline weight) after the 9-month intervention. Of note, physical activity was not significantly associated with this degree of weight loss. The study suggests that dietary factors seem to have a greater impact than exercise, at least in the short-term follow-up period (< 1 year), on weight reduction in NHPIs. Moreover, those individuals who succeed at early weight loss are more likely to maintain that weight over the next 6 months (Kaholokula *et al.* 2013). And that while physical activity remains an important component of an effective lifestyle program for weight reduction, it does not appear to be as strong a predictor of weight maintenance over a short-term follow-up period.

Environmental change

Community programs that seek to increase opportunities and promote supportive environments for physical activity have found success in several communities in Hawai'i. Moreover, higher levels of school and community connectedness may support physical activity behaviors in Pacific Islanders (Yang *et al.* 2014). For example, in urban Honolulu, a joint use agreement helped to increase physical activity opportunities in a public high school with a high proportion of Filipino, Native Hawaiian and Samoan students (Choy *et al.* 2008). Through the joint use agreement, the Honolulu Department of Parks and Recreation was able to offer fun, acceptable recreational activities, such as lunchtime volleyball and free after-school dance classes, to students, staff and community members using school facilities.

Another program in urban Honolulu focuses on promoting bicycling among Filipino, Native Hawaiian, Micronesian, Samoan and other youth who live in a low-income community. The Kalihi Valley Instructional Bike Exchange (KVIBE) program is an initiative of Kokua Kalihi Valley Comprehensive Family Services, a federally qualified health center. KVIBE is a bicycle repair and recycling program that gives youth the opportunity to earn a bicycle through community service. KVIBE also seeks to empower youth to advocate for better bike facilities, infrastructure and government policy (Kalihi Valley Instructional Bike Exchange 2016).

To address low rates of walking and bicycling to school among elementary school children in Hawai'i County, the HŌ'ALA research project aimed to institute Safe Routes to School programs in intervention schools. In the mostly rural county, researchers documented a lack of crosswalks, crossing aids, bicycle facilities, buffers between pedestrian paths and roadways and amenities such as benches and water fountains along roads that surrounded the elementary schools (Heinrich *et al.* 2011). The HŌ'ALA research project demonstrated the importance of working at public policy levels, such as having a community partner serve on the statewide Complete Streets Policy Task Force, to ensure that infrastructure changes would be made to support walking and bicycling among children at the intervention schools.

Finally, to decrease the prevalence of overweight in young children (between 2–8 years old) living in the U.S.-affiliated Pacific region, the Children's Healthy Living Project utilized the ANGELO (Analysis Grid for Environments/Elements Linked to Obesity) model to design a comprehensive intervention targeting nutrition, sedentary and physical activity behaviors (Braun *et al.* 2014). The ANGELO model allowed researchers to combine community preferences and evidence-based strategies into the intervention design to allow for greater cultural tailoring. Four cross-cutting functions targeted physical activity promotion: strengthening and implementing school wellness policies; partnering and advocating for environmental change; using role models to deliver healthy living messages; and building capacity by training the trainers. The intervention framework allowed each Pacific jurisdiction the flexibility to tailor the final intervention to fit its own culture, role models and resources. The Children's Healthy Living Project demonstrates that it is possible to design multilevel interventions in a culturally appropriate way for Native Hawaiian and Pacific Islander populations.

Implications for practice

In summary, national survey data have shown NHPI men and women's physical activity levels were relatively high in comparison to other ethnic/racial minority populations and comparable to Whites. Yet paradoxically, NHPIs are known to experience increased health inequalities in physical activity–related diseases such as overweight/obesity, DM, pre-DM and the metabolic syndrome. Although several studies with NHPIs have provided an understanding of their physical activity levels and health risks, there remain significant gaps in our knowledge on how changes in physical activity could decrease their disease risk, including what amount and types of physical activities and for what duration would be needed to significantly improve the health and lower decrease risks among NHPIs.

Also, there needs to be a better understanding of the types and amounts of physical activity that will engage NHPI populations and that will be sustainable for their body/physique (some may be too large for certain weight-bearing activities). NHPIs may also need to participate in physical activities appropriate to the environment where they live, such as the ocean (paddling, fishing, surfing) and other traditional activities that would be culturally relevant and be compatible with their island–ocean environment.

Studies that isolate physical activity as the focus would be needed to specify the role physical activity has in lowering disease risk in NHPI populations, particularly after their diet or other unhealthy behaviors had been taken into consideration (i.e. diet, obesity, smoking). Culturally relevant physical activities – such as hula dancing as well as athletic activities such as surfing, ocean voyaging, etc. – show initial promise of not only increasing physical activity/energy expenditure but also improving participation in and maintenance of the activities since they are culturally and ancestrally tied to the NHPI culture and their communities. Such studies are in their early development and testing but offer initial positive results among NHPIs, and they may be transferable to other high-risk populations who are seeking culturally relevant interventions to increase physical activity as a means to improve their own health and wellness.

Summary points

- NHPIs in the U.S. are one of the most racially diverse groups with 56% of its members ethnically identifying with more than one race and/or a NHPI subgroup.
- National survey data has shown NHPI adults' and teens' physical activity levels were relatively high in comparison to other ethnic/racial minority populations and comparable to Whites.
- NHPIs experience increased health disparities in physical activity–related diseases such as obesity/overweight, diabetes, metabolic syndrome and cancer.
- Traditional activities of NHPIs such as hula, surfing and ocean voyaging, to name a few, show initial promise of not only increasing energy expenditure but also improving participation in and maintenance of the activities because of the historical, cultural and ancestral significance of these activities to NHPI populations.

Critical thinking questions

1 How would you explain the apparent paradox where NHPI are found to have fairly high levels of physical activity yet are at increased risk for chronic diseases known to be reduced/modified by physical activity?

2   Why is there relatively little historical data on physical activity levels in NPHI prior to 1998?
3   How would you design a sustainable physical activity program for NHPI?

Acknowledgments

The authors would like to acknowledge Andrea Conching and Kara Saiki for their assistance with this chapter.

References

Ainsworth, B. E., Haskell, W. L., Herrmann, S. D., Meckes, N., Bassett, D. R., Jr., Tudor-Locke, C., Greer, J. L., Vezina, J., Whitt-Glover, M. C. and Leon, A. S. (2011). 'Compendium of physical activities: A second update of codes and MET values.' *Medicine and Science in Sports and Exercise*, 43: 1575–81.

Ainsworth, B. E., Haskell, W. L., Leon, A. S., Jacobs, D. R., Jr., Montoye, H. J., Sallis, J. F. and Paffenbarger, R. S., Jr. (1993). 'Compendium of physical activities: Classification of energy costs of human physical activities.' *Medicine and Science in Sports and Exercise*, 25: 71–80.

Ainsworth, B. E., Haskell, W. L., Whitt, M. C., Irwin, M. L., Swartz, A. M., Strath, S. J., O'brien, W. L., Bassett, D. R., Jr., Schmitz, K. H., Emplaincourt, P. O., Jacobs, D. R., Jr. and Leon, A. S. (2000). 'Compendium of physical activities: An update of activity codes and MET intensities.' *Medicine and Science in Sports and Exercise*, 32: S498–504.

Aluli, N. E., Jones, K. L., Reyes, P. W., Brady, S. K., Tsark, J. U. and Howard, B. V. (2009). 'Diabetes and cardiovascular risk factors in Native Hawaiians.' *Hawaii Medical Journal*, 68: 152–7.

Barrere, D. B. (1980). 'The hula in retrospect.' *In*: Barrere, D. B., Pukui, M. K. and Kelley, M. (eds.) *Hula Historical Perspectives, Pacific Anthropological Records*. Honolulu, Hawai'i: Department of Anthropology, Bernice Pauahi Bishop Museum.

Behrens, G. and Leitzmann, M. F. (2013). 'The association between physical activity and renal cancer: Systematic review and meta-analysis.' *British Journal of Cancer*, 108: 798–811.

Behrens, T. K., Moy, K., Dinger, M. K., Williams, D. P. and Harbour, V. J. (2011). 'Objectively assessed physical activity among Tongans in the United States.' *Research Quarterly in Exercise and Sport*, 82: 565–9.

Bitton, A., Zaslavsky, A. M. and Ayanian, J. Z. (2010). 'Health risks, chronic diseases, and access to care among US Pacific Islanders.' *Journal of General Internal Medicine*, 25: 435–40.

Black, N., Nabokov, V., Vijayadeva, V. and Novotny, R. (2011). 'Higher percent body fat in young women with lower physical activity level and greater proportion Pacific Islander ancestry.' *Hawai'i Medical Journal*, 70: 43–6.

Boyle, T., Keegel, T., Bull, F., Heyworth, J. and Fritschi, L. (2012). 'Physical activity and risks of proximal and distal colon cancers: A systematic review and meta-analysis.' *Journal of the National Cancer Institute*, 104: 1548–61.

Braun, K. L., Nigg, C. R., Fialkowski, M. K., Butel, J., Hollyer, J. R., Barber, L. R., Bersamin, A., Coleman, P., Teo-Martin, U., Vargo, A. M. and Novotny, R. (2014). 'Using the ANGELO model to develop the children's healthy living program multilevel intervention to promote obesity preventing behaviors for young children in the U.S.-affiliated Pacific Region.' *Child Obesity*, 10: 474–81.

Bungum, T. J., Landers, M., Azzarelli, M. and Moonie, S. (2012). 'Perceived environmental physical activity correlates among Asian Pacific Islander Americans.' *Journal of Physical Activity and Health*, 9: 1098–104.

Centers for Disease Control and Prevention, National Center for Chronic Disease Prevention and Health Promotion and Division of Population Health. (2015). '*BRFSS Prevalence and Trends Data* [Online].' Available: www.cdc.gov/brfss/brfssprevalence/ (Accessed January 23 2016).

Chiem, B., Nguyen, V., Wu, P. L., Ko, C. M., Cruz, L. A. and Sadler, G. R. (2006). 'Cardiovascular risk factors among Chamorros.' *BMC Public Health*, 6: 298.

Choy, L. B., Mcgurk, M. D., Tamashiro, R., Nett, B. and Maddock, J. E. (2008). 'Increasing access to places for physical activity through a joint use agreement: A case study in urban Honolulu.' *Preventing Chronic Disease*, 5: A91.

Chung-Do, J. J., Davis, E., Lee, S., Jokura, Y., Choy, L. and Maddock, J. E. (2011). 'An observational study of physical activity in parks in Asian and Pacific Islander communities in urban Honolulu, Hawai'i, 2009.' *Preventing Chronic Disease*, 8: A107.

Danaei, G., Ding, E. L., Mozaffarian, D., Taylor, B., Rehm, J., Murray, C. J. and Ezzati, M. (2009). 'The preventable causes of death in the United States: Comparative risk assessment of dietary, lifestyle, and metabolic risk factors.' *Public Library of Science Medicine*, 6: e1000058.

Emerson, N. B. (1909). 'Unwritten literature of Hawai'i.' *Smithsonian Institution Bureau of American Ethnology Bull*, Washington, D.C.: United States Government Printing Office: 38.

Emerson, N. B. (1915). *Pele and Hiiaka*. Honolulu, HI: Honolulu Star-Bulletin Press.

Geller, K. S., Nigg, C. R., Ollberding, N. J., Motl, R. W., Horwath, C. and Dishman, R. K. (2015). 'Access to environmental resources and physical activity levels of adults in Hawai'i.' *Asia Pacific Journal of Public Health*, 27: NP288–98.

Grandinetti, A., Chang, H. K., Mau, M. K., Curb, J. D., Kinney, E. K., Sagum, R. and Arakaki, R. F. (1998). 'Prevalence of glucose intolerance among Native Hawaiians in two rural communities.' Native Hawaiian Health Research (NHHR) Project. *Diabetes Care*, 21: 549–54.

Grandinetti, A., Liu, D. M. and Kaholokula, J. K. (2015). 'Relationship of resting heart rate and physical activity with insulin sensitivity in a population-based survey.' *Journal of Diabetes and Metabolic Disorders*, 14: 41.

Haskell, W. L., Lee, I. M., Pate, R. R., Powell, K. E., Blair, S. N., Franklin, B. A., Macera, C. A., Heath, G. W., Thompson, P. D. and Bauman, A. (2007). 'Physical activity and public health: Updated recommendation for adults from the American College of Sports Medicine and the American Heart Association.' *Medicine and Science in Sports and Exercise*, 39: 1423–34.

Hawai'i Health Data Warehouse, S. O. H. (2016). '*Youth Risk Behavior Survey Module, Meet Physical Activity Guidelines in Hawai'i, by School Type, State, Gender, Grade Level, and DOH Race-Ethnicity, for the Years 2005–2015* [Online].' Available: http://hhdw.org/wp-content/uploads/YRBS_HealthyLifestyles_IND_00021.pdf.

Hawai'i Health Data Warehouse, S. O. H., Hawai'i State Department of Health. (2009). '*Physical Activity (Archive) – Moderate Physical Activity Risk Factor, Aggregrated Two Year Data: 2001–2005* [Online].' Available: http://hhdw.org/wp-content/uploads/BRFSS_Physical-Activity_AGG3_00005.pdf (Accessed May 3, 2016).

Heinrich, K. M., Dierenfield, L., Alexander, D. A., Prose, M. and Peterson, A. C. (2011). 'Hawaii's Opportunity for Active Living Advancement (HO'ALA): Addressing childhood obesity through safe routes to school.' *Hawai'i Medical Journal*, 70: 21–6.

Hixson, L., Hepler, B. B. and Kim, M. O. (2012). '*The Native Hawaiian and Other Pacific Islander Population, 2010* [Online].' Available: www.census.gov/prod/cen2010/briefs/c2010br-12.pdf (Accessed May 17 2016).

Jokura, Y., Heinrich, K. M., Chung-Do, J. J., Lee, S., Choy, L. and Maddock, J. (2010). 'Disparities in features, amenities and incivilities of physical activity resources in urban

Honolulu parks by neighborhood income.' *3rd International Congress on Physical Activity and Public Health*. Toronto, Canada.

Kaeepler, A. L. (1993). *Hula Pahu*. Honolulu: Bishop Museum Press.

Kaholokula J. K., Look, M., Mabellos, T., Zhang, D., De Silva, M., Yoshimura, S. R., Wills, T., Seto, T. and Sinclair, K. (2017). 'Cultural Dance Program Improves Hypertension Management for Native Hawaiians and Pacific Islanders: a Pilot Randomized Trial.' *Journal Racial Ethnic Health Disparities*, 4 (1): 35-46.

Kaholokula, J. K., Townsend, C. K., Ige, A., Sinclair, K., Mau, M. K., Leake, A., Palakiko, D. M., Yoshimura, S. R., Kekauoha, P. and Hughes, C. (2013). 'Sociodemographic, behavioral, and biological variables related to weight loss in native Hawaiians and other Pacific Islanders.' *Obesity (Silver Spring)*, 21: E196–203.

Kalihi Valley Instructional Bike Exchange. (2016). '*What Is KVIBE? Blog* [Online].' Available: http://k-vibe.blogspot.se/ (Accessed February 17 2016).

Kanahele, G. S. (1993). 'Hula Pahu.' *Bishop Museum Bulletin in Anthropology*, 3: 289.

Kanaka'ole, N. (1997). 'Chapter 26.' *In*: Itagaki, J. M. and Lependu, L. (eds.) *Nana i na Loea Hula (Look to the Hula Resources)*. Honolulu: Kalihi-Palama Culture and Arts Society.

Kim, S. K., Gignoux, C. R., Wall, J. D., Lum-Jones, A., Wang, H., Haiman, C. A., Chen, G. K., Henderson, B. E., Kolonel, L. N., Le Marchand, L., Stram, D. O., Saxena, R. and Cheng, I. (2012). 'Population genetic structure and origins of Native Hawaiians in the multiethnic cohort study.' *PLoS One*, 7: e47881.

Klimentidis, Y. C., Chen, Z., Arora, A. and Hsu, C. H. (2014). 'Association of physical activity with lower type 2 diabetes incidence is weaker among individuals at high genetic risk.' *Diabetologia*, 57: 2530–4.

Knowler, W. C., Barrett-Connor, E., Fowler, S. E., Hamman, R. F., Lachin, J. M., Walker, E. A., Nathan, D. M. and Diabetes Prevention Program Research Group. (2002). 'Reduction in the incidence of type 2 diabetes with lifestyle intervention or metformin.' *New England Journal of Medicine*, 346: 393–403.

Kolonel, L. N., Henderson, B. E., Hankin, J. H., Nomura, A. M., Wilkens, L. R., Pike, M. C., Stram, D. O., Monroe, K. R., Earle, M. E. and Nagamine, F. S. (2000). 'A multiethnic cohort in Hawai'i and Los Angeles: Baseline characteristics.' *American Journal of Epidemiology*, 151: 346–57.

Latino-Martel, P., Cottet, V., Druesne-Pecollo, N., Pierre, F. H., Touillaud, M., Touvier, M., Vasson, M. P., Deschasaux, M., Le Merdy, J., Barrandon, E. and Ancellin, R. (2016). 'Alcoholic beverages, obesity, physical activity and other nutritional factors, and cancer risk: A review of the evidence.' *Critical Reviews in Oncology and Hematology*, 99: 308–23.

Liu, Y., Hu, F., Li, D., Wang, F., Zhu, L., Chen, W., Ge, J., An, R. and Zhao, Y. (2011). 'Does physical activity reduce the risk of prostate cancer? A systematic review and meta-analysis.' *European Urology*, 60: 1029–44.

Look, M. A., Kaholokula, J. K., Carvhalo, A., Seto, T. and De Silva, M. (2012). 'Developing a culturally based cardiac rehabilitation program: The HELA study.' *Progress in Community Health Partnerships*, 6: 103–10.

Maskarinec, G., Grandinetti, A., Matsuura, G., Sharma, S., Mau, M., Henderson, B. E. and Kolonel, L. N. (2009). 'Diabetes prevalence and body mass index differ by ethnicity: The multiethnic cohort.' *Ethnicity and Disease*, 19: 49–55.

Mau, M. K., Grandinetti, A., Arakaki, R. F., Chang, H. K., Kinney, E. K. and Curb, J. D. (1997). 'The insulin resistance syndrome in native Hawaiians: Native Hawaiian Health Research (NHHR) Project.' *Diabetes Care*, 20: 1376–80.

Mau, M. K., Keaweaimoku, K. J., West, M. R., Leake, A., Efird, J., Rose, C., Palakiko, D. M., Yoshimura, S. R., Kekauoha, B. K. and Gomes, H. (2010). 'Translating the Diabetes

Prevention into Native Hawaiian and Pacific Islander communities: The PILI "Ohana pilot project".' *Progress in Community Health Partnerships*, 4: 7–16.

Mau, M. K., Wong, K. N., Efird, J., West, M., Saito, E. P. and Maddock, J. (2008). 'Environmental factors of obesity in communities with native Hawaiians.' *Hawaii Medical Journal*, 67: 233–6.

Miller, B. A., Chu, K. C., Hankey, B. F. and Ries, L. A. (2008). 'Cancer incidence and mortality patterns among specific Asian and Pacific Islander populations in the U.S.' *Cancer Causes and Control*, 19: 227–56.

Moy, K. L., Sallis, J. F. and David, K. J. (2010a). 'Health indicators of Native Hawaiian and Pacific Islanders in the United States.' *Journal of Community Health*, 35: 81–92.

Moy, K. L., Sallis, J. F., Ice, C. L. and Thompson, K. M. (2010b). 'Physical activity correlates for Native Hawaiians and Pacific Islanders in the mainland United States.' *Journal of Health Care for the Poor and Underserved*, 21: 1203–14.

Nicolotti, N., Chuang, S. C., Cadoni, G., Arzani, D., Petrelli, L., Bosetti, C., Brenner, H., Hosono, S., La Vecchia, C., Talamini, R., Matsuo, K., Müller, H., Muscat, J., Paludetti, G., Ricciardi, G., Boffetta, P., Hashibe, M. and Boccia, S. (2011). 'Recreational physical activity and risk of head and neck cancer: A pooled analysis within the International Head and Neck Cancer Epidemiology (INHANCE) consortium.' *European Journal of Epidemiology*, August 28; 26: 619–28.

Pate, R. R., Pratt, M., Blair, S. N., Haskell, W. L., Macera, C. A., Bouchard, C., Buchner, D., Ettinger, W., Heath, G. W., King, A. C., Kriska A., Leon, A.S., Marcus, B.H., Morris, J., Paffenbarger, R.S., Patrick, K., Pollock, M.L., Rippe, J.M., Sallis, J., Wilmore, J.H. (1995). 'Physical activity and public health: A recommendation from the Centers for Disease Control and Prevention and the American College of Sports Medicine.' *JAMA*, 273: 402–7.

Pukui, M. K. and Korn, A. L. (1973). *The Echo of Our Song*. Honolulu: University of Hawaii Press.

Schmid, D., Behrens, G., Jochem, C., Keimling, M. and Leitzmann, M. (2013). 'Physical activity, diabetes, and risk of thyroid cancer: A systematic review and meta-analysis.' *European Journal of Epidemiology*, 28: 945–58.

Shai, I., Jiang, R., Manson, J. E., Stampfer, M. J., Willett, W. C., Colditz, G. A. and Hu, F. B. (2006). 'Ethnicity, obesity, and risk of type 2 diabetes in women: A 20-year follow-up study.' *Diabetes Care*, 29: 1585–90.

Steinbrecher, A., Erber, E., Grandinetti, A., Nigg, C., Kolonel, L. N. and Maskarinec, G. (2012). 'Physical activity and risk of type 2 diabetes among Native Hawaiians, Japanese Americans, and Caucasians: The multiethnic cohort.' *Journal of Physical Activity and Health*, 9: 634–41.

Sun, J. Y., Shi, L., Gao, X. D. and Xu, S. F. (2012). 'Physical activity and risk of lung cancer: A meta-analysis of prospective cohort studies.' *Asian Pacific Journal of Cancer Prevention*, 13: 3143–7.

Torre, L. A., Sauer, A. M., Chen, M. S., Jr., Kagawa-Singer, M., Jemal, A. and Siegel, R. L. (2016). 'Cancer statistics for Asian Americans, Native Hawaiians, and Pacific Islanders, 2016: Converging incidence in males and females.' *CA Cancer Journal Clinics*, 66: 182–202.

Usagawa, T., Look, M., De Silva, M., Stickley, C., Kaholokula, J. K., Seto, T. and Mau, M. (2014). 'Metabolic equivalent determination in the cultural dance of hula.' *International Journal of Sports Medicine*, 35: 399–402.

Vermaete, N. V., Wolter, P., Verhoef, G. E., Kollen, B. J., Kwakkel, G., Schepers, L. and Gosselink, R. (2013). 'Physical activity and risk of lymphoma: A meta-analysis.' *Cancer Epidemiology and Biomarkers Prevention*, 22: 1173–84.

Wada, R., Glaser, D., Bantu, E., Orimoto, T., Steffen, A. D., Elia, J. and Albright, C. (2013). 'Hawaii's multiethnic adolescent and young adult survivors of childhood cancer: Are their health behavior risks similar to state and national samples?' *Hawai'i Journal of Medicine and Public Health*, 72: 380–6.

Wu, Y., Zhang, D. and Kang, S. (2013). 'Physical activity and risk of breast cancer: A meta-analysis of prospective studies.' *Breast Cancer Research and Treatment*, 137: 869–82.

Yang, F., Tan, K. A. and Cheng, W. J. (2014). 'The effects of connectedness on health-promoting and health-compromising behaviors in adolescents: Evidence from a statewide survey.' *Journal of Primary Prevention*, 35: 33–46.

Zou, Y., Zhang, M. and Maddock, J. E. (2012). 'Assessing physical activity and related correlates among adults in Hawaii.' *Hawai'i Journal of Medicine and Public Health*, 71: 310–8.

9

PHYSICAL ACTIVITY AMONG LOW-INCOME POPULATIONS

Wendell C. Taylor

All racial and ethnic minority groups and other subpopulations discussed in this text (e.g., rural, LGBT, veterans) include low-income people. Therefore, low-income populations are an essential high-priority group to study and promote physical activity. Understanding the physical activity patterns and trends, influences, and intervention successes in this population has the potential to affect all other target populations. In this chapter, definitions, patterns and trends, influences, evidence-based strategies, and implications for practice are presented.

Understanding the low-income population

Definitions of low income

Depending on the source, "low income" has been defined in a variety of ways. According to the United States Department of Housing and Urban Development's (2016) definition, there are three levels of low income: low, very low, and extremely low. The levels are derived from county statistics using median income and the Fair Market Rent Document, which averages rental prices in each specific county. For example, to be classified as "low income," the household must earn 80% or lower of the median income of the county; there are average amounts for 1- to 8-person households. Similarly, to be classified as "very low income," the household must earn 50% or less of the median income for the number of people per household for the county. Correspondingly, to be classified as "extremely low income," the household must earn 30% or less of the median income for the county. To calculate county statistics for each state, the United States Department of Housing and Urban Development has a website, the HUD Income Limits Documentation System.

The United States Department of Education has a different approach to classify low income. The term "low-income individual" means an individual whose family's taxable income for the preceding year did not exceed 150% of the poverty level amount. A family is defined as all persons living in the same household who are related by blood, marriage, or adoption. Adult children who continue to live at home and dependent children living outside of the home (e.g., students living in a dormitory or other student housing) are considered to be part of the family for the purpose of determining family income (United States Department of Health and Human Services 2016).

Based on poverty guidelines published by the United States Department of Health and Human Services in the Federal Register on January 25, 2016, the Department of Education published a table showing low income for the 48 contiguous states, Washington, D.C., and outlying jurisdictions, Alaska, and Hawaii (Table 9.1) (United States Department of Health and Human Services 2016).

As an example, for a family of four, the family incomes classified as low income for the 48 contiguous states, Alaska, and Hawaii, respectively, are $36,450, $45,570, and $41,925. Table 9.1 displays low family incomes and family sizes (one through eight) for the 48 contiguous states, Washington, D.C., and outlying jurisdictions, Alaska, and Hawaii.

Another perspective is advocated by Columbia University's National Center for Children in Poverty (2016) in which families and children are defined as low income if the family income is less than twice the federal poverty threshold. The rationale is that on average, families need an income of about twice the federal poverty threshold to meet their most basic needs. Children living in families with incomes below this level – $48,016 for a family of four with two children in 2014 – are referred to as low income.

TABLE 9.1 Federal TRIO Programs current-year low-income levels

Size of Family Unit	48 Contiguous States, D.C., and Outlying Jurisdictions	Alaska	Hawaii
1	$17,820	$22,260	$20,505
2	$24,030	$30,030	$27,645
3	$30,240	$37,800	$34,785
4	$36,450	$45,570	$41,925
5	$42,660	$53,340	$49,065
6	$48,870	$61,110	$56,205
7	$55,095	$68,880	$63,345
8	$61,335	$76,680	$70,515

Note: For family units with more than eight members, add the following amount for each additional family member: $6,240 for the 48 contiguous states, the District of Columbia, and outlying jurisdictions; $7,800 for Alaska; and $7,170 for Hawaii.
Source: United States Department of Health and Human Services (2016)

In summary, low income is defined by a variety of different metrics. To advance the field, agreement on a common metric for low income in physical activity research would enable consistency of comparisons among studies and over time. In most cases, for the research cited in this chapter, the authors explicitly defined the parameters for the threshold of low income.

Demographics of low-income populations

Fundamental to understanding any population is to identify patterns by subgroups within the population based on demographic characteristics. Demographic characteristics include weight status, income level, education, socioeconomic status (combining income and education), racial and ethnic identity, gender, age, geographic location, and sexual identity. In the following section, we examine socioeconomic status, racial and ethnic identity, and geographic location.

Health disparities and inequities among low-income populations

In examining the obesity epidemic (Wang and Beydoun 2007), researchers found the associations of obesity and socioeconomic status were complex and dynamic. Nonetheless, low-socioeconomic-status groups (i.e., combining income and education) were disproportionately affected by obesity at all ages (i.e., greater obesity levels). However, the association between socioeconomic status and obesity varied by ethnicity. In contrast, the relationship between income and life expectancy was clear and straightforward. A recent study (Chetty *et al.* 2016) found that life expectancy increased with income level. For example, between the top 1% and bottom 1% of the income distribution, life expectancy differed by 15 years for men and 10 years for women. Also, life expectancy varied among local areas. Given the geographic variation in life expectancy, the authors concluded that policy interventions should focus on changing health behaviors (e.g., increasing physical activity and reducing smoking rates) among low-income households. Life expectancy was positively correlated with physical activity and negatively correlated with smoking rates.

Physical activity among low-income populations

For any population, the patterns of physical activity and inactivity over time are important to know. The following section describes patterns of physical activity among low-income populations over time from a variety of sources.

Physical activity levels among low-income populations

In 1996, there was the first Report of the Surgeon General for Physical Activity and Health. In 2016, data were published based on the National Health Interview Survey, United States, 2014. During this 20-year period, the findings are consistent.

Low-income populations report lower levels of physical activity compared to higher-income populations. In 1996, the Surgeon General's Report found that, for the most part, the prevalence of physical inactivity was greater among persons with lower levels of education and income. "For example, there was twofold to threefold more inactivity from lowest to highest income categories: only 10.9 to 17.8 percent of participants with an annual family income of $50,000 or more reported no leisure-time physical activities, whereas 30.3 to 41.5 percent of those with an income less than $10,000 reported this" (p. 177). Twenty years later, based on the United States National Health Interview Survey, there is a clear, linear trend for the percentage of adults who met federal guidelines for aerobic activity and income levels (Morbidity and Mortality Weekly Report 2016). The poverty statuses were as follows: < 100%, 100%–199%, 200%–399%, 400%–599%, and > 600% of poverty threshold. The overall pattern was that physical activity increased as family income increased. For those with family incomes < 100% of the poverty level (i.e., low income), 34.8% met federal guidelines for aerobic physical activity. In contrast, of those with family incomes ≥ 600% of poverty level (high income), 66.8% met federal guidelines for aerobic physical activity (Figure 9.1). The basic conclusion was that income levels and physical activity levels are positively correlated. There are not comparable, extensive data analyzing sedentary behavior and income levels. However, obesity, life expectancy, and income levels have been studied.

Overall, based on the current evidence, low-income populations compared to middle- and high-income populations have lower levels of physical activity, higher

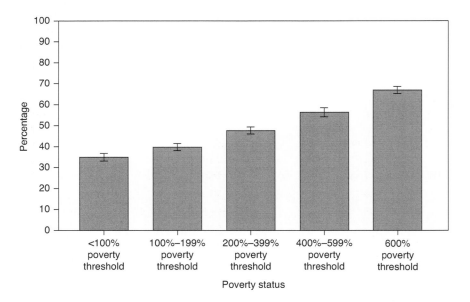

FIGURE 9.1 Percentage of adults who met federal guidelines for aerobic physical activity, by poverty status

rates of obesity, and lower rates of life expectancy. The next section examines influences on physical activity in low-income populations.

Common barriers and facilitators to physical activity among low-income populations

To promote physical activity and develop effective programs and interventions to increase physical activity, factors (referred to as correlates and determinants) most related to increasing and hindering physical activity should be identified. Ecological models are particularly well suited for studying physical activity, because physical activity happens in specific places. Studying characteristics of places that facilitate or hinder physical activity is a priority (Sallis *et al.* 2006). Levels included in ecological models of physical activity are intrapersonal (biological, psychological), interpersonal/cultural, organizational, physical environment (built, natural), and policy (laws, rules, regulations, codes) (Sallis *et al.* 2006). A recent commentary on physical activity recommended that interactions among factors 'within' or 'between' levels of the ecological model should be examined (Atkin *et al.* 2016). Based on the ecological model, the following section examines the physical environment (built environment), interpersonal (social capital), and intrapersonal (behavioral economics) levels related to physical activity and low-income populations.

Built environment, physical activity, and low-income populations

The built environment is defined as characteristics of one's surroundings, particularly neighborhood infrastructures that are human-made or modifiable, such as residential or commercial buildings, sidewalks, streets, transportation infrastructures, and parks or other open spaces (Lovasi *et al.* 2009). For example, the built environment includes neighborhood streets, walking and biking trails, parks, and exercise facilities such as gymnasiums or pools.

A major concern is the extent to which the built environment influences the physical activity patterns of low-income populations. From a historical perspective, environmental justice principles have been codified in federal law. The term "environmental justice" refers to efforts to address the disproportionate exposure to and burden of harmful environmental conditions experienced by low-income and racial/ethnic minority populations. Environmental justice is concerned with fair treatment and meaningful involvement of all people (regardless of race, ethnicity, income, national origin, or educational level) in the development, implementation, and enforcement of environmental laws, regulations, and policies (Taylor *et al.* 2006). "Fair treatment" means that no population, due to policy or economic disempowerment, is forced to bear a disproportionate burden of the negative human-health impacts. These impacts include air and water pollution and other environmental consequences resulting from industrial, municipal, and commercial operations or the execution of federal, state, local, and tribal programs and policies. Meaningful involvement is known as "procedural justice," which means that all segments of the community should participate in the decision-making process related to the placement of toxic waste sites and any other environmental hazards. The environmental justice movement has been well documented (Taylor 2000).

A second wave of the environmental justice movement has been proposed and advocated. This research agenda would specifically address environmental justice concerns with regard to improving physical activity, dietary habits, and weight patterns among disadvantaged populations (Floyd *et al.* 2009; Greenberg and Renne 2005; Taylor *et al.* 2006; Taylor *et al.* 2007a). A basic concern is expressed by the term "deprivation amplification," which is a pattern defined as follows: in places where people have fewer resources the local facilities that enable people to lead healthy lives are poorer compared to non-impoverished and non–socially deprived areas (Macintyre 2000, 2007). The term "deprivation amplification" is an extension of the "inverse care law" which postulates that places that have the fewest physicians have the greatest healthcare needs and the healthiest communities have the most physicians. Related to physical activity and low-income communities, the expectation is that there are fewer open green spaces where people can walk, jog, or take their children to play; children's playgrounds are less attractive; there are more perceived threats (e.g., litter, graffiti, youth gangs, assaults) in the environments (Macintyre 2000, 2007). This perspective is in line with the socio-environmental theories of health disparities outlined in Chapter 2. The conclusion is that residents living in poorer areas are less likely to engage in physical activity because of unfavorable features of the physical environment.

A research study conducted in the fourth-largest county in the United States directly tested the deprivation amplification principle by comparing the physical activity friendliness of low-, middle-, and high-income neighborhoods (Taylor *et al.* 2012). All block groups in the county were stratified into low-, middle-, and high-income levels according to tertiles of median household income. The median household income was $41,922, and 16.8% of the population was below the poverty level. Block groups were randomly selected from each income strata. Pairs of students and professors completed comprehensive walking audits of the selected block groups and evaluated each block group on several dimensions of physical activity friendliness.

Physical activity friendliness of each neighborhood was evaluated by four Ds which have been empirically related to physical activity (Taylor *et al.* 2012). The four Ds are population *density* (defined as the number of people per square mile, apportioned to the size of the block); land use *diversity* (defined as the mix of commercial destinations and residential land uses in an area); street *design* (defined as the extent to which neighborhoods are pedestrian- and bicycle-friendly, e.g., by having sidewalks, bicycle lanes, traffic calming features, etc.); and physical *disorder*/incivilities (defined as the extent to which litter, graffiti, stray dogs, and other unpleasant attributes are present in the environment). The best environment for promoting physical activity has population density, land use diversity, and street design conducive to activity and low levels of physical disorder/incivilities (Taylor *et al.* 2012).

To further clarify the meaning of the four Ds, the more people visible outside in a neighborhood, the more likely others will walk outside and feel safe. The more bicycle lanes; wide and connected sidewalks; and traffic-calming infrastructures such as stop signs and speed bumps, the more likely residents will be physically active. The evidence suggests that the less automobile traffic and the slowing of existing automobile traffic encourage residents to be physically active. Diversity is mixed use of an area wherein homes and business are in close proximity. For example, residents can walk to nearby restaurants, coffee shops, grocery stores, bookstores, libraries, post offices, and parks. The opposite of mixed land use (i.e., diversity) is a suburb which is automobile-dependent. Discord refers to cleanliness of streets, safety, and aesthetics of the environment (scenery, pleasantness of surroundings, grass, flowers, shrubbery, etc.).

The findings of the study (Taylor *et al.* 2012) to test deprivation amplification found that two of the four Ds (density and diversity) favored the low-income populations. One D favored the high-income population (discord); street design and income were not related. The study findings were consistent with a review (Lovasi *et al.* 2009) that reported low-income populations had greater physical and social disorder but had advantages related to greater walkability as commonly measured.

The obvious question is that if the built environment favors low-income populations for physical activity why do low-income populations report lower rates of physical activity? This discrepancy has been referred as the "urban paradox" (Lopez and Hynes 2006). First, "deprivation amplification" was revisited by the original author (Macintyre 2007) because empirical studies show that place does not always disadvantage poorer neighborhoods, which is consistent with the findings from Taylor *et al.* (2012). The revised "deprivation amplification" emphasized that the quality, meaning, perceived accessibility, and relevance of resources as well as perceived safety from crime and traffic may be more important than the presence or absence of physical activity resources and walkability (Macintyre 2007). An alternative explanation is that the weaker associations of the built environment and physical activity among low-income populations may reflect life circumstances in which more basic needs eclipse the influence of the built environment (Lovasi *et al.* 2009; Taylor *et al.* 2007). For example, if you are a "captive walker" dependent on transit without access to an automobile, the features of the built environment are less salient and related to physical activity (Lovasi *et al.* 2009).

Lopez and Hynes (2006) addressed the "urban paradox" by proposing other factors of the urban, built, and physical environment that undermine any positive features of the environment that facilitate, in principle, being physically active in low-income communities. The other factors include documented health risks such as the stress of poverty, racism, and violence; discrimination in health services; and food insecurity.

As noted, there are several explanations for the "urban paradox." However, most important, any interventions and changes to the built environment and parks should include prior to program implementation a careful assessment of the impact on low-income populations. Retrofitting the environment and building walking and bicycle trails that exacerbate physical activity disparities should be carefully recon-sidered. On the other hand, there are strategies to evaluate the environment that can increase the physical activity levels of low-income populations (Dolash *et al.* 2015).

Social capital, physical activity, and low-income populations

Social capital represents various collective aspects of a social environment – such as trust, shared values, willingness to intervene against unacceptable behavior, will-ingness to do favors, and access to information (Broyles *et al.* 2011). In a study, among adult park users, communities with higher levels of social capital had parks with greater daily numbers of observed park users and had more energy expended within the park than communities with lower levels of social capital. The authors concluded that interventions to improve the social environments in which parks reside should be conducted to promote increased physical activity among park users (Broyles *et al.* 2011). The social environment can be a critical factor to promote physical activity in low-income populations.

In another study, parents of fifth graders were surveyed about perceptions of their neighborhood social processes and systematic observations of the physical envi-ronment were analyzed (Franzini *et al.* 2010). Higher-poverty neighborhoods and non-White neighborhoods had better accessibility for physical activity; however, these neighborhoods were less safe, less comfortable, and less pleasurable for outdoor physical activity, and had less favorable social processes (i.e., collective efficacy, col-lective socialization of children, and satisfaction with neighborhood). The authors concluded that interventions to reduce disparities in physical activity should address not only the physical environment, but also social processes favorable to physical activity (Franzini *et al.* 2010).

Behavioral economics, physical activity, and low-income populations

Behavioral economics has been defined as the application of psychology to eco-nomics to better understand the boundaries of rational decision making and factors that lead to suboptimal behavioral choices (Leonard *et al.* 2013). For example, in an economic experiment to measure time preferences, participants chose between receiving a smaller amount of money now or a larger amount of money six months from now. Participants who chose the six-month option were classified as having a patient time preference (Leonard *et al.* 2013).

Two studies directly investigated behavioral economics and physical activ-ity among low-income populations. In one study (Leonard *et al.* 2013) with low-income individuals (median household income – $19,939), based on actual economic experiments, the authors found that individuals who were more tolerant of financial risks and had more patient time preferences were more likely to report physical activity. The authors concluded that higher levels of financial risk aversion and lower levels of patient time preferences can represent a barrier for engaging in physical activity for low-income populations. With a group of low-income individuals (median household income − $19,939), another study (Shuval *et al.* 2015) examined the relationship between time preferences and physical activity. The authors found that individuals who had more patient time preferences were more likely to engage in physical activity. Specifically, those with a future orientation were 29% more likely to meet physical activity guidelines; those with checking/savings accounts were more than twice as likely to meet physical activity guidelines, controlling for income and other potential confounders. Using behavioral economics to promote physical activity in low-income populations is an emerging area of study (Zimmerman 2009).

Healthy Weight Disparity Index

In research on physical activity, obesity, and other health indices, analysis by income levels should be a priority. For example, a recent study (Taylor *et al.* 2015) illustrated that the typical obesity rankings by state can be misleading in terms of which states are the best exemplars. The authors applied a Healthy Weight Disparity Index based on an algorithm that identified differences by income levels and obesity rates. Categories of household income were designated as low (less than $35,000 per year), middle ($35,000 to less than $75,000), and high ($75,000 or more). The BMI rankings and Healthy Weight Disparity Index rankings when applied to all 50 states and Washington, D.C., were discordant. For example, Washington, D.C., had the 9th lowest BMI ranking and the 49th worse index ranking, which means there was substantial disparity among the high-, middle-, and low-income populations related to obesity (Taylor *et al.* 2015). This study highlights the importance of analyzing income-related disparities to better identify geographic variability related to health and physical activity.

Intervention strategies

Three reviews have examined the evidence of physical activity interventions among low-income populations. The first review (Taylor *et al.* 1998) concluded that more focused and consistent theory-based research is needed to advance the field. Also, long-term evaluations and an infrastructure to sustain the intervention should be priorities. Another review (Chaudhary and Kreiger 2007) recommended that intervention strategies for low-income groups should address barriers to health behavior change such as literacy, accessibility, knowledge, skill level, and lack of time and money. A third review (Cleland *et al.* 2012) reported that 9 of the 14 effective studies were informed by a theoretical framework of behavior change (e.g., Social Cognitive Theory and Socio-Ecological Model). Several studies reported that transportation may be necessary to provide for participants if the intervention site is beyond walking distance from home, school, or place of work (Cleland *et al.* 2012). Frequent contact over longer periods was associated with effectiveness; without frequent contact, physical activity declined after six months. This review (Cleland *et al.* 2012) found evidence for the effectiveness of adult group-based and community-based interventions to increase physical activity in socioeconomically disadvantaged communities. Interventions delivered to groups of children and adolescents were found to be ineffective. The authors concluded that some programs have demonstrated increases in physical activity but no unique recipe for success was identified. Based on these reviews, research with physical activity interventions among low-income populations is sparse and replete with methodological limitations.

In addition to the reviews, recent empirical studies have investigated a variety of approaches to promote physical activity in low-income populations with various levels of success. These approaches have included school-based health promotion; low-cost, in-home education-based intervention; motivational interviewing; community-based physical activity intervention; intervention based on Health Promotion Model and Self Determination Theory for middle school girls; a stair-climbing intervention; and a community/school-based program to promote walking and running among low-income, elementary school children (Bastian *et al.* 2015; Davis *et al.* 2013; Everson-Hock *et al.* 2013; Hardcastle *et al.* 2012; Robbins *et al.* 2013; Ryan *et al.* 2011; Springer *et al.* 2012). In summary, much more research is needed among low-income populations and physical activity. The majority of effective interventions were based on behavioral sciences theories. More high-quality studies with longer-term follow-up are required. A test of the effectiveness of an intervention is the RE-AIM model which assesses reach, effectiveness-efficacy, adoption, implementation, and maintenance (Glasgow *et al.* 1999). As new interventions are developed to promote physical activity in low-income populations, the RE-AIM model is a useful framework.

BOX 9.1   EVIDENCE FOR PRACTICE: LOW-INCOME, PREDOMINANTLY HISPANIC COMMUNITIES PROMOTING PHYSICAL ACTIVITY IN PARKS

There is an absence of data related to what park features are associated with physical activity among predominantly low-income Hispanic neighborhoods. The purpose of the study was to assess factors associated with park use and physical activity among park users in predominantly low-income Hispanic neighborhoods.

The authors used a mixed-methods approach to identify what features in the park promote and hinder physical activity in low-income Hispanic neighborhoods. Importantly, in addition to audits of park features and observations of physical activity in the parks (i.e., estimates of physical activity energy expenditure per kcal/kg/minute per person), the authors conducted park user interviews with Hispanic neighborhood residents to assess motivators and barriers to park use. Six parks were studied. The authors found that parks that were renovated had greater physical activity energy expenditure scores than non-renovated parks. Basketball courts had a significantly greater number of vigorously active park users than tennis courts. Thematic analysis of park user interviews was conducted collectively and by each park. Thematic analysis of qualitative data revealed four recurrent themes: motivation to be physically active, using the play spaces in the park, parks as the main place for physical activity, and social support for using parks.

Renovations to park amenities, such as increasing basketball courts and trail availability, could potentially increase physical activity among low-socioeconomic-status Hispanic populations. Notably, the findings from this study can guide park renovations and identify what features are important in the development of new parks to promote physical activity. In addition, this mixed-methods approach can be used to identify similarities and differences by age, gender, and family composition (number and ages of children) within the target population to promote physical activity at parks (Dolash *et al.* 2015).

Implications for practice

The health benefits of physical activity are dose-related; so compared to no physical activity, individuals who are physically active at half the recommended levels of physical activity have a 14% lower risk of coronary heart disease (Sattelmair *et al.* 2011). Careful evaluations of future physical activity interventions among low-income populations are needed to provide evidence of best practice. Physical activity interventions to increase physical activity should strive to eliminate barriers based on social, cultural, educational, and economic situations and capitalize on resources, assets, and resilience that reside within the community. One approach, based on this principle, is Community Based Participatory Research (CBPR).

Community Based Participatory Research (CBPR)

Community Based Participatory Approaches represent a true and synergistic partnership between researchers and community members to develop effective and sustainable interventions to increase physical activity in a target community. This approach is helpful for tailoring to the population (constituent-involving) and involves some of the formative research outlined in Chapter 3. These strategies combine qualitative and quantitative procedures to understand and summarize the perceptions and beliefs of community members and exemplify the effectiveness of participatory approaches.

New York City is a walkable city given the transit and subway systems, connected and walkable street patterns, and people walking all the time. Given this setting, what environmental changes would low-income, racial, and ethnic minority women recommend to promote physical activity? Using formative research strategies, a study found that low-income African American and Latina women reported that more police protection, cleaner streets, removal of drugs from streets, more street lights, and no unleashed dogs such as Pit Bulls and Rottweilers would promote a more physical activity–friendly environment in their New York City neighborhoods (Taylor *et al.* 2007). Involving residents in all stages of initiating, developing, and implementing a physical activity intervention can increase effectiveness and sustainability.

Community Energy Balance Framework

We need to better understand how high-priority groups, including low-income communities, adapt to and function in the surrounding community. The Community Energy Balance Framework can help achieve this objective (Kumanyika *et al.* 2012). This framework advocates that researchers, practitioners, and community organizers working with high-priority groups should contextualize their food- and physical activity–related sociocultural perspectives by accounting for relevant historical, political, and structural contexts. Importantly, the health consequences of cultural-contextual stressors and accommodating these stressors are emphasized. For intervention development, the Community Energy Balance Framework identifies several factors and elements in three broad domains: cultural-contextual influences, intervention settings and agents, and intervention targets (Kumanyika *et al.* 2012). In summary, this framework recognizes current sociocultural factors as well as historical influences on physical activity patterns of high-priority groups and can be used for program or intervention development.

Policy and ordinance decision making

Urban planning policies and ordinances can have a broad impact on the built environment, physical activity, and healthy eating. An environmental justice issue is whether policy development includes representatives from all segments of the community. A central concern is whether low-income and racial/ethnic minority populations fully participate in policy decisions (i.e., procedural justice) that affect their neighborhoods and health of residents (Taylor *et al.* 2006).

There is no single, simple strategy for eliminating physical activity–related disparities among low-income populations. We need innovative, comprehensive, and multifaceted strategies emanating from Community Based Participatory Approaches such as reported in Taylor *et al.* (2007) and theoretical and conceptual frameworks such as the Community Energy Balance Framework (Kumanyika *et al.* 2012). As noted at the beginning of the chapter, low-income populations are a crucial high-priority group. Therefore, comprehensive and rigorous research to promote physical activity in this population has the potential to carry over to all target groups.

Summary points

- Compared to high- and middle-income populations, low-income populations report lower rates of physical activity.

- Built environment features are insufficient to account for the lower rates of physical activity among low-income populations.
- Low income has not been consistently defined in the literature on physical activity and low-income populations.
- Community Based Participatory Approaches are recommended to initiate, implement, and sustain interventions in low-income communities.
- Interventions based on behavioral sciences theoretical frameworks have been the most effective in low-income populations.
- More rigorous research is needed to promote physical activity among low-income populations.

Critical thinking questions

1 Would financial assistance increase physical activity and improve health among low-income populations?
2 What changes in the physical environment can be implemented to reduce health disparities rather than exacerbate health disparities related to physical activity and low-income populations?
3 Would you focus on income, education, or racial and ethnic identity to understand physical activity patterns and how to increase physical activity?
4 Think about the neighborhood you grew up in. How would you describe it from an environmental justice perspective?

Acknowledgments

The author acknowledges Helena VonVille, MLS, MPH, Director of the Library, The University of Texas Health Science Center at Houston, School of Public Health, for her assistance in searching and retrieving literature from several electronic databases. Also, the author acknowledges the helpful assistance of Karen L. Pepkin, MA, in reviewing and critiquing the chapter.

References

Atkin, A. J., Sluijs, E. M. F. van, Dollman, J., Taylor, W. C. and Stanley, R. M. (2016). 'Identifying correlates and determinants of physical activity in youth: How can we advance the field?'. *Preventive Medicine*, 87: 167–169.

Bastian, K. A., Maximova, K., McGavock, J. and Veugelers, P. (2015). 'Does school-based health promotion affect physical activity on weekends? and, does it reach those students most in need of health promotion?'. *PLoS One*, 10(10): e0137987.

Broyles, S., Mowen, A., Theall, K., Gustat, J. and Rung, A. (2011). 'Integrating social capital into park use and active living framework'. *American Journal of Preventive Medicine*, 40: 522–529.

Chaudhary, N. and Kreiger, N. (2007). 'Nutrition and physical activity interventions for low-income populations'. *Canadian Journal of Dietetic Practice and Research*, 68: 201–206.

Chetty, R., Stepner, M., Abraham, S., Lin, S., Scuderi, B., Turner, N., Bergeron, A. and Cutler, D. (2016). 'The association between income and life expectancy in the United States, 2001–2014', *JAMA*, 315(16): 1750–1766. Published online April 10, 2016.

Cleland, C. L., Tully, M. A., Kee, F. and Cupples, M. E. (2012). 'The effectiveness of physical activity interventions in socio-economically disadvantaged communities: A systematic review'. *Preventive Medicine*, 54: 371–380.

Columbia University's National Center for Children in Poverty. (2016). *National data were calculated from the 2014 American community survey, representing information from 2014*, State data were calculated from the 2010–2014 American Community Survey, representing information from the years 2010 to 2014.

Davis, A. M., Gallagher, K., Taylor, M., Canter, K., Gillette, M. D., Karen, K. and Nelson, E. (2013). 'An in-home intervention to improve nutrition, physical activity and knowledge among low-income teen mothers and their children: Results from a pilot study'. *Journal of Developmental Behavioral Pediatrics*, 34(8): 609–615. October, 34.

Dolash, K., He, M., Yin, Z. and Sosa, E. T. (2015). 'Factors that influence park use and physical activity in predominantly Hispanic and low-income neighborhoods'. *Journal of Physical Activity and Health*, 12: 462–469.

Everson-Hock, E. S., Johnson, M., Jones, R., Woods, E., Goyder, E., Payne, N. and Chilsott, J. (2013). 'Community-based dietary and physical activity interventions in low socioeconomic groups in UK: A mixed methods systematic review'. *Preventive Medicine*, 56: 265–272.

Floyd, M. F., Taylor, W. C. and Whitt-Glover, M. C. (2009). 'Measurement of park and recreation environments that support physical activity in low-income communities of color: Highlights of challenges and recommendations'. *American Journal of Preventive Medicine*, 36: s156–s160.

Franzini, L., Taylor, W. C., Elliott, M. N., Cuccaro, P., Tortolero, S. R., Gilliland, M. J., Grunbaum, J. and Schuster, M. A. (2010). 'Neighborhood characteristics favorable to outdoor physical activity: Disparities by socioeconomic and racial/ethnic composition'. *Health & Place*, 16: 267–274.

Glasgow, R. E., Vogt, T. M. and Boles, S. M. (1999). 'Evaluating the public health impact of health promotion interventions: The REAIM framework'. *American Journal of Public Health*, 89: 1322–1327.

Greenberg, M. and Renne, J. (2005). 'Where does walkability matter the most? An environmental justice interpretation of New Jersey data'. *Journal of Urban Health*, 82: 90–100.

Hardcastle, S., Blake, N. and Hagger, M. S. (2012). 'The effectiveness of a motivational interviewing primary-care based intervention on physical activity and predictors of change in a disadvantaged community'. *Journal of Behavioral Medicine*, 35: 318–333.

Kumanyika, S., Taylor, W. C., Grier, S. A., Lassiter, V., Lancaster, K. J., Morssink, C. B. and Renzaho, A. M. N. (2012). 'Community energy balance: A framework for contextualizing cultural influences on high risk of obesity in ethnic minority populations'. *Preventive Medicine*, 55: 371–381.

Leonard, T., Shuval, K., Oliveira, A., Skinner, S. C., Eckel, C. and Murdoch, J. C. (2013). 'Health behavior and behavioral economics: Economic preferences and physical activity stages of change in a low-income African American community'. *American Journal of Health Promotion*, 27: 211–221.

Lopez, R. P. and Hynes, P. (2006). 'Obesity, physical activity, and the urban environment: Public'. *Environmental Health: A Global Access Science Source*, 5: 25.

Lovasi, G. S., Hutson, M. A., Guerra, M. and Neckerman, K. M. (2009). 'Built environments and obesity in disadvantaged populations'. *Epidemiologic Reviews*, 31: 7–20.

Macintyre, S. (2000). 'The social patterning of exercise behaviours: The role of personal and local resources'. *British Journal of Sports Medicine*, 34: 6.

Macintyre, S. (2007). 'Deprivation amplification revisited; or, is it always true that poorer places have poorer access to resources for healthy diets and physical activity'. *International Journal of Behavioral Nutrition and Physical Activity*, 4: 32.

Morbidity and Mortality Weekly Report. (2016). 'Percentage★ of adults who met federal guidelines for aerobic physical activity, by poverty status: National health interview survey, United States, 2014.' 65: No. 17 459. US Department of Health and Human Services/ Centers for Disease Control and Prevention 6.

Robbins, L. B., Pfeiffer, K. A., Vermeesch, A., Resnicow, K., You, Z., An, L. and Wesolek, S. M. (2013). '"Girls on the move" intervention protocol for increasing physical activity among low-active underserved urban girls: A group randomized trial'. *BMC Public Health*, 13: 474.

Ryan, J., Lyon, K., Webb, O. J., Eves, F. F. and Ryan, C. G. (2011). 'Promoting physical activity in a low socioeconomic area: Results from an intervention targeting stair climbing'. *Preventive Medicine*, 52: 352–354.

Sallis, J. F., Cervero, R. B., Ascher, W., Henderson, K. A., Kraft, M. K. and Kerr, J. (2006). 'An ecological approach to creating active living communities'. *Annual Review of Public Health*, 27: 297–322.

Sattelmair, J., Pertman, J., Ding, E. L., Kohl, H. W., 3rd, Haskell, W. and Lee, I. M. (2011). 'Dose response between physical activity and risk of coronary heart disease: A meta-analysis'. *Circulation*, 124: 789–795.

Shuval, K., Si, X., Nguyen, B. and Leonard, T. (2015). 'Utilizing behavioral economics to understand adherence to physical activity guidelines among a low-income urban community'. *Journal of Physical Activity and Health*, 12: 947–953.

Springer, A. E., Kelder, S. H., Ranjit, N., Hochberg-Garrett, H., Crow, S. and Delk, J. (2012). 'Promoting physical activity and fruit and vegetable consumption through a community-school partnership: The effects of marathon kids® on low-income elementary school children in Texas'. *Journal of Physical Activity and Health*, 9: 739–753.

Taylor, D. E. (2000). 'The rise of the environmental justice paradigm: Injustice framing and the social construction of environmental discourses'. *American Behavioral Scientist*, 43: 508–580.

Taylor, W. C., Baranowski, T. and Young, D. R. (1998). 'Physical activity interventions in low-income, ethnic minority, and populations with disability'. *American Journal of Preventive Medicine*, 15: 334–343.

Taylor, W. C., Floyd, M. F., Whitt-Glover, M. C. and Brooks, J. (2007a). 'Environmental justice: A framework for collaboration between public health and parks and recreation fields to study disparities in physical activity'. *Journal of Physical Activity and Health*, 4: s50–s63.

Taylor, W. C., Franzini, L., Olvera, N., Poston, W. S. C. and Lin, G. (2012). 'Environmental audits of friendliness toward physical activity in three income levels'. *Journal of Urban Health*, 89: 296–307.

Taylor, W. C., Paxton, R. J., Fischer, L. S. and Bellows, L. L. (2015). 'The healthy weight disparity index: Why we need it to solve the obesity crisis'. *Journal of Health Care for the Poor and Underserved*, 26: 1186–1199.

Taylor, W. C., Poston, W. S. C., Jones, L. and Kraft, M. K. (2006). 'Environmental justice: Obesity, physical activity, and healthy eating'. *Journal of Physical Activity & Health*, 3: s30–s54.

Taylor, W. C., Sallis, J. F., Lees, E., Hepworth, J. T., Feliz, K., Volding, D. C., Cassels, A. and Tobin, J. N. (2007b). 'Changing social and built environments to promote physical activity: Recommendations from low income, urban women'. *Journal of Physical Activity & Health*, 4: 54–65.

United States Department of Health and Human Services. (1996). '*Physical activity and health: A report of the surgeon general.*' Atlanta, GA: U.S. Department of Health and Human Services, Centers for Disease Control and Prevention, National Center for Chronic Disease Prevention and Health Promotion.

United States Department of Health and Human Services. (2016). '*The poverty guidelines* [Online].' published in the Federal Register on January 25, 2016, United States Government Publishing Office, Washington District of Columbia US. Available: www.gpo.gov/fdsys/pk (Accessed May 24 2016).

United States Department of Housing and Urban Development. (2016). '*HUD: 2016 low income documentation system* [Online].' Available: www.huduser.gov/portal/datasets/il/il16/index.html (Accessed May 24 2016).

Wang, Y. and Beydoun, M. A. (2007). 'The obesity epidemic in the United States: Gender, age, socioeconomic, racial/ethnic, and geographic characteristics: A systematic review and meta-regression analysis'. *Epidemiologic Reviews*, 29: 6–28.

Zimmerman, F. J. (2009). 'Using behavioral economics to promote physical activity'. *Preventive Medicine*, 49: 289–291.

10

PHYSICAL ACTIVITY AMONG RURAL POPULATIONS

Deborah H. John and Katherine B. Gunter

Understanding rural populations

In the U.S., the health and habits of nearly 60 million people are greatly influenced by the rural context (U.S. Census Bureau 2012) and culture where they live, travel, learn, work, and play. Compared with their urban counterparts, rural populations experience higher rates of chronic disease (Meit *et al.* 2014); preventable conditions such as obesity, diabetes, and injury (Eberhardt and Pamuk 2004); unhealthy lifestyle behaviors such as smoking, physical inactivity, and poor diet (Hartley 2004); as well as automobile reliance and longer commutes (Zhang *et al.* 2014). Whether through the physical attributes of the rural landscapes, structural features of the rural built environment, or the culture and composition of their rural communities, including the distribution of intersecting social determinants – gender, age, race and ethnicity, SES, and family type – rural populations are at greater risk of health problems for which physically active rural living may be the solution.

One of the challenges facing an examination of health and physical activity in rural populations is how to define and appropriate the notion of rurality. For example, "rural" may provoke images of people and/or places: farming families and farms, ranch hands riding the open range, fisherwomen and coastal habitats, country folk in historic villages and small towns, retirees living in planned developments, even sparsely populated expanses of forests, deserts, mountains, wetlands, or seashores. Rural as a group classification is socially and contextually constructed (Trussell and Shaw 2009), as are other demographic categories such as race, gender, and (dis)ability (refer to Chapter 2). In addition to being aware of the intersection of demographic categories when considering rural people, understanding how a definition of "rural" is applied has significant implications for studying and promoting physical activity in this priority population.

ꞓientific literature, conceptual definitions of rural include (1) low
⌐ ur low population density, (2) reliance on agriculture and extractive
⌐ɑral resource industries, (3) a residual condition of "not being urban" (Crosby
et al. 2012). Population thresholds used to classify communities as rural (versus
urban) range from 2,500 up to 50,000, depending on the definition source. At the
county-level, the U.S. Department of Agriculture (USDA) scales rural–urban on a
nonmetropolitan to metropolitan continuum, or by the degree of urban influence.
In both cases "rural" is being characterized by population size, degree of urbanization, and adjacency to an urban metro area (Cromartie and Parker 2016) with
smaller populations, less urbanization, and located farther from an urban center
being characteristics typical of "rural" communities. Nonetheless, inconsistently
applied definitions and classifications make comparisons across scientific studies and
identification of effective strategies challenging. Whatever definition is identified,
research findings must be interpreted considering differences across rural communities with regard to land use, natural amenities, and proximity to resources, in
addition to demographic variables already discussed. In this chapter, we accept the
definitions of rural presented by the authors of all literature cited, and acknowledge
the inherent limitations.

Demographic characteristics

The rural areas of the U.S. for the 2010 Census contain 19.3% of the population
compared to the 80.7% contained in urban areas. Approximately 78% of the rural
population, about 60 million people, are White and non-Hispanic, compared to 64%
of the population in the nation as a whole. Rural minority populations include Hispanics (9.3%), African Americans (8.2%), and Native Americans (< 2%), although
more than half of all Native Americans reside in rural areas. Compared with their
urban counterparts, rural populations experience higher rates of chronic and preventable disease and injury, tobacco use, physical inactivity, poor diet, and less access
to preventative and health service (Meit *et al.* 2014). Minority populations in rural
areas have significantly lower levels of educational attainment and higher poverty
when compared to the White and non-Hispanic rural populations, and are more
likely to live in substandard and cost-burdened housing. Many rural minorities are
clustered geographically in regions closely tied to historical, social, and economic
dynamics, and may especially experience in communities that have large minority
populations social and economic conditions that continue to lag far behind those of
their White counterparts and urban populations overall (Stern 2014).

Health disparities and inequities among rural populations

"Rurality" is recognized by *Healthy People 2020* (US ODPHP 2014) as one of 14
health disparities in the United States. Rural U.S. residents face a unique combination of factors that contribute to inequalities in health, preventive services, and
medical care not observed in urban areas. In this chapter, we discuss how the rural

context – cultural and social norms, educational attainment, economic weakening, lack of political attention, and assumptions of accessible material resources despite the isolation of living in rural and remote landscapes – conspires to make it harder for rural individuals, families, groups, and populations to live healthy, active life-styles. While access to health care remains the highest priority for rural people (Bolin *et al.* 2010), nutrition and unhealthy weight status rose to second (from tenth in 2000) highest priority. In 2010 a new rural health priority emerged – physical activity. Ranked as seventh in importance to rural populations, this priority area is closely linked to other rural priorities, including nutrition and obesity, heart disease, diabetes, and a plethora of chronic conditions (Bolin *et al.* 2010). The *Rural Healthy People 2020* initiative focus on physical activity and health includes a review of the significant health benefits of physical activity. A variety of options available to rural populations for age groups ranging from older adults to children is presented, as are rural-specific barriers to increasing physical activity that may require alternative strategies and interventions (Bolin *et al.* 2010). Despite being informed by data representing geographically diverse rural stakeholders' priorities (West, Midwest, South, Northeast), the report neglects to address health disparities within rural populations that may be determined not only by geographic location but by intersecting categories of difference within rural people, such as gender, race/ethnicity, socio-economics, and ability with age. For example, older adults were ranked as the eighth priority by rural stakeholders' poll; yet within the older adult category, diversity and disparities exist that may differently determine accessibility of preventive care, community resources, and active living programs. For instance, different solutions may be warranted to support physical activity in older rural populations who are African American or Latina women and poor versus White and poor, regardless of their attitude, ability, or as advised by their healthcare provider. Acknowledging diversity within and among rural communities, including the aging of rural America, and income, racial/ethnic inequalities (Berry and Kirschner 2013) as well as regional cultural and geographic differences, should serve as a reminder that not all rural communities are the same and that there is no "one-size-fits-all" approach to addressing physical activity disparities and inactivity in rural populations. Understanding the influence of intersectionality and social determinants of health provides a lens through which physical activity influences in rural populations and evidence-based strategies for promoting physical activity among this population are examined and understood as culturally and contextually appropriate.

Metabolic health

Obesity is of epidemic proportions worldwide. Despite national attention, obesity rates in the U.S. have risen significantly among youth and adults over the last three decades (Ogden *et al.* 2014). While the rise in prevalence among all youth seems to have stabilized over the past decade (Ogden *et al.* 2016), rural youth experience higher prevalence of unhealthy weight and have 26% greater odds of obesity compared to non-rural youth (Johnson and Johnson 2015). The obesity epidemic

ed by consistent lower daily and weekly energy expenditure in comparison to higher dietary energy intake that has sustained over time. Obesity and obesity-related behaviors, specifically physical inactivity, are also associated with significantly increased risk of a plethora of chronic diseases and health conditions that have devastating consequences, including co-morbidities, disability, and increased mortality (Trivedi *et al.* 2015). Beyond the significant toll on life quality and quantity, obesity and related health complications are driving up healthcare costs, threatening workforce productivity, and employers' bottom lines.

Many risk factors have been associated with obesity, including rural residency (Befort, Nazir, and Perri 2012; Johnson and Johnson 2015). Approximately 20% of the population lives in the rural geographies that encompass over 70% of the U.S. landscape (Kusmin 2015). Rural residents have higher rates of obesity and chronic diseases than urban residents (Jones *et al.* 2009). Physical inactivity is associated with higher rates of chronic diseases and obesity (Trivedi *et al.* 2015), and some research suggests that rural residents are less physically active than urban residents (Fan, Wen, and Kowaleski-Jones 2014). When compared to their urban counterparts, rural adults report higher physical inactivity and limitation in activity due to chronic health conditions (Eberhardt and Pamuk 2004), many of which are associated with insufficient physical activity and mostly preventable through healthy lifestyle behavioral patterns sustained over the lifespan. Wu and associates (2011) suggest that individually focused interventions, like behavioral counseling, effectively impact targeted behaviors but are costly. Furthermore, even the most cost-effective individual-level treatments are ineffective in achieving broad and enduring behavioral outcomes or public health impact, relying on individuals to maintain health actions despite disparate demographic conditions (Beauchamp *et al.* 2014). Instead, interventions that change the environmental context to make healthy behaviors the default, regardless of socioeconomic or geographic conditions, require less individual effort and have great potential for public health impact.

Rural contexts

Rural community contexts pose unique challenges for rural folks and families to develop and maintain good health and sustain health-promoting and protective lifestyle habits that differ from those faced by people residing in more urban settings. Rural families have higher rates of poverty, fewer community resources, less access to preventive services and health care, greater geographic dispersion, and more transportation challenges (e.g., lack of public transit, greater travel distance) than urban residents (Sumaya 2012). To help to meet the chronic disease burden in the U.S., and promote healthy communities, the CDC *Partnerships to Improve Community Health* program builds on a body of knowledge developed through previously funded CDC programs, and supports implementation of evidence-based strategies to improve the health of communities and reduce the prevalence of chronic disease (CDC 2016). *Partnership* communities are implementing population-based strategies, tailored to individual community needs, across various settings (community institutions/organizations, healthcare facilities, schools, and worksites), to create greater access to healthier environments and address risk factors that contribute to tobacco use and exposure, poor nutrition, physical inactivity, and lack of equitable access to opportunities for chronic disease prevention, risk reduction, and disease management. Establishment of community conditions to support healthy behaviors and promote effective management of chronic conditions will deliver healthier students to schools, healthier workers to employers and businesses, and a healthier population to the healthcare system (Bauer *et al.* 2014). Although this collaborative approach is intended to improve health equity and prevent chronic diseases by building communities that promote a culture of health (Lavizzo-Mourey 2014) rather than disease, have more accessible and direct health care and preventive services, and focus the health system on improving population health, there is little of the evidence supporting population approaches or policy, systems, and environmental strategies that is derived from rural people or places (Kahn *et al.* 2002).

Physical activity among rural populations

Nearly one-quarter of the U.S. population lives in rural places. Lower levels of physical activity among rural relative to urban residents have been suggested as an important contributor to rural-urban health disparity; however, empirical evidence is sparse. Physical inactivity is associated with higher rates of chronic diseases and obesity (Trivedi *et al.* 2015), and some research suggests that rural residents are less physically active (Fan, Wen, and Kowaleski-Jones 2014) compared to urban residents. It is often assumed that rural populations can engage in physical activity more than their urban counterparts because of the expansive amounts of green space and natural environmental amenities. Additionally, popular thought is that many rural occupations are conducive to physical activity, such as those in the agriculture, forestry, mining, fishing, or natural amenity–based recreation industries, which may hold true for a population subgroup, or proportion of the rural labor force, and apply seasonally. Attributes of rural places reportedly make it difficult for residents to safely and actively transport to and from destinations, including school, access a variety of affordable recreation facilities, regularly utilize public trails and parks, and sustainably resource exercise and recreational physical activity programs (Umstattd Meyer *et al.* 2016a).

Adult physical activity

Fan, Wen, and Kowaleski-Jones (2014) examined rural-urban differences in physical activity measured both objectively (examining intensity by time in exercise bout) and subjectively (total, leisure, household, and transportation) in a nationally representative adult sample. They further organized the sample into urban and two types of rural categories to analyze urban-rural and within-rural differences in physical activity. They found adults residing in rural areas compared to urban were less active in long-bout (10 minutes or longer), high-intensity physical activity, but the urban-rural difference disappeared at the lower-intensity activity threshold measured using accelerometers. However, rural residents self-reported more total physical activity than urban residents with differences primarily attributed to household physical activity. Within the rural category, residents in smaller (less than 10,000 persons) rural areas were more active than residents in larger (10,000–49,999 persons) rural areas, indicating that physical activity did not vary in line with degree of rurality as defined (Fan, Wen, and Kowaleski-Jones 2014). Parks, Housemann, and Brownson (2003) found suburban, higher-income adults were more than twice as likely to meet physical activity recommendations compared to rural, lower-income residents. Older rural residents are less likely to meet the U.S. recommendations for physical activity (US ODPHP 2008) in comparison to their urban counterparts, and report unique challenges to aging actively in rural places (Hunter *et al.* 2009; John and Gunter 2015). On closer examination, John and colleagues (2014) found older people living in rural versus suburban communities had lower odds of walking around their neighborhoods, which were less supportive of walking for exercise or transportation. Healthy, older women of higher income had higher odds of participating in strength and balance exercise; however, community-based options were under-resourced or not available in rural communities (John, Abi Nader, Ghavami, and Gunter 2014). Rural women compared to men, especially those residing in southern states, were reported to be more sedentary than urban women, and being inactive among rural women was positively associated with being older age, less educated, and American Indian/Alaskan Native, and African American (Wilcox *et al.* 2000).

Youth physical activity

Studies comparing physical activity in rural compared to urban youth provide a variety of findings. In a narrative review of the existing literature comparing rural and urban youth in the U.S., McCormack and Meendering (2016) found differences despite inconsistencies in the criteria used to define and measure physical activity and rural. When compared to urban youth, nine studies showed rural youth to be generally more active, three studies showed rural youth to be more sport involved, and three showed rural youth engaged in more sedentary screen time, although another indicated no rural-urban categorical differences. In this same analysis, five studies using objective measures of physical activity showed no difference in MVPA, weekly energy expenditure, sedentary time, or meeting PA recommendations between rural and urban youth (McCormack and Meendering 2016). On the other hand, rural children have been found to engage in less MVPA activity when compared to urban children (Davis *et al.* 2008; Moore *et al.* 2013). Gender differences between rural, suburban, and urban youth were also studied. Moore and colleagues (2013) found while no differences emerged between boys based on rurality, there was an inverse relationship between boys' daily MVPA and school grade. Rural girls accumulated more daily MVPA than suburban or urban girls and were more likely to accumulate > 60 minutes MVPA per day. In a study using objective measures with a large sample of rural elementary school students,

Gunter, Abi Nader, and John (2015) found more MVPA was associated with lower BMI, independent of sex, grade, or device wear time; MVPA was higher in healthy-weight rural children when compared to obese children; and no rural children were meeting the recommendations for MVPA (Gunter, Abi Nader, and John 2015).

Common barriers and facilitators to physical activity for rural populations

Individual and social

Research suggests that the social ecological model (outlined in Chapter 1) is a relevant framework for understanding common barriers and enablers to physical activity for rural populations, although individual-level factors in rural populations are similar to those emerging generally. For example, Jahns and colleagues (2014) found rural-dwelling, Native American adults reported knowledge of health benefits of physical activity and the perception of physical activity as enjoyable, including feeling good when working out, as facilitators to following physical activity recommendations. Physical activity barriers were identified as lack of knowledge of how to fit physical activity into a daily schedule, work, caring for family members, and prioritizing sedentary activities (Jahns *et al.* 2014). In another study, women residing in rural areas reported contradictory barriers and facilitators to PA, and those barriers and facilitators were found to differ by age groups (Zimmermann, Carnahan, and Peacock 2016). Across all age groups, knowledge about or experiences with the benefits of physical activity emerged as an individual facilitator to physical activity. Individual-level barriers included lack of awareness about the importance of physical activity or how to be physically active (all age groups), personal health challenges (women older than 30), and motivation difficulty in maintaining a routine (women older than 50). Social facilitators shared across age groups included women motivating one another. Other facilitators emerged and differed by age group, such as desire to be a role model for or spend time with one's children (women younger than 50), and for older women (over 50) desire to do things for or with one's family and social support. Shared barriers to physical activity emerged as competing priorities, caretaking responsibilities, and lack of time. Sedentary society emerged as a barrier but only for younger women (Zimmermann, Carnahan, and Peacock 2016). In a comparison of urban and rural youth, researchers suggested that interpersonal level (safety, social/peer interactions, and supervision) had the greatest impression on youth as facilitators and barriers in addition to organizational (school) level policies, yet when compared to urban, rural youth perceived and related to social and physical environments differently (Moore *et al.* 2010).

Environmental

Participation in physical activity is not just a matter of people's biological, psychological, and demographic factors. Bandura's (1985) Social Cognitive Theory posits that personal factors, environmental factors, and behaviors reciprocally, dynamically, and continuously interact. Frost and colleagues (2010) found positive associations among physical activity and rural community attributes, including pleasant aesthetics, trails, safety/crime, parks, and walkable destinations. Research has shown that the physical activity context differs greatly between rural and urban places (Hansen and Hartley 2015). When compared to urban and suburban environments, rural communities offer fewer and less variety of indoor physical activities and provide fewer structural supports for walking and biking to destinations, including work and school. Fewer indoor physical activity options may be offset by easier access to the great outdoors and no-/low-cost activity options on public lands, parks, and trails for some rural residents (Edwards *et al.* 2014). However, geographic features, such as deserts, mountains, and wetlands, as well as spatial and seasonal weather accessibility influences and few indoor options, hinder physical activity choices, development and maintenance of physically active lifestyle patterns for many rural people (John *et al.* 2016). Physical layout and attributes of rural places contribute to automobile reliance, make it difficult for residents to safely and actively transport to and from destinations, access a variety of affordable recreation facilities, regularly utilize public trails and parks, and sustainably resource exercise and recreational physical activity programs (John, McCahan, and Gaulocher 2012; Hansen and Hartley 2015; Umstattd Meyer *et al.* 2016b; John *et al.* 2017). The CDC, to help lead the nation toward active living, recommends the strategies to create environments that encourage physical activity, such as enhancing infrastructures to support walking and bicycling for transportation and recreation, locating schools within easy walking distance of residential areas, improving access to public transportation and recreational facilities, and supporting mixed-use development within neighborhoods, which are more applicable to urban and non-rural suburban settings (Kahn *et al.* 2002). Rural communities are understudied prompting a call for public health efforts targeting rural communities for physical activity promotion (Dobbins *et al.* 2009) and active living research (Umstattd Meyer *et al.* 2016a).

Intervention strategies

In a 2010 national survey conducted to inform *Rural Healthy People 2020* (Bolin *et al.* 2010), rural stakeholders ranked "Physical Activity and Health" as the seventh-highest priority for rural Americans. This percentage was highest in the U.S. Census Bureau Midwest region (48%) compared to the South, Northeast, and West regions (41%). Aiming to reduce the prevalence of low physical activity levels in the U.S., the *National Physical Activity Plan* (Chapter 1) describes and recommends the use of strategies organized by sectors, including 'Business and Industry'; 'Education'; 'Health Care'; 'Mass Media'; 'Community, Recreation, Fitness and Parks'; 'Sports'; 'Public Health'; 'Transportation, Land Use, and Community Design'; and 'Faith-based settings' (NPAP Alliance 2016). When considering engaging sector partners in rural places to plan, implement, and evaluate evidence-based strategies for promoting physical activity in rural populations, it is important to consider the needs and intersection of subgroups within the population, including minorities, older adults, individuals with disabilities, children and others, and their different experiences of the rural environmental, programmatic, and policy features as supporting or hindering rural active living at multiple levels of ecological influence.

BOX 10.1   EVIDENCE FOR PRACTICE: GENERATING RURAL OPTIONS THROUGH COMMUNITY PARTNERSHIPS

In a large-scale effort to engage rural-sector stakeholders, consider the diverse resource needs of rural people, and to better understand the environmental context that contributes to rural obesity disparities, the chapter authors employed participatory action research. Rural communities ($n = 21$) across six Western U.S. states were engaged with two objectives: (1) involve residents in photomapping local resources that they encountered as supporting or hindering weight-healthy lifestyles; (2) involve sector stakeholders with residents to determine community readiness to implement population strategies that would sustainably change the rural context. The ultimate goal was to ecologically model the environmental factors that obstruct weight-healthy lifestyle patterns for some people more than others, and to strategize how to best improve the rural context to optimize all residents' healthy dietary and physical activity patterns as the behavioral defaults. Our research revealed across all rural communities, thematic supports for physical activity emerged as a variety of resources, both indoors and outdoors, that were locally available, easily accessible year-round, and affordable (no/low cost); barriers emerged as spatial and temporal inaccessibility or distance to resource deterring daily use, resource quality, maintenance and safety issues, and usage/participation fees. Applying the Community Readiness Model (Stanley *et al.* 2014), we found overall rural community readiness to address resource gaps to be at the Preplanning stage (M = 3.68, SD = 0.47). Across all communities, readiness dimension scores ranged from lowest (2; denial/resistance) in Leadership to highest (6; initiation) in both Current Efforts and Available Resources dimensions (John *et al.* 2016). In a subset of six communities in Oregon, "easy" spatial access was defined by rural families with children in the household relative to walking and driving to destinations, and analyzed using various distance and drive-time metrics, which showed similar patterns. In all rural communities, less than 50% of households had "easy" access to either food or physical activity resources (John *et al.* 2017). Our work provides additional evidence as to the importance of engaging and mobilizing rural populations, particularly priority subgroups, and multi-sector leaders to build solidarity in intervention actions that are informed by those most affected by the environmental inequities that contribute to physical activity disparities within rural populations and among rural communities.

Acknowledgment: This material is based upon work that is supported by the National Institute of Food and Agriculture, U.S. Department of Agriculture, under award number 2011–68001–30020. Any opinions, findings, conclusions, or recommendations expressed in this publication are those of the author(s) and do not necessarily reflect the view of the U.S. Department of Agriculture (USDA).

Environmental and policy approaches

Evidence supports the effectiveness of population approaches, that is, policy, systems, and environmental strategies, to increase the proportion of people in the U.S. that meet physical activity recommendations as a prevention strategy and promote health equity. In 2009, the CDC recommended a total of 24 community-based strategies for planning and monitoring obesity-related policy and environmental changes. Of the 24 strategies, 12 focused on physical activity with four strategies specifically encouraging physical activity or limiting inactivity among youth and eight strategies aimed at creating safe, physical activity supportive communities (CDC 2009). A systematic review of the physical activity–related literature published (2002–2013) specific to rural communities synthesized the evidence on rural implementation success relative to the 12 CDC strategies (Umstattd Meyer *et al.* 2016b). The study team found only 26 distinct studies that successfully implemented one of the 12 physical activity–related strategies recommended by the CDC. The subset of seven strategies, including all four youth-focused strategies – requiring physical education, increasing physical activity time during physical education, increasing opportunities for extracurricular physical activity, and reducing screen time in childcare settings – and three community strategies – improving access to outdoor recreational facilities, increasing infrastructure supporting bicycling and supporting walking – were deemed most applicable in rural communities. The team suggested that further research is needed using robust study designs and measurement to better ascertain implementation success and effectiveness of recommended and emerging strategies in rural communities (Umstattd Meyer *et al.* 2016b). Nonetheless, there are strategies for promoting active living in rural settings that have been studied and shown to be effective in some contexts and populations.

Interventions for rural adults

Examining effective interventions aimed at increasing physical activity in rural adults can be organized according to individual, social group, or population approaches. Various approaches can be implemented at multiple ecological levels and in various contexts where adult physical activity occurs, such as at home and in the neighborhood, at work, in and around the community, and when actively transporting to/from these places and others.

Individually-tailored behavioral and home-based strategies

In a 2016 review of effective interventions to increase intentional physical activity in rural adult populations, researchers found interventions that were specifically personalized or tailored to individuals or treatment groups, and/or included high-dose intervention contacts, including face-to-face delivery followed by indirect contacts via postal mail, telephone, and/or electronic delivery modes, were found most effective (Cai and Richards 2016). The review noted that the majority of participants in the eight studies meeting all criteria for inclusion in their analyses were younger midlife (mean ages from 35 to 58 years), White women living in the Midwest and not representative of rural populations overall. Rural minority, lower-income, older, less educated, and/or people living in the South were under-represented in these trials. Consequently, the physical activity promotion strategies determined to be most effective from these analyses will not generalize across group differences within rural populations. Among these interventions, effective individual-level physical activity strategies were guided by social and behavioral theories, and mainly included (a) enhancing motivation and social support, (b) providing group-based exercise and educational classes, and (c) mail- or web-based activity promotion messages. Most trials were of shorter duration, while six targeted physical activity as a component of chronic disease prevention and management interventions (Cai and Richards 2016).

Healthy People 2020 includes a goal to increase the proportion of healthcare providers that include physical activity education or counseling as a prevention strategy. Nonetheless, a majority of rural healthcare providers reported little or no PA counseling comfort due to either the lack of knowledge of PA recommendations or individual challenges in being physically active (Miller and Beech 2009). Despite global efforts driven by organizations such as the American College of Sports Medicine to institutionalize a focus on physical activity counseling into healthcare systems through initiatives like Exercise is Medicine® (ACSM), little is known about the effectiveness of such efforts for rural health centers and rural providers (Bobo *et al.* 2014). It is also likely in rural areas that economic, socio-cultural, political, geographic, and structural environments may obstruct some residents' and population groups' ability to fill their physical activity prescription more than others. Thus, interventions aimed at increasing physical activity in adults must be examined using the intersection of rural geography with other social determinants of health, such as gender, race, (dis)ability, and/or SES. Only then will the complexities and inequalities embedded in rural contexts and cultures that determine, influence, and reinforce adults' disparate physical activity motivations, behaviors, levels, and patterns be seen as strategic rural priorities for improving population health.

Worksite strategies

Meeting recommendations for physical activity may be difficult for low-income, rural adults with limited access to supportive conditions. Considering that rural workers spend more than half of their awake hours at or transporting to/from work, worksites may be key sites for implementing strategies that support physical activity in adults. Dodson *et al.* (2008) examined the association of rural worksite policies and incentives to workers' physical activity. They found that worksites with multiple supports, specifically the presence of safe and accessible stairways and personal coaching/counseling services, were associated with meeting physical activity recommendations through moderate or vigorous activity. Meeting recommendations through walking was associated with worksite support for exercise, having exercise facilities (gym, locker, shower), and equipment (treadmill, weights).

According to the USDA Economic Research Service (2016), rural worksites include those that specialize in resource-based activities such as agriculture, forestry, mining, or natural amenity–based recreation; manufacturing, including processing food, wood, and mining products; public sector; service and retail industries, which have emerged in the literature as accounting for most job growth in rural America over the past few decades. A large proportion of rural worksites are small, employing less than 50 workers, and over-represent minority and immigrant populations (USDA ERS 2016). In a qualitative study with rural workers (*n* = 30) from small worksites (Escoffery *et al.* 2011), participants explained they are physically active at work. Strong themes emerged from their narratives, included walking at work and performing various types of physical labor activities required by the job, including lifting items, climbing ladders or stairs, loading trucks, working on a farm, landscaping, shoveling and sweeping, painting, doing laundry, operating tools or equipment. Almost all of the respondents reported no exercise facilities were provided at work, which was an additional strong theme. Many reported doing no additional physical activity on days that they worked, citing lack of time and being tired as key reasons (Escoffery *et al.* 2011).

Community-based strategies

In a 2010 report examining active transportation principles in rural places, the authors classified half of those places as classic farm/ranch country, about one-quarter as exurban (economically and culturally connected to a nearby urban metro area), and about one-quarter as tourism or recreation destinations (Shoup and Homa 2010). Shoup and Homa (2010) further contend that the largest population growth in rural places is occurring in exurban and tourism/recreation areas, and that these rural populations include groups, including young families, retirees, and outdoor enthusiasts, that have an interest in walking and biking for recreation and transportation. The Rails to Trails Conservancy (2011) *Active Transportation Beyond Urban Centers* report provides a comprehensive analysis of the 2009 National Household Travel Survey and success stories through the lens of "rural" America, which claims to debunk "the myth that walking and bicycling are prevalent only in big cities" (p. 22). The size and type of rural communities highlighted in this report range from small cities hosting a large, public university (Eugene, OR; pop. 156,185) to the tiny town of Ohiopyle, PA (pop. 82), a tourist/outdoor recreation destination that hosts over 1.5 million annual visitors. Consistent across all communities included in this report is the strong understanding that investments in active transportation-friendly rural places result in healthier communities, people, economies, and environments.

Interventions for rural youth

Examining effective interventions aimed at increasing physical activity in rural youth can be organized according to the contexts and levels where youth physical activity occurs, such as at home and neighborhood, during school, after school and in other community locales, and when actively transporting to/from these places and others.

Family home strategies

Rural households and neighborhoods may differently influence physical activity in younger compared to older youth. Younger children engage in more sedentary activities indoors at home after school because of parents' concerns for their safety if playing outdoors, especially if parents aren't at home (Hansen *et al.* 2015). Despite the dearth of evidence, even less with a rural focus, for the long-term effectiveness of family involvement methods or parental components in promoting children's physical activity at home, face-to-face, telephone, or web-based interactions with parents that provide parent training, family counseling, or preventive messages appear to offer some promise (O'Connor, Jago, and Baranowski 2009). In addition to parental support for physical activity, more fixed play equipment, fewer bedroom media devices have been associated with higher at-home MVPA and lower overall sedentary behavior in children (Tandon *et al.* 2014). Rural parents/family caregivers revealed, during semi-structured focus group interviews conducted in six rural communities, their perceptions of factors that influence physical activity behaviors in the family home. Family physical activity and screen use emerged as thematic factors that influence family physical activity behaviors. Thematic environmental factors influencing children's physical activity emerged as internal and external to the home, including seasonal variation, features of home and property, distance from neighborhood resources, family policies limiting screen time, financial and schedule constraints, and outdoor safety (Jackson 2015). Thus, when considering how to tailor strategies aimed at increasing physical activity and decreasing sedentary patterns in rural youth, it is important to understand how to navigate the challenges specific to rural people and rural areas – the interplay of child- and family-level factors with rural family home and community factors – as interactive influences on intervention effectiveness.

School-based strategies

Schools are critical settings for rural children to be physically active, particularly in rural communities with fewer and spatially dispersed resources. In rural communities, public schools are widely recognized as a central hub, and perhaps the best venue for physical activity for youth and adults of every age. Despite trends to consolidate schools and reorganize districts, in many rural communities, public schools are the only physical activity facility locally available. In the rural elementary school context, multi-pronged approaches with elements sustained over time (> 2 years), including physical education, classroom physical activity, professional development and health promotion for teachers and families, and strengthening wellness policies and family/community partnerships), significantly improved students' objectively measured daily physical activity (King and Ling 2015). Nonetheless, with regard to rural youth and schools implemented strategies have shown varying degrees of intervention effectiveness. Policies requiring physical education in schools, strategies increasing the amount of physical activity during physical education and availability and access to extracurricular physical activity and outdoor recreational facilities, and enhancing infrastructures to support walking and bicycling to/from schools have shown little impact on physical activity (Umstattd Meyer *et al.* 2016b).

Community-based strategies

There are also few studies documenting the effectiveness of interventions improving rural community places, such as parks, fields and courts, community pools and centers, community gardens and farms; increasing public access to natural resources, such as rivers, lakes, trails, and boulders; or utilizing community places for changes in the physical activity program system on promoting physical activity in youth. In an effort to understand the role of easy physical activity access on rural high school girls' daily physical activity, Trilk and colleagues (2011) examined the association between the number of facilities within an easy walking distance (0.75-mile buffer) of school and self-reported physical activity. Overall, having ≥ 5 facilities within the buffer was positively associated with girls' physical activity with rural students reporting about 12% more daily physical activity than girls who attended rural schools with < 5 facilities. No physical activity difference existed for girls in urban/suburban schools with ≥ 5 or < 5 facilities (Trilk *et al.* 2011). Perry *et al.* (2011) found park use was positively associated with youths' younger age, participation in an after-school activity, and being on a team. The odds of being sedentary in the park was associated with being older aged and using alcohol. Their results also showed that boys and Latinos had greater odds of being active in the park, and that use of higher-quality court and field parks was associated with organized team activities in and after school and being Latino. This study exemplifies how attributes of place, such as organized programs and resource quality, interplay with attributes of people, such as race/ethnicity, to contextualize physical activity experiences among diverse rural populations. Strategies improving pedestrian and bicycle safe transportation routes for youth are challenging to implement in rural places (NADO 2015). Nonetheless, an innovative partnership model in Minnesota enabled school districts and local communities served by regional development organizations to successfully implement the Safe Routes to School (SRTS) program in 76 rural Minnesota communities reaching all corners of the state (Minnesota SRTS 2015).

Implications for practice

Rural areas continue to experience population loss, higher poverty rates, and lower educational attainment than urban areas. According to *Rural America at a Glance: 2015 Edition*, between 2010 and 2014, about two of three rural counties lost population, resulting in a net increase in the proportion of older people and a "graying" of rural places. Rural poverty rates are highest for children and among minority racial and ethnic groups. Single-parent families, especially if headed by a woman, are more likely to be in poverty. While educational attainment has increased in both rural and urban areas, educational attainment rates are lower for rural Black, Hispanic, and Native American than for White populations. Rural child poverty rates are higher in counties with a higher proportion of the population with low educational attainment (Kusmin 2015). Considering the complex intersectional relationships among social determinants of health (refer to Chapter 1) – income status, race and ethnicity, education, gender, age, and so on – and physical activity and inactivity, it is clear that an ecologically grounded, social justice lens (Lee and Cubbin 2009) is necessary to identify highest-priority rural populations and communities to target for intervention if we are to be successful in moving the dial toward meeting recommendations for physical activity, reduce disparities, and achieve physical activity equity among rural populations.

Rural active living researchers in a Call to Action (Umstattd Meyer *et al.* 2016a) specified eight areas to focus discovery and translational efforts (Table 10.1). Active Living by Design (ALbD) encourages the use of a "5P" community action model that includes strategies for preparation and partnerships, promotion, programs, policy, and physical projects. In analyses of implementation across five ALbD rural community cases, four factors emerged in each of the communities: (1) the culture, (2) implementation of the 5P strategies, (3) assets and challenges experienced, and (4) additional insight that can inform future work. Not surprising, innovative strategies were required to encourage physical activity, including events that drew people to markets and town assets, and thus promoted economic development and cultural pride as a value-added incentive. Two rural insights emerged from these analyses, both related to local resources: (1) planning for future place-based development must be deliberate in locating community resources in relation to other amenities; and (2) while people are a valuable and valued resource, rural human resources may be under-capitalized simply because there are fewer people per geographic area to carry the load (Schwantes 2010).

TABLE 10.1 Rural Active Living Research Call to Action Areas of Focus

1	System for conceptualizing rurality for empirical applications
2	Consider the unique social, cultural, and environmental contexts are as critical to treatments as being less populated
3	Center that diversity exists within the continuum of rurality
4	Include qualitative and mixed-methods studies to better characterize the unique interplay among variables
5	Develop, test, and validate rural-specific environmental assessments
6	Measure objectively to assess physical activity and sedentary behaviors of rural residents
7	Employ ecological models to guide the rural-specific evidence base and active living domains
8	Partner with government, school and other sectors to optimize natural experiments, specific environmental or policy changes, when the opportunities present

Source: Umstattd Meyer *et al.* (2016b)

In conclusion, we suggest that expanding "Rural Active Living Call to Action" beyond the research community and obvious partnerships to include "Rural Active Living by Design" across the diversity of rural resources and novel partners – residents and subgroups, stakeholders (including visitors), social networks, volunteer and non-profit organizations, and business communities – is a mechanism to strengthen our charge. Intentionally bringing communities together that have a diverse voice and stake in creating rural places that are activity friendly for all, and that have a shared value for both a comprehensive knowledge base and solutions focused on assuring rural living is healthy, active, and just, will help catalyze changes to the rural community context that are equitable and enduring, and create opportunities to address physical activity and health disparities in U.S. rural populations.

Summary points

- Rural is a socially constructed population category that is inconsistently or poorly defined for comparison in the scientific literature, and constitutes a challenge for physical activity scholarship and practice.
- Rural populations are heterogeneous. Health and physical activity disparities exist within rural populations as well as between rural populations when compared to urban or suburban counterparts.
- Rural residency is generally associated with lower rates of physical activity than residing in urban or suburban areas.
- Rural residents have unique and often more pronounced barriers to physical activity due to socioeconomic, sociocultural, geographic, environmental, and political contextual factors.

- Rural contexts are highly variable within communities and between communities within counties, states, and geographic regions. Thus, supporting active rural living among all rural populations requires practitioners to engage diverse people, and solicit sector partners in finding creative, multi-level solutions that are matched to the unique contexts, cultures, and capacities of their rural place.

Critical thinking questions

1   Why does diversity within rural populations and among rural communities contribute to challenges in planning and implementing effective strategies to increase the proportion of rural adults and youth that meet the physical activity recommendations to address rural health disparities?
2   How does the application of intersectionality theory and social justice lens reveal opportunities for research and practice that will prioritize rural populations for physical activity interventions?
3   How does access to and affordability of available physical activity resources in rural communities differ experientially, that is, as supportive or obstructive of developing and maintaining physically active lifestyle patterns, by various segments of the local population?

How would you use this understanding to plan, implement, and evaluate strategies that make physical activity the easy choice for all? What strategies and measurements would you suggest, and why?

References

Bandura, A. (1985). *Social Foundations of Thought and Action: A Social Cognitive Theory* (7th ed.). Englewood Cliffs, N. J: Prentice-Hall.

Bauer, U. E., Briss, P. A., Goodman, R. A. and Bowman, B. A. (2014). 'Prevention of chronic disease in the 21st century: Elimination of the leading preventable causes of premature death and disability in the USA.' *The Lancet*, 384: 45–52.

Beauchamp, A., Backholer, K., Magliano, D. and Peeters, A. (2014). 'The effect of obesity prevention interventions according to socioeconomic position: A systematic review.' *Obesity Reviews*, 15: 541–554.

Befort, C. A., Nazir, N. and Perri, M. G. (2012). 'Prevalence of obesity among adults from rural and urban areas of the United States: Findings from NHANES (2005–2008).' *The Journal of Rural Health*, 28: 392–397.

Berry, E. H. and Kirschner, A. (2013). 'Demography of rural aging.' In N. Glasgow and E. H. Berry (Eds.), *Rural Aging in 21st Century America* (pp. 17–36). New York: Springer Dordrecht.

Bobo, C., Buie, R., Culbertson, M., Dobberstein, L., Duke, K., Gray, M., Hamlett, B., Huckabee, O., Hyder, E., Jones, C., Spearman, L., Stilwell, W., Szabo, J., Martens, C., McGowans, S., Patton, R., Prosser, K., Hughes, L. and Williams, J. (2014). 'Exercise is medicine in rural health centers and federally qualified health centers [Online].' Available: http://tigerprints.clemson.edu/foci/54 (Accessed October 25 2016).

Bolin, J. N., Bellamy, G., Ferdinand, A. O., Kash, B. A. and Helduser, J. W. (Eds.). (2010). 'Rural healthy people 2020 [Online].' Available: http://sph.tamhsc.edu/srhrc/rhp2020.html (Accessed October 25 2016).

Cai, Y. and Richards, E. A. (2016). 'Systematic review of physical activity outcomes of rural lifestyle interventions.' *Western Journal of Nursing Research*, 38: 909–927.

CDC, Centers for Disease Control and Prevention. (2009). 'Recommended community strategies and measurements to prevent obesity in the United States [Online].' Available: www.cdc.gov/mmwr/preview/mmwrhtml/rr5807a1.htm (Accessed October 25 2016).

CDC, Centers for Disease Control and Prevention. (2016). 'Partnerships to Improve Community Health (PICH) [Online].' Available: www.cdc.gov/nccdphp/dch/programs/partnershipstoimprovecommunityhealth/index.html (Accessed October 25 2016).

Cromartie, J. and Parker, T. (2016). 'USDA ERS: What is rural? [Online].' Available: www.ers.usda.gov/topics/rural-economy-population/rural-classifications/what-is-rural.aspx (Accessed October 25 2016).

Crosby, R. A., Wendel, M. L., Vanderpool, R. C. and Casey, B. R. (2012). *Rural Populations and Health: Determinants, Disparities, and Solutions*. San Francisco: Jossey-Bass.

Davis, A. M., Boles, R. E., James, R. L., Sullivan, D. K., Donnelly, J. E., Swirczynski, D. L. and Goetz, J. (2008). 'Health behaviors and weight status among urban and rural children.' *Rural and Remote Health*, 8: 810.

Dobbins, M., DeCorby, K., Robeson, P., Husson, H. and Tirilis, D. (2009). 'Cochrane review: School-based physical activity programs for promoting physical activity and fitness in children and adolescents aged 6–18.' *Evidence-Based Child Health: A Cochrane Review Journal*, 4: 1452–1561.

Dodson, E. A., Lovegreen, S. L., Elliott, M. B., Haire-Joshu, D. and Brownson, R. C. (2008). 'Worksite policies and environments supporting physical activity in midwestern communities'. *American Journal of Health Promotion*, 23: 51–55.

Eberhardt, M. S. and Pamuk, E. R. (2004). 'The importance of place of residence: Examining health in rural and nonrural areas.' *American Journal of Public Health*, 94: 1682–1686.

Edwards, M. B., Theriault, D. S., Shores, K. A. and Melton, K. M. (2014). 'Promoting youth physical activity in rural southern communities: Practitioner perceptions of environmental opportunities and barriers.' *The Journal of Rural Health*, 30: 379–387.

Escoffery, C., Kegler, M. C., Alcantara, I., Wilson, M. and Glanz, K. (2011). 'A qualitative examination of the role of small, rural worksites in obesity prevention.' *Preventing Chronic Disease*, 8: A75.

Fan, J. X., Wen, M. and Kowaleski-Jones, L. (2014). 'Rural – Urban differences in objective and subjective measures of physical activity: Findings from the National Health and Nutrition Examination Survey (NHANES) 2003–2006.' *Preventing Chronic Disease*, 1–11.

Frost, S. S., Goins, R. T., Hunter, R. H., Hooker, S. P., Bryant, L. L., Kruger, J. and Pluto, D. (2010). 'Effects of the built environment on physical activity of adults living in rural settings.' *American Journal of Health Promotion*, 24: 267–283.

Gunter, K. B., Abi Nader, P. and John, D. (2015). 'Physical activity levels and obesity status of Oregon rural elementary school children.' *Preventive Medicine Reports*, 2: 478–482.

Hansen, A. and Hartley, D. (2015). 'Promoting active living in rural communities [Online].' Available: www.activelivingresearch.org (Accessed October 25 2016).

Hansen, A., Umstattd Meyer, Y., Lenardson, M. and Hartley, R. (2015). 'Built environments and active living in rural and remote areas: A review of the literature.' *Current Obesity Reports*, 4: 484–493.

Hartley, D. (2004). 'Rural health disparities, population health, and rural culture.' *American Journal of Public Health*, 94: 1675–1678.

Hunter, R., Sharkey, J., Bryant, L., Hunter, W. and Skeele, M., (2009). 'Overcoming challenges to active aging in rural and small town America.' *Gerontologist*, 49: 134.

Jackson, J. (2015). *Associations between Family Nutrition and Physical Activity, Food Security, and Childhood Obesity in Rural Oregon*, PhD Thesis, Oregon State University, Corvallis, OR.

Jahns, L., McDonald, L. R., Wadsworth, A., Morin, C. and Liu, Y. (2014). 'Barriers and facilitators to being physically active on a Rural U.S. Northern Plains American Indian Reservation.' *International Journal of Environmental Research and Public Health*, 11: 12053–12063.

John, D. H., Abi Nader, P., Ghavami, A. and Gunter, K. (2014). 'Using mixed methods to explore physical activity attributes of older residents and their community place.' *Medicine and Science in Sports and Exercise*, 46: 122–125.

John, D. H. and Gunter, K. (2015). 'EngAGE in community: Using mixed methods to mobilize older people to elucidate the age-friendly attributes of urban and rural places.' *Journal of Applied Gerontology*, 35: 1095–1120.

John, D. H., Gunter, K., Hystad, P., Langellotto, G. and Manore, M. (2016). 'Generating rural options for weight healthy kids and communities: Outcomes and impacts.' *Journal of Nutrition Education and Behavior*, 48: S122.

John, D. H., McCahan, B. and Gaulocher, S. (2012). 'Partnering to enable active rural living: PEARL project.' *Journal of Rural Social Sciences*, 27: 74–101.

John, D. H., Winfield, T., Hystad, P., Langellotto, G., Manore, M. and Gunter, K. (2017). 'Community-engaged attribute mapping: Exploring resources and readiness to change the rural context for obesity prevention.' *Progress in Community Health Partnerships: Research, Education, and Action,* 11 (2): in press.

Johnson, J. A. and Johnson, A. M. (2015). 'Urban-rural differences in childhood and adolescent obesity in the United States: A systematic review and meta-analysis.' *Child Obesity*, 11: 233–241.

Jones, C., Parker, T., Ahearn, M., Mishra, A. and Variyam, J. (2009). 'Health status and health care access of farm and rural populations [Online].' Available: www.ers.usda.gov/publications/eib-economic-information-bulletin/eib57.aspx (Accessed October 25 2016).

Joseph, R. P., Ainsworth, B. E., Keller, C. and Dodgson, J. E. (2015). 'Barriers to physical activity among African American women: An integrative review of the literature.' *Women and Health*, 55: 679–699.

Kahn, E. B., Ramsey, L. T., Brownson, R. C., Heath, G. W., Howze, E. H., Powell, K., Stone, E., Rajab, M. and Corso, P. (2002). 'The effectiveness of interventions to increase physical activity: A systematic review 1 and 2.' *American Journal of Preventive Medicine*, 22: 73–107.

King, K. M. and Ling, J. (2015). 'Results of a 3-year, nutrition and physical activity intervention for children in rural, low-socioeconomic status elementary schools.' *Health Education Research*, 30: 647–659.

Kusmin, L. (2015, November 30). 'USDA ERS: Rural America at a glance [Online].' Available: www.ers.usda.gov/publications/pub-details/?pubid=44016 (Accessed October 23 2016).

Lavizzo-Mourey, R. (2014, February 10). 'Building a culture of health: 2014 president's message [Online].' Available: www.rwjf.org/content/rwjf/en/library/annual-reports/presidents-message-2014.html (Accessed October 25 2016).

Lee, R. E. and Cubbin, C. (2009). 'Striding toward social justice: The ecologic milieu of physical activity.' *Exercise and Sport Sciences Reviews*, 37: 10–17.

McCormack, L. A. and Meendering, J. (2016). 'Diet and physical activity in rural vs urban children and adolescents in the United States: A narrative review.' *Journal of the Academy of Nutrition and Dietetics*, 116: 467–480.

Meit, M., Knudson, A., Gilbert, T., Tzy-Chyi Yu, A., Tanenbaum, E., Ormson, E., TenBroeck, S., Bayne, A. and Popat, S. (2014, December 9). 'The 2014 update of the rural-urban Chartbook [Online].' Available: www.ruralhealthresearch.org/webinars/rural-urban-chartbook (Accessed October 25 2016).

Miller, S. T. and Beech, B. M. (2009). 'Rural healthcare providers question the practicality of motivational interviewing and report varied physical activity counseling experience.' *Patient Education and Counseling*, 76: 279–282.

Minnesota SRTS. (2015). '5 year strategic plan [Online].' Available: www.dot.state.mn.us/ saferoutes/index.html (Accessed October 25 2016).

Moore, J. B., Brinkley, J., Crawford, T. W., Evenson, K. R. and Brownson, R. C. (2013). 'Association of the built environment with physical activity and adiposity in rural and urban youth.' *Preventive Medicine*, 56: 145–148.

Moore, J. B., Jilcott, S. B., Shores, K. A., Evenson, K. R., Brownson, R. C. and Novick, L. F. (2010). 'A qualitative examination of perceived barriers and facilitators of physical activity for urban and rural youth.' *Health Education Research*, 25: 355–367.

NADO, National Association of Development Organizations. (2015). 'Rural safe routes to school planning [Online].' Available: http://ruraltransportation.org/rural-safe-routes-to-school-planning/ (Accessed October 25 2016).

National Physical Activity Plan Alliance. (2016). 'About the plan [Online].' Available: www. physicalactivityplan.org/theplan/about.html (Accessed October 25 2016).

O'Connor, T. M., Jago, R. and Baranowski, T. (2009). 'Engaging parents to increase youth physical activity.' *American Journal of Preventive Medicine*, 37: 141–149.

Ogden, C. L., Carroll, M. D., Kit, B. K. and Flegal, K. M. (2014). 'Prevalence of childhood and adult obesity in the United States, 2011–2012.' *JAMA*, 311: 806.

Ogden, C. L., Carroll, M. D., Lawman, H. G., Fryar, C. D., Kruszon-Moran, D., Kit, B. K. and Flegal, K. M. (2016). 'Trends in obesity prevalence among children and adolescents in the United States, 1988–1994 through 2013–2014.' *JAMA*, 315: 2292.

Parks, S. E., Housemann, R. A. and Brownson, R. C. (2003). 'Differential correlates of physical activity in urban and rural adults of various socioeconomic backgrounds in the United States.' *Journal of Epidemiology and Community Health*, 57: 29–35.

Perry, C. K., Saelens, B. E. and Thompson, B. (2011). 'Rural Latino youth park use: Characteristics, park amenities, and physical activity.' *Journal of Community Health*, 36: 389–397.

Rails to Trails Conservancy. (2011). 'Active transportation beyond urban centers report | rails-to-trails conservancy [Online].' Available: www.railstotrails.org/resource-library/ resources/active-transportation-beyond-urban-centers-report/ (Accessed October 25 2016).

Schwantes, T. (2010, February). 'Using active living principles to promote physical activity in rural communities [Online].' Available: http://activelivingresearch.org/using-active-living-principles-promote-physical-activity-rural-communities (Accessed October 25 2016).

Shoup, L. and Homa, B. (2010). 'Principles for improving transportation options in rural and small town communities [Online].' Available: http://t4america.org/wp-content/ uploads/2010/03/T4-Whitepaper-Rural-and-Small-Town-Communities.pdf (Accessed October 25 2016).

Stanley, L., Oetting, E., Plested, B., Edwards, R. and Jumper Thurman, P. (2014). 'Tri-ethnic center community readiness handbook, 2nd Ed. [Online].' Available: Community Readiness, http://triethniccenter.colostate.edu/communityReadiness_home.htm (Accessed October 25 2016).

Stern, D. (2014). 'Race and ethnicity in rural America: Housing assistance council [Online].' Available: www.ruralhome.org/sct-information/mn-hac-research/rural-rrb/484-rrn-race-and-ethnicity (Accessed October 25 2016).

Sumaya, C. (2012). 'Foreword.' In R. Crosby, M. Wendel and R. Vanderpool (Eds.), *Rural Populations and Health: Determinants, Disparities, and Solutions* (pp. xiii–xiv). Somerset, US: Jossey-Bass.

Tandon, P., Grow, H. M., Couch, S., Glanz, K., Sallis, J. F., Frank, L. D. and Saelens, B. E. (2014). 'Physical and social home environment in relation to children's overall and home-based physical activity and sedentary time.' *Preventive Medicine*, 66: 39–44.

Trilk, J. L., Ward, D. S., Dowda, M., Pfeiffer, K. A., Porter, D. E., Hibbert, J. and Pate, R. R. (2011). 'Do physical activity facilities near schools affect physical activity in high school girls?' *Health and Place*, 17: 651–657.

Trivedi, T., Liu, J., Probst, J., Merchant, A., Jhones, S. and Martin, A. B. (2015). 'Obesity and obesity-related behaviors among rural and urban adults in the USA.' *Rural Remote Health*, 15: 3267.

Trussell, D. E. and Shaw, S. M. (2009). 'Changing family life in the rural context: Women's perspectives of family leisure on the farm.' *Leisure Sciences*, 31: 434–449.

Umstattd Meyer, M. R., Moore, J. B., Abildso, C., Edwards, M. B., Gamble, A. and Baskin, M. L. (2016a). 'Rural active living.' *Journal of Public Health Management and Practice*, 22(5): E11-20.

Umstattd Meyer, M. R., Perry, C. K., Sumrall, J. C., Patterson, M. S., Walsh, S. M., Clendennen, S. C., Hooker, S., Evenson, K., Goins, K., Heinrich, K., Tompkins, N., Eyler, A., Jones, S., Tabak, R. and Valco, C. (2016b). 'Physical activity: Related policy and environmental strategies to prevent obesity in rural communities: A systematic review of the literature, 2002–2013.' *Preventing Chronic Disease*, 1–13.

U.S. Census Bureau. (2012). '2010 census urban and rural classification and urban area criteria [Online].' Available: www.census.gov/geo/reference/ua/urban-rural-2010.html (Accessed October 25 2016).

U.S. Department of Agriculture Economic Research Service, USDA ERS. (2016). 'State fact sheets [Online].' Available: www.ers.usda.gov/data-products/state-fact-sheets/ (Accessed October 25 2016).

U.S. Office of Disease Prevention and Health Promotion, ODPHP. (2008). 'Guidelines index: 2008 physical activity guidelines[Online].' Available: https://health.gov/paguidelines/guidelines/ (Accessed October 25 2016).

U.S. Office of Disease Prevention and Health Promotion, ODPHP. (2014). 'Healthy people 2020: Disparities [Online].' Available: www.healthypeople.gov/2020/about/foundation-health-measures/Disparities (Accessed October 25 2016).

Wilcox, S., Castro, C., King, A., Housemann, R. and Bownson, R. (2000). 'Determinants of leisure time physical activity in rural compared with urban older and ethnically diverse women in the United States.' *Journal of Epidemiology and Community Health*, 54: 667–672.

Wu, S., Cohen, D., Shi, Y., Pearson, M. and Sturm, R. (2011). 'Economic analysis of physical activity interventions.' *American Journal of Preventive Medicine*, 40: 149–158.

Zhang, X., Holt, J. B., Lu, H., Onufrak, S., Yang, J., French, S. P. and Sui, D. Z. (2014). 'Neighborhood commuting environment and obesity in the United States: An Urban – Rural stratified multilevel analysis.' *Preventive Medicine*, 59: 31–36.

Zimmermann, K., Carnahan, L. R. and Peacock, N. R. (2016). 'Age-associated perceptions of physical activity facilitators and barriers among women in rural southernmost Illinois.' *Preventing Chronic Disease*, 1–13.

11

PHYSICAL ACTIVITY AMONG LESBIAN, GAY, BISEXUAL AND TRANSGENDER POPULATIONS

Danielle R. Brittain and Mary K. Dinger

Understanding lesbian, gay, bisexual and transgender populations

Although often grouped together, lesbian, gay, bisexual and transgender (LGBT) individuals constitute four distinct populations. Before beginning a discussion on the health of LGBT populations, there needs to be a clear understanding of important terminology, including (a) sex; (b) gender; (c) gender identity; and (d) sexual orientation.

- *Sex* refers to a person's biological status and is typically categorized as male, female or intersex (i.e., atypical combinations of features that usually distinguish male from female). There are a number of indicators of biological sex, including sex chromosomes, gonads, internal reproductive organs and external genitalia.

  (American Psychological Association [APA] 2012, p. 11)

- *Gender* refers to the attitudes, feelings, and behaviors that a given culture associates with a person's biological sex. Behavior that is compatible with cultural expectations is referred to as gender normative; behaviors that are viewed as incompatible with these expectations constitute gender nonconformity.

  (APA 2012, p. 11)

- *Gender identity* refers to "one's sense of oneself as male, female, or transgender" (APA 2012, p. 11). When one's gender identity and biological sex are not congruent, the individual may identify as transsexual or as another transgender category (APA 2012, p. 11). Cisgender is used to refer to people whose sex assigned at birth is aligned with their gender identity.

  (APA 2015)

- *Sexual orientation* refers to an enduring pattern of or disposition to experience sexual or romantic desires for, and relationships with, people of one's same sex, the other sex or both sexes (Institute of Medicine [IOM] 2011). Sexual orientation includes three components: identity (e.g., self-identification as heterosexual, gay, lesbian, bisexual, queer), attraction (e.g., tendency for attraction to persons of the same sex, opposite sex or both sexes) and behavior (e.g., engagement in sexual contact with a person of the same sex, opposite sex, or both sexes).

(IOM 2011)

Demographic characteristics

Challenges to assessment of LGBT demographic information

Assessment of accurate demographic information for LGBT populations has historically been, and continues to be, very challenging. The three main issues to the assessment of LBGT demographic information include: (a) a lack of sexual orientation and gender identity measures on the majority of national- and state-level health surveys; (b) views that sexuality and gender exist on a broad spectrum (e.g., not identifying with one sexual orientation or gender) and thus, are difficult to measure; and (c) fear of negative repercussions for disclosing sexual orientation and gender identity. Although each of these challenges is due to a multitude of factors, the most influential has been socially conservative values in the American culture, particularly religious-based definitions of morality (Flores 2014). It wasn't until the past few years that we have seen a shift in the percentage of Americans who believe lesbian and gay relations are morally acceptable. According to the 2016 Gallup Poll, 60% of Americans polled believe lesbian and gay relations are morally acceptable, which is a 20% increase from the rate reported in 2001 (40%).

An important result of this societal attitude shift has been improved efforts by the federal government to understand LGBT demographics and health status. In 2011, the United States Department of Health and Human Services (USDHHS) developed a plan to incorporate sexual orientation and gender identity questions into all USDHHS national health surveys. A portion of this plan was the development and inclusion of the first-ever Healthy People 2020 objectives targeting LGBT health (Office of Disease Prevention and Health Promotion 2016). The two objectives developed for HP2020 are to improve population-based monitoring of LGBT health through the inclusion of sexual orientation and gender identity questions on state- and national-level health surveys. Through these federal-level efforts, the assessment and monitoring of LGBT demographic and health information will be dramatically improved.

Population estimates

Based on the results of research conducted by Gates (2014) examining the years 2010–2014, LGBT individuals constituted 2.2–4.0% of the total United States population which equated to 5.2–9.5 million adults aged 18 years and older. More specifically, lesbian and gay adults constituted 1.4–1.6%, bisexual adults constituted 0.6–1.6% and transgender adults constituted 0.36–0.95% of the total adult population (Flores *et al.* 2016; Gates 2014). Additionally, 2.2–4.1% of female adults in the United States and 2.2–3.9% of male adults identified as LGBT. Overall, among those who identified as LGBT, females were more likely to identify as bisexual (68–77%) and less likely to identify as lesbian or gay (41–49%) when compared to males (23–32% bisexual and 51–59% gay). These population estimates were based on the analysis of national health surveillance survey data (i.e., National Survey of Family Growth, General Social Survey, National Health Interview Survey, Behavioral Risk Factor Surveillance System [BRFSS]) and Gallup Poll data. It should be noted that only one survey (BRFSS) included a specific measure assessing gender identity.

According to Gates (2014), younger adults in the United States aged 18–29 years were more likely to identify as LGBT (3.5–7.2%) when compared to adults aged 60 years and older (1–2.1%). The majority of those who identified as LGBT were White, non-Hispanic (60–69%), 13–20% were Hispanic, 11–16% were African American, 2–4% were Asian, 1% were American Indian/Alaska Native, and 2–4% were multi-racial/other. Approximately 36% of adults who identified as bisexual also identified with a race/ethnicity other than White, non-Hispanic whereas only 30–32% of those who identified as lesbian/gay also identified as a racial minority. When examining educational attainment, 35–45% of LGBT adults aged 25 years and older had a college degree. More specifically, 46–52% of those who identified as lesbian/gay and 33–38% who identified as bisexual had a college degree.

Health disparities and inequities among LGBT populations

Across the life-course, LGBT compared to heterosexual and/or cisgender populations disproportionately experience cultural discrimination, minority stress (i.e., stress associated with being a member of a sexual minority, Meyer 2003), victimization and violence, which has resulted in health disparities (Andersen *et al.* 2015; Burton *et al.* 2013; Fredriksen-Goldsen *et al.* 2013b; Lick *et al.* 2013; Mustanski *et al.* 2016) and higher all-cause mortality among LGBT (Cochran *et al.* 2016). In 2011, the Institute of Medicine (IOM) released the most extensive health report to date regarding LGBT populations, entitled *The Health of Lesbian, Gay, Bisexual, and Transgender People: Building a Foundation for Better Understanding*. Based on this report LGBT compared to heterosexual and/or cisgender populations experience mental, physical, risk and protective, and health services disparities from adolescence to adulthood.

This section of the chapter includes findings from the IOM report, as well as additional research findings published since the release of the IOM report. Criteria used for the inclusion of study findings in this section included: (a) comparisons between LGBT and heterosexual or cisgender populations; (b) larger samples sizes (typically national or state level); and (c) examination of multiple health disparities (e.g., mental and physical).

Physical health

While most physical health disparities (i.e., cardiovascular disease, cancer [breast and anal], arthritis, asthma, HIV, overall worse health) have been identified among LGBT adults (Boehmer *et al.* 2014; Cochran *et al.* 2016; Fredriksen-Goldsen *et al.* 2013a; IOM 2011), there are also physical health disparities identified earlier in the life-course that extend into adulthood. For example, while adult lesbian and bisexual females compared to heterosexual females have higher rates of obesity, this health disparity has also been identified among female adolescents and college students (Brittain and Dinger 2015; Eliason *et al.* 2015; Fredriksen-Goldsen *et al.* 2013b; IOM 2011; VanKim *et al.* 2014). Additionally, lesbian, gay and bisexual adolescents and college students have higher rates of substance use (including smoking, alcohol consumption and binge drinking), a health disparity also identified among adults.

Mental health

Across the lifespan, LGBT populations experience numerous mental health disparities when compared to heterosexual and cisgender populations. Adolescents, college students and LGBT adults have an increased risk for depression, suicidal ideation, attempted suicide and suicide (Brittain and Dinger 2015; IOM 2011; Kann *et al.* 2011; Reisner *et al.* 2014). Higher rates of mood and anxiety disorders, stress, mental distress and poor mental health (Blosnich *et al.* 2014; Boehmer *et al.* 2014; Brittain and Dinger 2015; Cochran *et al.* 2016; Fredriksen-Goldsen *et al.* 2013b; IOM 2011) have also been identified among LGBT adults. Finally, higher rates of eating disorders have been identified among LGBT adolescents and adults (IOM 2011).

Understanding that LGBT populations experience a multitude of physical and mental health disparities when compared to heterosexual and cisgender populations, access to health care is critical to combatting these disparities. However, LGBT populations have less access to and utilization of healthcare services, particularly those that provide LGBT appropriate care (Blosnich *et al.* 2014; Cochran *et al.* 2016; Dickey *et al.* 2016; Grant *et al.* 2011; IOM 2011). Without equal access to health care, the role of behavioral strategies such as physical activity become even more essential to improving and maintaining a lifetime of good health. Particularly among LGBT, many of the mental and physical health disparities identified in the previous section may be mitigated through regular participation in physical activity (USDHHS 2008).

Physical activity among LGBT populations

Only a few research studies have been conducted to examine physical activity among LGBT populations (Gorczynski and Brittain 2016) with mixed results reported. Some studies indicate a significant difference in physical activity participation rates between LGBT and heterosexual and/or cisgender populations and other studies show no differences between any of the groups. The next section includes an overview of a portion of the research studies in which participation in aerobic physical activity was examined between LGB and heterosexual populations and transgender and cisgender populations. Criteria used for the majority of studies reviewed in this section of the chapter included: (a) comparisons between LGBT and heterosexual or cisgender populations and (b) larger sample sizes (typically national or state level).

Physical activity participation among specific LGBT groups

Adolescence

Beginning with adolescents, Kann and colleagues (2011) reported that LGB high school students compared to heterosexual high school students had lower median rates of daily participation in 60 minutes of moderate to vigorous physical activity on seven days each week (Figure 11.1). However, Rosario and colleagues (2014) reported that only gay and bisexual male high school students significantly differed in rates of moderate to vigorous physical activity on five days each week when compared to heterosexual male students. Lesbian, bisexual and heterosexual female high school students did not differ in participation rates in the Rosario et al. (2014) study.

College years

Among college students, Brittain and Dinger (2015) reported that gay males had significantly lower rates of participation in moderate to vigorous aerobic physical

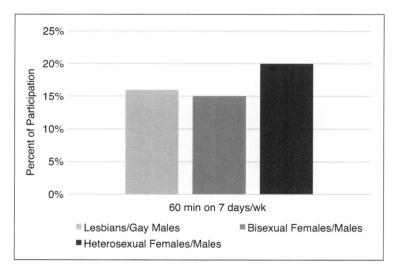

FIGURE 11.1 Median percentage of adolescents by sexual orientation participating in moderate to vigorous physical activity

Source: Kann et al. (2011)

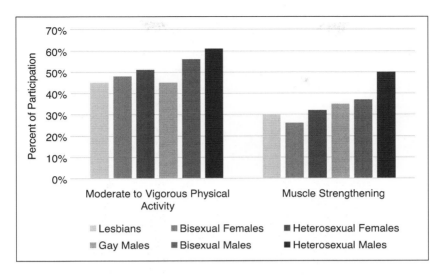

FIGURE 11.2 Rates of participation in moderate to vigorous physical activity and muscle strengthening among college students by sexual orientation

Source: Brittain and Dinger (2015)

activity when compared to heterosexual males, while bisexual and heterosexual males had similar physical activity participation rates. Further, bisexual males were less likely to participate in strength training than their heterosexual peers. Finally, lesbian, bisexual and heterosexual female college students did not differ in rates of aerobic physical activity or strength training (Figure 11.2).

Laska and colleagues (2015) reported slightly different results when examining physical activity participation rates among Minnesota college students. Bisexual females and gay and bisexual males had lower rates of participation in aerobic physical activity compared to heterosexuals while rates among lesbians and heterosexual females did not differ. In addition, VanKim and colleagues (2014) reported that transgender students were less likely to engage in moderate to vigorous aerobic physical activity and muscle strengthening when compared to cisgender students.

Adulthood

While the results of studies comparing participation in physical activity between lesbian, bisexual and heterosexual adult females have been varied, the majority have shown no differences in physical activity participation rates (Boehmer and Bowen 2009; Dilley *et al.* 2010; Fredriksen-Goldsen *et al.* 2013b). Among gay, bisexual and heterosexual adult males, the majority of study results have been similar in that no differences in physical activity rates have been identified between groups (Dilley *et al.* 2010; Fredriksen-Goldsen *et al.* 2013b). One exception was reported by Dilley *et al.* (2010) in which they found that bisexual males had lower rates of participation in sufficient amounts of moderate to vigorous physical activity when compared to heterosexual males (56% vs. 67%).

Additional research findings identified differences in physical activity between LGBT and heterosexual and/or cisgender populations. Boehmer and colleagues (2012) conducted age-stratified analyses to examine physical activity between sexual orientation groups. Based on comparisons with heterosexuals: (1) lesbians had higher rates of participation in moderate physical activity, but only at ages 50 years and younger, (2) bisexual females and gay males had higher rates of participation in strength training, but only at ages 50 years and younger, and (3) bisexual males had higher rates of participation in vigorous physical activity, but only at ages 50 years and younger. These age-stratified results may provide valuable insight for the design, implementation and evaluation of future physical activity interventions.

Finally, among the minimal research conducted on transgender adults, Muchicko *et al.* (2014) found no significant differences in physical activity between transgender and cisgender adults. However, Fredriksen-Goldsen and colleagues (2013a) reported significant differences in physical activity among transgender and cisgender adults aged 50 years and older. Only 15% of transgender individuals engaged in sufficient amounts of moderate physical activity compared to 23% of cisgender individuals.

As indicated in the previous section, only minimal research has been conducted examining participation in physical activity among LGBT populations (Gorczynski and Brittain, 2016). There are several reasons for this lack of research, including but not limited to a lack of national-level funding for LGBT-focused research on physical activity and a lack of sexual orientation and gender-identity questions on national-level surveillance surveys. Only recently has the federal government created national health objectives (Healthy People 2020) to increase the number of population-based surveys that include sexual orientation and gender-identity questions (e.g., BRFSS) as a way to monitor and understand the health of LGBT populations (e.g., physical activity, health disparities) (Office of Disease Prevention and Health Promotion 2016). Currently, most studies on LGBT populations have been based on state-specific data (i.e., Washington, California, Minnesota) and not national-level samples (Boehmer *et al.* 2012; Laska *et al.* 2015). Further, many studies have combined sexual orientation groups (e.g., lesbians/gays; bisexual females/males; lesbians/bisexuals; gay/bisexual males) due to small sample sizes and thus, information on physical activity is often limited to these combined groups (Fredriksen-Goldsen *et al.* 2013b; Kann *et al.* 2011). Regardless of these limitations with previous research, the information that does exist provides some indication of physical activity trends among LGBT populations and suggests that a large number of individuals are not engaging in sufficient amounts of physical activity to achieve health benefits. Thus, it is imperative to continue the pursuit of understanding factors that hinder or stop participation in physical activity.

Common barriers and facilitators to physical activity among LGBT populations

This section will include an overview of factors (i.e., correlates) associated with participation in physical activity among LGBT populations. Identification of correlates of physical activity is imperative to the design of evidence-based culturally appropriate interventions to increase participation in physical activity. The majority of correlate research has included an examination of general (i.e., experienced by multiple populations) and sexual orientation–specific (i.e., specific to LGB or heterosexual populations) barriers to engaging in physical activity. Barriers can also be delineated into one of five ecological categories which represent potential influences on health (e.g., physical activity behavior): (a) intrapersonal (i.e., factors internal to the individual); (b) interpersonal (i.e., social networks and social support systems); (c) institutional (i.e., rules and regulations within institutions); (d) community (i.e., relationships between organizations and institutions; geographic areas of defined boundaries); and (e) public policy (i.e., local, state and national laws and policies) (McLeroy *et al.* 1988).

The majority of barriers research has targeted adult lesbians; however, information will be presented for all LGBT groups across the lifespan. Due to the minimal amount of barriers research among LGBT populations, adolescents and college students have been combined and no transgender-specific barriers have been identified.

Unique influences among specific LGBT populations

Adolescence/college years

Of the research among LGB adolescents and college students, general intrapersonal and sexual orientation–specific institutional barriers associated with participation in physical activity have been identified. General intrapersonal barriers included low athletic self-esteem, gender non-conformity (Calzo *et al.* 2014), being overweight, inaction toward weight loss and being a current smoker (McElroy and Jordan 2014).

In terms of sexual orientation–specific institutional barriers, discrimination and sexual prejudice within sport and physical activity settings (i.e., gyms, locker rooms, Physical Education (PE) class) excludes many LGBT adolescents and college students from engaging in physical activity (Gill *et al.* 2010; Griffin 1998; Messner 1992). Due to this sexual prejudice, many LGBT students often do not feel safe to engage in sport or physical activity for fear of violence, outing and overall oppression.

Adulthood

Due to the majority of barriers research being conducted on adults, general and sexual orientation–specific barriers in all ecological categories (i.e., intrapersonal, interpersonal, institutional, community, public policy) have been identified (Table 11.1). Among lesbians, gay males and bisexual female and male populations

TABLE 11.1 Barriers to physical activity among LGBT populations

---

Barriers to Physical Activity

Intrapersonal – General

Lack of time

Laziness or lack of motivation

Physical body limitations/fatigue (e.g., injury, older age issues, being overweight/obese)

Self-reported health status as poor

Distractions at home/other priorities

Cost/lack of financial resources

Lack of opportunity for women

Low athletic self-esteem/physical self-perception

Lack of knowledge about physical activity (e.g., goal setting)

General depression/anxiety

Gender non-conformity

Body image issues (e.g., being overweight, not satisfied with body)

Currently smoking

Low drive for muscularity

Low desire to control weight/workout for appearance-related reasons

Low desire to express masculinity

Lower personal eating disorder concerns

Higher level of body satisfaction

Intrapersonal – Sexual orientation–specific

Level of sexual orientation public disclosure

Interpersonal – General

Caregiving responsibilities

Lack of an exercise partner

Lack of social support (e.g., friends, family, partner)

Uncomfortable exercising around other people

Interpersonal – Sexual orientation–specific

Lack of others' acceptance of a lesbian sexual orientation

Lack of out lesbians in certain physical activity opportunities

Lack of desire to participate on sport teams comprising primarily lesbians

Institutional – General

Work-related issues

School-related issues (e.g., homework)

Lack of role models in the family

Institutional – Sexual orientation–specific

Lack of the acceptance of lesbian sexual orientation by religious institutions

Barriers to Physical Activity

Fitness facilities not allowing family memberships for same-sex couples

Lack of the acceptance of sexual minorities by the military

Negative attitudes/homophobia toward LGBT in sport and physical activity settings (Physical Education class, gyms, locker rooms)

Community/Public Policy – General

Safety issues (e.g., violence and physical/built environment)

Outdoor physical environment (e.g., inclement weather, time of day/dark outside)

Too many stoplights on street intersections

Living in a rural area

Cultural/community acceptance of a larger body type

Community/Public Policy – Sexual orientation–specific

Lack of sport teams or physical activity opportunities in community for sexual orientation minorities/subgroups

Expectation that all lesbians are athletic

Lack of fitness facility membership coverage within workplace domestic partner benefits

Sources: Barefoot *et al.* (2015); Bowen *et al.* (2006); Brittain *et al.* (2006); Brittain *et al.* (2013); Brittain *et al.* (2008); Calzo *et al.* (2014); Cary *et al.* (2015); Garbers *et al.* (2015); Gill *et al.* (2010); Griffin (1998); McElroy and Jordan (2014); Messner (1992); Muchicko *et al.* (2014)

several general barriers that hinder or stop participation in physical activity included: (a) a lack of motivation; (b) physical health limitations (e.g., injury); (c) poor self-rated health; (d) lack of social support; (e) work- and school-related issues; (f) living in a rural area; (g) personal safety concerns (e.g., violence) and (h) physical environment concerns (e.g., inclement weather) (Barefoot *et al.* 2015; Bowen *et al.* 2006; Brittain *et al.* 2006; Brittain *et al.* 2013; Cary *et al.* 2015; Garbers *et al.* 2015).

In terms of sexual orientation–specific barriers, the majority of research has targeted adult lesbians (Table 11.1). Sexual orientation–specific barriers included: (a) the expectation of having to be "out" to participate on lesbian sport teams; (b) concerns regarding being seen exercising with a lesbian partner; (c) discomfort while participating on sport teams primarily consisting of lesbian participants; (d) perception that heterosexual females will be uncomfortable sharing the locker room in a fitness facility with a lesbian; (e) the lack of same-sex partner family memberships at exercise facilities; (f) the expectation that all lesbians are athletic and enjoy sports; and (g) the perception that the lesbian community is accepting of larger body types (Bowen *et al.* 2006; Brittain *et al.* 2006; Brittain *et al.* 2008; Garbers *et al.* 2015).

Among transgender populations, only one study to date has examined factors that hinder or stop participation in physical activity (Muchicko *et al.* 2014). Based on this study, transgender individuals when compared to cisgender individuals had lower social support and lower self-perception regarding physical activity abilities, which helped to explain a portion of the non-significant differences in physical activity rates between the groups (Muchicko *et al.* 2014).

Intervention strategies

To date, few evidence-based and culturally appropriate physical activity interventions designed specifically for LGBT populations have been published (Brittain and Dinger 2014; Fogel *et al.* 2016; McElroy *et al.* 2016). All of these interventions have targeted adult lesbian and bisexual females, which is not surprising considering that the majority of research examining factors (e.g., barriers) associated with participation in physical activity has targeted these populations (Bowen *et al.* 2006; Brittain *et al.* 2006; Brittain *et al.* 2008; Garbers *et al.* 2015). Physical activity interventions have primarily been designed for adult lesbian and bisexual females for at least two other reasons: (a) sufficient evidence has identified obesity health disparities among adult lesbian and bisexual females when compared to heterosexuals (Eliason *et al.* 2015) and (b) federal funding was provided by the United States Department of Health and Human Services Office on Women's Health to create evidence-based culturally appropriate programs targeting weight-related behaviors (i.e., physical activity, nutrition) among adult lesbian and bisexual females (Fogel *et al.* 2016). The remainder of this section will highlight the evidence-based interventions designed to increase participation in physical activity among adult lesbian and bisexual females.

BOX 11.1 EVIDENCE-BASED PRACTICE: HEALTHY WEIGHT IN LESBIAN AND BISEXUAL WOMEN: STRIVING FOR A HEALTHY COMMUNITY

Healthy Weight in Lesbian and Bisexual Women: Striving for a Healthy Community (HWLB) is a coordinated national initiative to address obesity disparities among middle-aged to older adult lesbian and bisexual females. This coordinated initiative consisted of five unique yet related 12- to 16-week community-based or clinic-based group interventions designed and implemented in 10 cities across the United States: (a) Doing It For Ourselves; (b) Living Out, Living Actively; (c) Strong, Healthy, Energized; (d) Making Our Vitality Evident; and (e) Women's Health and Mindfulness. The overall goal of each intervention was to improve the health of adult lesbian and bisexual females by targeting healthy weight-related behaviors (i.e., physical activity, dietary intake [alcohol consumption; reduced sugar-sweetened beverages]).

A total of 333 females aged 40–84 years participated in the HWLB interventions. Overall, 57% of participants in the intervention groups increased their total weekly minutes of physical activity by 20%, and 38% of intervention group participants were considered sufficiently active or higher. The success of the HWLB interventions was in part due to the targeting of deep and surface structure dimensions of cultural sensitivity including: (a) the inclusion of lesbian and bisexual female community members in the design, implementation and evaluation of the interventions; (b) self-identified lesbian and bisexual females leading weekly intervention group meetings; (c) use of lesbian-specific images in the design of study-related materials and incentives; (d) not using the term *lesbian* on any publically displayed intervention-related signs; (e) choosing incentives from lesbian-friendly businesses; (f) choosing centrally located safe spaces for group meetings; and (g) use of recruitment strategies targeting local lesbian or LGBT businesses, online and in-person LGBT social groups, churches and publications.

Barriers to Engaging in Physical Activity Among Lesbians intervention

Barriers to Engaging in Physical Activity Among Lesbians (BE-PALS) was an eight-week community-based pilot intervention designed to increase participation in moderate physical activity among adult lesbians (Brittain and Dinger 2014). The intervention combined principles of social cognitive theory and group dynamics (Bandura 1986) in which 16 participants (intervention group = 10; comparison group = 6) participated in weekly group meetings that included an educational session (30 minutes) and a moderate physical activity session (30-minute walk). During the educational sessions, participants in the intervention group engaged in self-regulatory skill learning and practicing and participants in the comparison group were provided information on health topics not related to physical activity, but were specific to lesbian health. Self-regulatory skills highlighted in the weekly educational sessions included goal setting, self-monitoring (tracking physical activity, assessing whether goals have been met and readjusting them if necessary) and relapse prevention (identifying and using coping strategies to address barriers) (Meichenbaum and Turk 1987).

At baseline and the end of the intervention all participants completed demographic and self-regulatory efficacy (i.e., belief in one's abilities to overcome barriers and engage in physical activity, Bandura 1997) measures and wore an accelerometer (Brittain and Dinger 2014). No significant between-group differences in physical activity or self-regulatory efficacy at end-intervention were identified, which may be attributed to the small sample size. Although no significant differences between the groups were identified, the intervention curtailed declines in both moderate physical activity and self-regulatory efficacy among adult lesbians, which were both promising trends for conducting a larger intervention.

Healthy Weight in Lesbian and Bisexual Women: Striving for a Healthy Community initiative

In 2012, the United States Department of Health and Human Services, Office on Women's Health (OWH), provided funding for a coordinated national initiative to address obesity disparities among lesbian and bisexual females. The initiative was titled "Healthy Weight in Lesbian and Bisexual Women: Striving for a Healthy Community (HWLB)" (Fogel *et al.* 2016). This coordinated initiative was the first time national-level funding was provided to specifically assess evidence-based and culturally appropriate approaches to improve the overall health of lesbian and bisexual females. This national initiative was distinct in that five unique yet related 12- to 16-week community-based or clinic-based group interventions were designed and implemented in 10 cities across the United States: (a) Doing It For Ourselves; (b) Living Out, Living Actively; (c) Strong, Healthy, Energized; (d) Making Our Vitality Evident; and (e) Women's Health and Mindfulness.

Each intervention followed community-based participatory research principles in which LGBT community organizations, lesbian and bisexual females in their respective communities and a research team were involved with each intervention design, implementation and evaluation (Fogel *et al.* 2016). The overall goal of each intervention was to improve the health of adult lesbian and bisexual females by targeting healthy weight-related behaviors (i.e., physical activity, dietary intake [alcohol consumption; reduced sugar-sweetened beverages]). To achieve the overall goal, objectives for physical activity were: (a) a 20% increase in total weekly minutes of physical activity; (b) a 20% increase in the number of participants engaging in recommended amounts of moderate to vigorous physical activity (> 150 minutes of moderate to vigorous or > 75 minutes of vigorous physical activity each week); and (c) a 25% increase in participants exceeding the recommended levels of moderate to vigorous physical activity (McElroy *et al.* 2016). Physical activity was measured using self-report surveys. Criteria for participation in the interventions included: (a) aged > 40 years; (b) self-identification as a lesbian or bisexual female; and (c) having a BMI of > 25 kg/m² or self-identifying as being overweight.

Doing It For Ourselves intervention

Doing It For Ourselves (DIFO) was a 12-week community-based group intervention that included an intervention group and a comparison group (Fogel *et al.* 2016). The DIFO intervention components included: (a) participation in weekly 2-hour sessions in which participants engaged in a 15-minute physical activity routine (targeting core strength, spine mobility and body awareness) and (b) mindfulness-based discussions on nutritional intake and various health topics specific to lesbian and bisexual females (e.g., minority stress; coming out to healthcare providers). Participants also engaged in weekly homework activities regarding the topics covered in the group sessions. The physical activity objective for the DIFO program was a 20% increase in minutes of physical activity/week for 75% of the enrolled participants.

Living Out, Living Actively intervention

Living Out, Living Actively (LOLA) was a 16-week community-based intervention that consisted of two different intervention groups (i.e., full gym group; pedometer group) and a comparison group (Fogel *et al.* 2016). The full gym group intervention components included: (a) weekly support group meetings to discuss health topics both general (e.g., heart health) and unique to being a lesbian/bisexual female (e.g., legal protections for LGBTQ families); (b) 12 personal training sessions (45–60 minute duration); (c) a 12-month gym membership; (d) an individualized exercise training plan; and (e) four additional support group meetings to discuss nutritional intake. All participants in the pedometer group received a Fitbit Zip to track physical activity and participated in weekly support group meetings to discuss general and lesbian/bisexual health-related topics. The pedometer group participants were also eligible to participate in four optional sessions on nutritional intake. To control for interventionist contact time, the comparison group participated in weekly educational sessions regarding female health topics. The physical activity objective for all intervention groups was a 75% increase in participants engaging in > 150 minutes of moderate to vigorous or > 75 minutes of vigorous physical activity each week.

Strong, Healthy, Energized intervention

Strong, Healthy, Energized (SHE) was a 12-week community-based intervention that included weekly 90-minute group sessions with the following components: (a) a 30-minute TheraBand resistance training bout (could be completed standing or sitting); (b) a stress reduction activity; (c) a nutritional intake discussion; (d) a discussion session to address participants' experiences regarding barriers and coping strategies for physical activity, nutrition and stress reduction; and (e) a group walk (optional but strongly encouraged) (Fogel *et al.* 2016). The physical activity objective for the SHE intervention was to increase average daily steps by 2,000 from baseline to post-intervention and thus, each participant was provided a Fitbit to monitor steps. All participants had a weekly objective of increasing steps by 10%, with the ultimate objective of achieving an average of 10,000 steps each day.

Making Our Vitality Evident intervention

Making Our Vitality Evident (MOVE) was a 12-week clinic- and community-based intervention that included 90-minute weekly group sessions (Fogel *et al.* 2016). The main intervention components included: (a) weekly health-related discussions (e.g., nutrition, stress management, mindfulness and health topics related to lesbian/bisexual female health [e.g., body image]; (b) a 1-hour nutrition consultation with a registered dietician; (c) a 4-month membership to a local gym with 18 branches (intervention leaders strongly encouraged group workout sessions following each weekly meeting); (d) a SMART Health Walking Fit timekeeper; and

(e) strong encouragement to use the MyFitnessPal app for self-monitoring physical activity and nutritional intake. The physical activity objective for the MOVE intervention participants was to engage in 150 minutes of moderate or 75 minutes of vigorous physical activity each week by the end of the intervention.

Women's Health and Mindfulness intervention

Women's Health and Mindfulness (WHAM) was a 12-week clinic-based intervention that consisted of two groups, the immediate intervention group and delayed start group (served as the comparison group) (Fogel *et al.* 2016). The WHAM intervention consisted of the following components: (a) weekly 2- to 3-hour group mindfulness-based discussion/practice sessions on health-related topics (e.g., nutrition, physical activity, stress reduction and lesbian/bisexual female–specific topics); (b) four 10- to 15-minute individual or small group meetings with a personal trainer and a nutritionist; and (c) weekly mindfulness-based homework activities. The physical activity objective for the WHAM program included a 30% increase in weekly minutes of moderate physical activity.

Results: Healthy Weight in Lesbian and Bisexual Women: Striving for a Healthy Community initiative

While the HWLB initiative included five unique, yet related interventions, the results of the initiative have been reported collectively and by intervention protocol (i.e., gym membership, pedometer use, mindfulness approach) (McElroy *et al.* 2016). A total of 333 females aged 40–84 years (intervention group [$n = 266$]; comparison group [$n = 67$]) participated in the HWLB initiative. Overall, at the end of the interventions, 57% of participants in the intervention groups increased their total weekly minutes of physical activity by 20%, and 38% of intervention group participants were considered sufficiently active or higher.

In terms of the intervention protocol, the pedometer interventions seemed to be most effective (McElroy *et al.* 2016). Specifically, a significantly higher percentage of participants who engaged in a pedometer (70%) or a mindfulness-based intervention group (58%) compared to a comparison group (42%) had a 20% increase in total weekly minutes of physical activity. A significantly higher percentage of participants who engaged in a pedometer intervention group (60%) compared to a comparison group (28%) were considered sufficiently active or higher. Finally, total weekly minutes of walking was higher among participants in a pedometer intervention group (416 minutes) compared to those who were not (183 minutes).

Overall, the interventions highlighted in this section are examples of evidence-based culturally appropriate approaches to increasing physical activity among lesbian and bisexual adult female populations. All interventions comprised targeted strategies to address both surface and deep dimensions of cultural sensitivity (Chapter 3, Resnicow *et al.* 1999), which will be discussed in the "Implications for practice" section of this chapter. The majority of interventions followed the National Physical

Activity Plan (2016) by utilizing community-based participatory research principles in the design, implementation and evaluation of each intervention. In addition, the interventions targeted behaviors that aid in the reduction or onset of obesity, which has been highlighted as a health disparity between lesbian, bisexual and heterosexual females (Office of Disease Prevention and Health Promotion 2016).

Implications for practice

Limited research suggests LGBT populations may experience multiple health disparities when compared to heterosexual and cisgender populations. A more thorough examination of multiple areas of health is still needed to identify and understand the unique health experiences of LGBT populations, including the role of physical activity in improving overall health (Gorczynski and Brittain 2016). Continued research efforts examining the health of LGBT populations should utilize various methodologies including: (a) sex- and gender-specific analyses; (b) sexual orientation–specific analyses; (c) comparative analyses between sexual orientations (i.e., LGB; heterosexual) and gender identities (i.e., transgender; cisgender); and (d) the collection and use of large national-level data samples.

Although limited, current research findings suggest that culturally sensitive interventions may successfully increase participation in physical activity among lesbian and bisexual females (Fogel et al. 2016; McElroy et al. 2016). Successful interventions designed for lesbian and bisexual females targeted both deep and surface structure dimensions of cultural sensitivity (Resnicow et al. 1999). Deep structure dimensions of cultural sensitivity included: (a) the use of focus groups to obtain information from target populations prior to the design and implementation of the interventions and (b) the inclusion of lesbian and bisexual female community members actively participating in the design, implementation and evaluation of the interventions (Brittain and Dinger 2014; Fogel et al. 2016). In addition, specific tactics to address surface structure components of cultural sensitivity included: (a) the inclusion of self-identified lesbian and bisexual females to lead weekly intervention group meetings; (b) use of lesbian-specific images (e.g., rainbow) in the design of educational and recruitment materials and incentives; (c) not using the term *lesbian* on any publically displayed intervention-related signs; (d) choosing incentives from lesbian-friendly businesses; (e) choosing centrally located safe spaces for group meetings (e.g., local public library, LGBT center); (f) use of recruitment strategies targeting local lesbian or LGBT businesses, online and in-person LGBT social groups, churches and publications; (g) assistance from local key stakeholders in the lesbian community to recruit participants; and (h) the use of specific language regarding the purpose of an intervention (i.e., the HWLB interventions were not designed to focus on weight loss, but rather participation in healthy behaviors).

Future inquiry on physical activity among LGBT populations should build upon the research presented in this chapter. While a foundation of information has been established, the unique experiences from one group may or may not transcend to other groups. However, what is important to consider is that by using deep and surface structure strategies to ensure cultural sensitivity, interventions may success-fully increase participation in physical activity.

Summary points

- LGBT populations experience multiple health disparities, potentially the result of cultural discrimination, minority stress, victimization and violence.
- Limited research has examined physical activity among LGBT populations.
- The majority of research comparing participation in physical activity between LGB and heterosexuals is mixed, in that some studies identify differences between the populations and others show no differences.
- Based on the results of minimal research, transgender individuals may have lower rates of participation in physical activity when compared to cisgender individuals.
- Research has shown that LGBT populations experience general barriers to physical activity and LGB populations experience sexual orientation–specific barriers to physical activity.
- Culturally sensitive interventions may successfully increase participation in physical activity among lesbian and bisexual females.

Critical thinking questions

1   Based on the multitude of gaps in research examining physical activity among LGBT populations, what gaps do you consider the most deserving of attention and why?
2   Understanding that transgender compared to cisgender individuals may have lower rates of physical activity, do you think transgender individuals experience unique barriers to engaging in physical activity? If yes, what might be some of those unique barriers?
3   If you were to design a culturally sensitive intervention to increase participation in physical activity among one of the LGBT populations, what are some impor-tant tactics you would consider when addressing deep and surface structure dimensions of cultural sensitivity?

References

American Psychological Association. (2012). 'Guidelines for psychological practice with les-bian, gay, and bisexual clients.' *American Psychologist*, 67: 10–42.
American Psychological Association. (2015). 'Guidelines for psychological practice with transgender and gender nonconforming people.' *American Psychologist*, 70: 832–864.
Andersen, J., Zou, C. and Blosnich, J. (2015). 'Multiple early victimization experiences as a pathway to explain physical health disparities among sexual minority and heterosexual individuals.' *Social Science & Medicine*, 133: 111–119.
Bandura, A. (1986). *Social foundations of thought and action*. New Jersey, NJ, Prentice Hall.

Bandura, A. (1997). *Self-efficacy: The exercise of control*. New York, NY, Freeman.

Barefoot, K., Warren, J. and Smalley, K. (2015). 'An examination of past and current influences of rurality on lesbians' overweight/obesity risks.' *LGBT Health*, 2: 154–161.

Blosnich, J., Farmer, G., Lee, J., Silenzio, V. and Bowen, D. (2014). 'Health inequalities among sexual minority adults evidence from ten U.S. states, 2010.' *American Journal of Preventive Medicine*, 46: 337–349.

Boehmer, U. and Bowen, D. (2009). 'Examining factors linked to overweight and obesity in women of different sexual orientations.' *Preventive Medicine*, 48: 357–361.

Boehmer, U., Miao, X., Linkletter, C. and Clark, M. (2012). 'Adult health behaviors over the life course by sexual orientation.' *American Journal of Public Health*, 102: 292–300.

Boehmer, U., Miao, X., Linkletter, C. and Clark, M. (2014). 'Health conditions in younger, middle, and older ages: Are there differences by sexual orientation?' *LGBT Health*, 1: 168–176.

Bowen, D., Balsam, K., Diergaarde, B., Russo, M. and Escamilla, G. (2006). 'Healthy eating, exercise, and weight: Impressions of sexual minority women.' *Women & Health*, 44: 79–93.

Brittain, D., Baillargeon, T., McElroy, M., Aaron, D. and Gyurcsik, N. (2006). 'Barriers to moderate physical activity in adult lesbians.' *Women & Health*, 43: 75–92.

Brittain, D. and Dinger, M. (2014). 'BE-PALS: An innovative theory-based intervention to promote moderate physical activity among adult lesbians.' *Women in Sport and Physical Activity Journal*, 22: 71–75.

Brittain, D. and Dinger, M. (2015). 'An examination of health inequities among college students by sexual orientation identity and sex.' *Journal of Public Health Research*, 4: 1–6.

Brittain, D., Dinger, M. and Hutchinson, S. (2013). 'Sociodemographic and lesbian-specific factors associated with physical activity among adult lesbians.' *Women's Health Issues*, 23: e103–e108.

Brittain, D., Gyurcsik, N. and McElroy, M. (2008). 'Perceived barriers to physical activity among adult lesbians.' *Women in Sport and Physical Activity Journal*, 17: 68–79.

Burton, C., Marshal, M., Chisolm, D., Sucato, G. and Friedman, M. (2013). 'Sexual minority-related victimization as a mediator of mental health disparities in sexual minority youth: A longitudinal analysis.' *Journal of Youth and Adolescence*, 42: 394–402.

Calzo, J., Roberts, A., Corliss, H., Blood, E., Kroshus, E. and Austin, S. (2014). 'Physical activity disparities in heterosexual and sexual minority youth ages 12–22 years old: Roles of childhood gender nonconformity and athletic self-esteem.' *Annals of Behavioral Medicine*, 47: 17–27.

Cary, M., Brittain, D., Dinger, M., Ford, M., Cain, M. and Sharp, T. (2015). 'Barriers to physical activity among gay men.' *American Journal of Men's Health*, 10: 408–417.

Cochran, S., Björkenstam, C. and Mays, V. (2016). 'Sexual orientation and all-cause mortality among us adults aged 18 to 59 years, 2001–2011.' *American Journal of Public Health*, 106: 918–920.

Dickey, L., Budge, S., Katz-Wise, S. and Garza, M. (2016). 'Health disparities in the transgender community: Exploring differences in insurance coverage.' *Psychology of Sexual Orientation and Gender Diversity*, 3: 275–282.

Dilley, J., Simmons, K., Boysun, M., Pizacani, B. and Stark, M. (2010). 'Demonstrating the importance and feasibility of including sexual orientation in public health surveys: Health disparities in the Pacific Northwest.' *American Journal of Public Health*, 100: 460–467.

Eliason, M., Ingraham, N., Fogel, S., McElroy, J., Lorvick, J., Mauery, D. and Haynes, S. (2015). 'A systematic review of the literature on weight in sexual minority women.' *Women's Health Issues*, 25: 162–175.

Flores, A. (2014). *National trends in public opinion on LGBT rights in the United States*. Los Angeles, CA: Williams Institute, UCLA School of Law.

Flores, A., Herman, J., Gates, G. and Brown, T. (2016). *How many adults identify as transgender in the United States?* Los Angeles, CA: Williams Institute, UCLA School of Law.

Fogel, S., McElroy, J., Garbers, S., McDonnell, C., Brooks, J., Eliason, M., Ingraham, N., Osborn, A., Rayyes, N., Redman, S., Wood, S. and Haynes, S. (2016). 'Program design for healthy weight in lesbian and bisexual women: A ten-city prevention initiative.' *Women's Health Issues*, 26: s7–17.

Fredriksen-Goldsen, K., Cook-Daniels, L., Kim, H., Erosheva, E., Emlet, C., Hoy-Ellis, C., Goldsen, J. and Muraco, A. (2013a). 'Physical and mental health of transgender older adults: An at-risk and underserved population.' *The Gerontologist*, 54: 488–500.

Fredriksen-Goldsen, K., Kim, H., Barkan, S., Muraco, A. and Hoy-Ellis, C. (2013b). 'Health disparities among lesbian, gay, and bisexual older adults: Results from a population- based study.' *American Journal of Public Health*, 103: 1802–1809.

Gallup Poll. (2016). '*Gay and lesbian rights* [Online].' Available: www.gallup.com/poll/1651/gay-lesbian-rights.aspx (Accessed October 1 2016).

Garbers, S., McDonnell, C., Fogel, S., Eliason, M., Ingraham, N., McElroy, J., Radix, A. and Haynes, S. (2015). 'Aging, weight, and health among adult lesbian and bisexual women: A metasynthesis of the multisite "Healthy Weight Initiative" focus groups.' *LGBT Health*, 2: 176–187.

Gates, G. (2014). *LGBT demographics: Comparisons among population-based surveys.* Los Angeles, CA: Williams Institute, UCLA School of Law.

Gill, D., Morrow, R., Collins, K., Lucey, A. and Schultz, A. (2010). 'Perceived climate in physical activity settings.' *Journal of Homosexuality*, 57: 895–913.

Gorczynski, P. and Brittain, D. (2016). 'Call to action: The need for an LGBT-focused physical activity research strategy.' *American Journal of Preventive Medicine*, 51: 527–530.

Grant, J., Mottet, L., Tanis, J., Harrison, J., Herman, J. and Keisling, M. (2011). *Injustice at every turn: A report of the national transgender discrimination survey.* Washington, DC: National Center for Transgender Equality and National Gay and Lesbian Task Force.

Griffin, P. (1998). *Strong women, deep closets.* Champaign, IL: Human Kinetics.

Institute of Medicine. (2011). *The health of lesbian, gay, bisexual, and transgender people: Building a foundation for better understanding.* Washington, DC: The National Academies Press.

Kann, L., O'Malley Olsen, E., McManus, T., Kinchen, S., Chyen, D., Harris, W. and Wechsler, H. (2011). 'Sexual identity, sex of sexual contacts, and health-risk behaviors among students in grades 9–12 – Youth Risk Behavior Surveillance, selected sites, United States, 2001–2009.' *Morbidity, Mortality, Weekly Report*, 60: 1–133.

Laska, M., VanKim, N., Erickson, D., Lust, K., Eisenberg, M. and Rosser, B. (2015). 'Disparities in weight and weight behaviors by sexual orientation in college students.' *American Journal of Public Health*, 105: 111–121.

Lick, D., Durso, L. and Johnson, K. (2013). 'Minority stress and physical health among sexual minorities.' *Perspectives on Psychological Science*, 8: 521–548.

McElroy, J., Haynes, S., Eliason, M., Wood, S., Gilbert, T., Toms Barker, L. and Minnis, A. (2016). 'Healthy weight in lesbian and bisexual women aged 40 and older: An effective intervention in 10 cities using tailored approaches.' *Women's Health Issues*, 26: s18–s35.

McElroy, J. and Jordan, J. (2014). 'Sufficiently and insufficiently active lesbian, bisexual, and questioning female college students: Sociodemographic factors among two age cohorts.' *Women's Health Issues*, 24: e243–e249.

McLeroy, K., Bibeau, D., Steckler, A. and Glanz, K. (1988). 'An ecological perspective on health promotion programs.' *Health Education & Behavior*, 15: 351–377.

Meichenbaum, D. and Turk, D. (1987). *Facilitating treatment adherence.* New York, NY: Plenum.

Messner, M. (1992). *Power at play.* Boston, MA: Beacon Press.

Meyer, I. (2003). 'Prejudice, social stress, and mental health in lesbian, gay, and bisexual populations: Conceptual issues and research evidence.' *Psychological Bulletin*, 129: 674–697.

Muchicko, M., Lepp, A. and Barkley, J. (2014). 'Peer victimization, social support and leisure-time physical activity in transgender and cisgender individuals.' *Leisure*, 38: 295–308.

Mustanski, B., Andrews, R. and Puckett, J. (2016). 'The effects of cumulative victimization on mental health among lesbian, gay, bisexual, and transgender adolescents and young adults.' *American Journal of Public Health*, 106: 527–533.

National Physical Activity Plan. (2016). '*National physical activity plan* [Online].' Available: www.physicalactivityplan.org (Accessed May 1 2016).

Office of Disease Prevention and Health Promotion. (2016). '*Lesbian, gay, bisexual, and transgender health: Healthy People 2020* [Online].' Available: www.healthypeople.gov/2020/topics-objectives/topic/lesbian-gay-bisexual-and-transgender-health (Accessed April 10 2016).

Reisner, S., White, J., Bradford, J. and Mimiaga, M. (2014). 'Transgender health disparities: Comparing full cohort and nested matched-pair study designs in a community health center.' *LGBT Health*, 1: 177–184.

Resnicow, K., Baranowski, T., Ahluwalia, J. and Braithwaite, R. (1999). 'Cultural sensitivity in public health: Defined and demystified.' *Ethnicity and Disease*, 9: 10–21.

Rosario, M., Corliss, H., Everett, B., Reisner, S., Austin, S., Buchting, F. and Birkett, M. (2014). 'Sexual orientation disparities in cancer-related risk behaviors of tobacco, alcohol, sexual behaviors, and diet and physical activity: Pooled youth risk behavior surveys.' *American Journal of Public Health*, 104: 245–254.

United States Department of Health and Human Services. (2008). '*2008 physical activity guidelines for Americans* [Online].' Available: www.health.gov/paguidelines/pdf/paguide.pdf (Accessed April 12 2016).

VanKim, N., Erickson, D., Eisenberg, M., Lust, K., Rosser, B. and Laska, M. (2014). 'Weight-related disparities for transgender college students. *Health Behavior and Policy Review*, 1: 161–171.

12

PHYSICAL ACTIVITY AMONG MILITARY VETERANS

David E. Goodrich and Katherine S. Hall

Understanding the veteran population

Military service is a formative life experience with few counterparts in civilian life. Upon entry into the service, individuals are assimilated into a unique institution with its own cultural and behavioral norms (Johnson *et al.* 2013) and as such, U.S. military veterans are diverse and may be considered a population with its own culture and subcultures (Olenick *et al.* 2015). A significant proportion of veterans constitute a medically complex and vulnerable health population due to the health risks that they took in service of their country. While military recruits and service members are healthier than nonveterans due to medical screening requirements and fitness standards, many veterans become insufficiently active and develop health problems soon after discharge from the military.

This chapter will help readers understand the surface and deep structural aspects of military culture that can guide culturally sensitive physical activity intervention efforts. We will provide an overview of the significant and complex health disparities seen in the veteran population compared to their civilian counterparts and examine the influences on physical activity from a multilevel, sociological perspective. We will then review current evidence-based strategies for promoting physical activity for veterans, focusing on the cultural implications for practice.

The average American is likely to be familiar with surface structures of veteran and military culture (Resnicow *et al.* 1999), which have been communicated regularly through news and entertainment media and which convey readily observable characteristics of military life such as military dress or language. With the end of compulsory military service in the 1970s, fewer Americans have direct contact with military culture compared to past generations (Olenick *et al.* 2015).

Demographic characteristics

The U.S. veteran population is diverse and consists of individuals who served during World War II and continuing through to the present operations Enduring Freedom, Iraqi Freedom, and New Dawn (OEF, OIF, OND) in Afghanistan, Iraq, and Libya, respectively. Yearly estimates of the total veteran population are based on the U.S. Census Bureau definition of veterans as, "men and women who have served (even for a short time), but are not currently serving, on Active Duty in the U.S. Army, Navy, Air Force, Marine Corps, or the Coast Guard, or who served in the U.S. Merchant Marine during World War II. People who served in the National Guard or Reserves are classified as veterans **only** if they were ever called or ordered to Active Duty, not counting the 4–6 months for initial training or yearly summer camps" (United States Census Bureau 2014).

In 2014, there were an estimated 21.9 million living American veterans (Bagalman 2014). Almost 92% of veterans were male with a median age of 64 years versus 41 years for a nonveteran civilian male (National Center for Veterans Analysis and Statistics March 2016). Nearly 78% of veterans were White, with minority veterans constituting 22% of the veteran population and broken out as the following: Black (11%), Hispanic (7%), Asian (2%), American or Alaskan Indian (1%), and two or more or other races (1%). Following discharge from the military, most veterans reside in urban or suburban locations, with 24% living in rural settings.

Recent social trends have resulted in dramatic changes in veteran demographics, including increased numbers of women and LGBT persons serving in the Armed Forces. During the Vietnam War, women represented only 2% of the total fighting force and had limited opportunities for promotion in rank (Boyd *et al.* 2013, Street *et al.* 2009). The implementation of the all-volunteer fighting force in the 1970s increased opportunities for women to serve, resulting in women becoming the fastest-growing demographic group among veterans (Conard and Armstrong 2015). Women veterans are significantly younger than their male counterparts, with a median age of 49 years, but older than the median age of 46 years for a nonveteran woman (National Center for Veterans Analysis and Statistics 2016). Between 2014 and 2040, it is projected that the proportion of women in the overall veteran population will more than double, from 8% to 18%.

In 2016, the LGBT subculture was officially acknowledged and endorsed as a result of the repeal of the Department of Defense's (DoD) "Don't Ask Don't Tell" (DADT) policy. Prior to the 2015 repeal of DADT, it was illegal for LGBT persons to openly serve in the Armed Forces. LGBT personnel were forced to hide their sexual orientation and endure discrimination, stigma, and the fear of punishment including early career termination and dishonorable discharge (Mattocks *et al.* 2015). Due to DADT, less is known about the prevalence and needs of this minority veteran subpopulation. However, one widely cited report estimated that lesbian, gay, and bisexual Americans represent 2.5% of Active Duty personnel (Burks 2011).

Military service

The branch of the Armed Forces in which a veteran served as well as the dates of service and length of time he/she spent in the military are structural elements of veteran culture. While *career* military individuals must stay in the military for a minimum of 20 years, the saliency of their participation may not be different than a soldier who saw one year of intense combat. Exercise professionals should also note that veterans who served in the Army and Marine Corps were likely to undergo more intensive physical training to prepare for ground combat than airmen and sailors who served in the Air Force, Navy, Coast Guard, or National Guard.

Active Duty service members are defined by their rank and the role that they performed in their service branch. In general, service ranks begin with enlisted personnel and progress to warrant officers and commissioned officers in a hierarchy that is positively correlated with educational training (Spelman *et al.* 2012). All personnel must go through a period of basic training (8–13) weeks followed by advanced training which lasts 6–12 weeks, followed by assignment to a specific unit for 2–3 years, a period in which they are likely to be deployed once. Additional specialized training is required for promotion, especially within the officer corps (Haibach *et al.* 2016). For exercise professionals, assessing a veteran's service, rank, what they did, and their combat or deployment history can help identify potential service-related health problems. Higher rank is generally a health protective factor closely associated with higher education, less risk for occupational/combat exposures, and better health status (Bagnell *et al.* 2013).

Military culture

Americans from a variety of different backgrounds join the Armed Forces, and they all undergo a process of transformation from a civilian to a military identity (Johnson *et al.* 2013). During Boot Camp/Basic Training and Officer Candidate School, recruits are indoctrinated in military culture which includes values, customs, norms, traditions, and standards of behavior (Olenick *et al.* 2015). Military core values include commitment, duty, honor, integrity, leadership and subordination, personal courage, respect, sacrifice, and service before self (Moss *et al.* 2015, Olenick *et al.* 2015). Military customs create the norms for unit camaraderie and are the foundation of good order, teamwork, and discipline. Recruits also learn the warrior ethos which emphasizes a constant readiness to complete the mission, stoicism, and loyalty to the team above self (Johnson *et al.* 2013).

Physical stamina and discipline are inherent aspects of military culture and service. All military personnel are required to maintain a high level of fitness as a job requirement, which is assessed at least once annually according to height, weight, and branch-specific tests. These tests include some measure of aerobic conditioning, muscular strength and endurance, and body composition (Littman *et al.* 2015). Failure to meet a fitness standard can result in involuntary separation from Active Duty, prevention of reenlistment, or adversely affect promotion opportunities. Hence, commanding officers have the incentive to make fitness a priority by allocating personnel time and resources for daily conditioning. Many enlisted personnel become accustomed to the extensive worksite health promotion practices afforded by a military job and the transition to being a veteran living in the community can be difficult without these environmental supports (Ahern *et al.* 2015, Jay *et al.* 2015b, Littman *et al.* 2015).

Veteran identity

Individuals develop a *veteran identity* during military service, which has been referred by Harada and colleagues as a self-concept derived from one's military experiences within a sociocultural context (Harada *et al.* 2002, Johnson *et al.* 2013). Table 12.1 summarizes a number of factors that serve to influence veteran identity over a lifetime including the service era or conflict in which a veteran served, deployment history, combat exposure, injury status, any service-related disabilities, exposure to

TABLE 12.1 Surface and deep structure dimensions for culturally sensitive interactions with veterans

Surface Structure Characteristics of Veteran Culture		
People	Demographics	Age, race, gender, LGBT status, rural vs. urban, U.S. region of residence (Northeast vs. Southwest)
Language	Military slang and acronyms	Dependent on service and service era
Music	Patriotic	Martial band music, American popular music
Clothing	Military attire	Uniforms, camouflage, medals, and clothing or hats remembering service branch and unit
Military service	Branch of service	Air Force, Army, Coast Guard, Marine Corps, Coast Guard, or National Guard or Reserve
	Assignment status	Military base, foreign country
	Time and status in military	Career military vs. draftee, rank, officer status
Channels	Current health care provider	VHA, Tricare, Military Healthcare Service, Medicaid, or private health provider
	Veteran Service Organizations and nonprofit foundations	Team Red, White & Blue; Foreign Legion, Veterans of Foreign Wars, etc.
	Community events	5K runs, parades, YMCA, sporting events
	Technology literacy	Smartphone vs. landline, social media vs. print, targeted technology by age/service era

(Continued)

TABLE 12.1 (Continued)

Deep Structure Characteristics of Veteran Culture

Military culture	Warrior Ethos values	Physical stamina, discipline, duty, honor, loyalty, respect, and commitment to comrades, unit, nation
	Hierarchy	Roles, and defined responsibilities in a structured routine; military provides health care
	Role of physical activity	Mandated physical activity and weight status as part of job description/ continued employment
Veteran identity	Service era/conflict	World War II, Korea, Vietnam, Gulf War, OEF/OIF
	Deployment history	Location of deployment status, combat status, how long deployed, number of deployments/tours (strain on family, jobs)
	Combat, occupational exposure	Saw combat, enemy fire, or casualties; musculoskeletal injury, weather extremes, excessive noise or vibration; sexual trauma
	Injury status	Veteran or comrades were wounded, injured, or hospitalized
	Service-related disability status	Traumatic brain injury, musculoskeletal injury, amputation, spinal cord injury, mental health diagnosis, shrapnel, etc.
Hazardous exposures	Exposure to environmental hazards	Chemicals, infectious diseases, radiation, or pollution (e.g., oil well smoke or burn pits)
	View of service experience	Positive or negative (military sexual trauma)
Post-deployment	Degree of public support	Strong anti-war view vs. broad public support
	Reintegration with family, work, and social network	Employment or housing status, sense of alienation/isolation, lack of purpose/ mission
	Self-efficacy to manage health	Confidence to do physical activity with respect to physical disability/health challenges; lack of autonomy and/ or physical and social environmental supports

certain hazards, and the veteran's perceived valence of their military experience. The strength and meaning of this identity are shaped by the salience of these factors and can vary across individuals.

Although service members generally have better overall health than nonveterans, the stresses of combat and deployment can undermine these advantages (Bagnell *et al.* 2013, Spelman *et al.* 2012). Deployment refers to movement of military personnel to temporary assignments away from their home installation and can last in duration from weeks to months for either peacekeeping or combat missions. Combat deployment is associated with a number of physical and psychological stressors. *Physical* combat and occupational stressors include coping with austere living conditions; poor physical and dental hygiene; extreme temperature variability; loud noises and vibrations from equipment, weapons, and ordnance; and among ground combat forces, the demands of carrying heavy combat equipment loads often over 100 pounds. Women service members are currently expected to use and carry the same equipment as men with no accommodations for body size. Combat deployment is *psychologically* stressful due to the anticipation of combat, separation from home and family, and the exposure to combat and noncombat-related trauma (Spelman *et al.* 2012). Combat increases the risk for unhealthy coping behaviors such as smoking, substance use, and heavy drinking as well as the onset of sleep problems and mental health disorders. Among women veterans, deployment is also associated with military sexual trauma (MST) due to physical/sexual assault or harassment, disproportionately affecting up to 41% of women versus 4% of men (Barth *et al.* 2016).

Veterans are at risk for service-related disabilities that may or may not have occurred in combat or during deployment. Rates of specific service-related disabilities differ by service era cohort based on the combat threats and/or work and

TABLE 12.2 Health and sociocultural factors affecting physical activity prescription in veterans

Health Factors	Sociocultural
Obesity	Older age
Unhealthy lifestyle behaviors	Race (non-White)
Substance use disorders	Gender
Mental health disorders	Sexual orientation
Sleep disorders	Rural vs. urban residence
Multiple medical morbidity	Poverty
Cognitive impairments	Homelessness
Traumatic brain disorders (TBI)	Unemployment/underemployment
Polytrauma (multiple injuries in 1 incident)	Literacy
Amputation and assistive devices	History of discrimination
Chronic pain	Isolation/lack of close social support
Environmental and chemical exposures	Inadequate physical activity programming

living conditions encountered. In prior wars, many combat wounds were more likely to be fatal (Geiling *et al.* 2012). However, improvements in protective combat armor, injury evacuation strategies, and medical care have decreased battlefield mortality rates but increased the morbidity among those surviving their injuries. Among OEF/OIF/OND veterans, explosions from improvised explosive devices (IEDs) and rocket-propelled grenades have resulted in complex lifelong injuries requiring multiple surgeries and rehabilitation periods (Gawande 2004, Johnson *et al.* 2013). Many OEF/OIF/OND veterans live with disabilities associated with multiple injuries sustained in the same incident (polytrauma) including amputations, severe burns, spinal cord injuries, and traumatic brain injuries (TBI) that put them at risk for cognitive impairments, mental health disorders, and addictions to pain medications (Johnson *et al.* 2013, Spelman *et al.* 2012).

Health disparities and inequities among the veteran population

Military veterans have been exposed to a range of individual, social, psychological, and physical stressors unique to training and combat. These stressors are often not germane to the general population and contribute to a disparate distribution of chronic disease and debilitating conditions among veterans. Considerable research has been conducted to understand these disparities among vulnerable veteran subpopulations. We briefly explore some of these health disparities here, focusing on their associations with physical activity.

Healthcare use and access

There is an important distinction between veterans who receive their health care within the Veterans Health Administration (VHA) and those who receive their care elsewhere. VHA is the largest integrated health system in the U.S. and is part of the Department of Veterans Affairs (VA). To be eligible for any kind of VA benefits, an individual must have participated in Active Duty military service with discharge for any reason other than dishonorable. To receive VA comprehensive *health benefits*, veterans must enroll in VHA and are assigned a priority level for services based on military service–connected *disability*, economic *need*, or special circumstances (e.g., prisoner of war).

Because of VHA eligibility criteria, veterans who use its services tend to be older, lower SES, minorities, to have been combat deployed, and more disabled by mental and physical health comorbidities than nonveterans or non-VHA users (Kizer and Dudley 2009). Figure 12.1 illustrates the burden of chronic health conditions born by VHA patients compared to other veterans and nonveterans. Notably, while VHA patients tend to be older than veterans who do not use it (52% are older than age 65 vs. 39% in nonusers), those who *rely* most heavily on VHA tend to be younger and from recent conflicts (Rand Health 2016). Compared to most community healthcare providers, VHA has specific programs designed to address patient needs

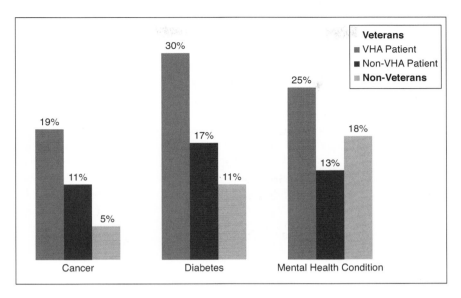

FIGURE 12.1 Prevalence rates of health conditions in nonveterans versus veterans who do or do not use VHA services

Source: Reprinted with permission from the Rand® Corporation, Santa Monica, CA (Rand Health 2016)

associated with military combat such as treatments for hearing loss, loss of limbs, traumatic brain injury (TBI), blindness, severe burns, and mental trauma, which endears VHA to the veterans who use it (Rand Health 2016).

Metabolic health

Veterans are at greater risk for overweight and obesity than nonveterans. In 2014, 42% of VHA patients were obese with combined prevalence rate of overweight/obesity of 78% (Department of Veterans Affairs and Department of Defense 2014). Comparatively, rates of overweight and obesity among U.S. adults were 67% and 35%, respectively (Ogden *et al.* 2014). While these disparities have been attributed to socio-demographic factors such as the older average age of veterans, studies of younger OEF/OIF/OND veterans indicate transition from the military as a critical period for weight gain (Maguen *et al.* 2013, Rosenberger *et al.* 2011). Within a couple of years of discharge, overweight/obesity rates range between 75% and 84% in this formerly active cohort (Rosenberger *et al.* 2011). This weight gain coincides with decreases in physical activity (Littman *et al.* 2015), particularly among veterans who are male, less educated, older, served in the Army or Navy, and report comorbid health conditions such as diabetes, chronic pain, and Post Traumatic Stress Disorder (PTSD) (Maguen *et al.* 2013, Rush *et al.* 2016).

Poor nutrition

Many veterans adopt unhealthy dietary practices during military service that persist into civilian life. As young adults, service members are encouraged to use exercise as the primary means to stay fit but are not taught principles of healthy eating by the military (Jay *et al.* 2015b). Active Duty personnel often have limited access to healthy foods whereas both fast food and highly processed foods are readily available. Moreover, unpredictable and long workdays encourage personnel to consume large quantities of food quickly (Ramsey *et al.* 2013, Smith *et al.* 2009). Male veterans of enlisted ranks are not only more likely to be obese but also to consume higher levels of red and processed meats and lower intake of fruits and vegetables compared to officers and nonveterans (Park *et al.* 2011). One in four OEF/OIF veterans from enlisted ranks report food insecurity in the past year (Widome *et al.* 2014). Finally, rates of subclinical binge-eating behaviors appear high among veterans (Litwack *et al.* 2014, Maguen *et al.* 2012). One VHA study reported 78% of candidates for weight management treatment endorsed binge-eating behavior, with higher rates among male versus female veterans (Higgins *et al.* 2013).

Behavioral health risk factors

The psychological and social stresses of military service significantly elevate alcohol, tobacco, and drug use among veterans. Current rates of smoking range between 21% and 27% among veterans compared to 19% to 20% in nonveterans (Centers for Disease Control and Prevention 2011, Kelly *et al.* 2016). However, approximately one-third of Active Duty personnel report smoking, with rates higher among troops who have been deployed (Institute of Medicine (IOM) 2009). A recent meta-analysis reported veterans have elevated annual diagnostic rates for alcohol use disorders compared to nonveterans (11% vs. 9%) as well as for drug use disorders (including prescription drugs) 5% compared to 2% (Lan *et al.* 2016). In recent years, prescription medications and alcohol abuse have become more urgent issues than illicit drugs, which were characteristic of earlier service eras. Substance use disorders greatly complicate medical and psychiatric treatment. The risk factors for these disorders are multifaceted and include biological risks but also include combat exposure, comorbid mental disorder, homelessness, history of trauma, low SES, sleep disorders, and difficulties integrating into civilian life (Department of Veterans Affairs and Department of Defense 2015).

Mental health

Mental health conditions are common and debilitating in military veterans. In 2015, nearly 25% of veterans using VHA primary care services had at least one mental illness (Trivedi *et al.* 2015) compared to 18% of nonveteran adults (Center for Behavioral and Health Statistics and Quality 2015). Rates of diagnosed mental disorders range between 10% to 13% in Active Duty service members who have been deployed compared to only 2.4% among new recruits who have never been deployed (Monahan *et al.* 2013, Office of the Surgeon General U.S. Army Medical Command *et al.* 2013). Depression is the most common mental health condition among veterans (13.5–16.7%), followed by PTSD (9.3%), anxiety disorders (4.8%), and serious mental illness (3.7%), with significant co-occurrence with other psychiatric diagnoses observed (Trivedi *et al.* 2015, Zivin *et al.* 2015). Suicide rates among veterans have exceeded U.S. population averages since 2001, with 18 to 22 veterans committing suicide daily (Kemp and Bossarte 2012). Notably, many mental health disorders are comorbid with a medical condition or combat injury. Finally, sleep disturbance is among the most common complaint of military personnel following deployment, with 64% of OEF/OIF veterans endorsing symptoms of insomnia upon their return which can indirectly undermine health behaviors like physical activity (Amin 2010).

Physical health disparities

Veteran patients often have poorer self-reported health status and more medical conditions than nonveterans (Kizer and Dudley 2009, Nelson *et al.* 2007). Some of these conditions may be linked to deployment-related exposures, while others may be associated with lifestyle factors. However, the prevalence of multiple cardiovascular risk factors is high in both male and female veterans aged 35–64 years, with increased frequency with increasing age (Vimalananda *et al.* 2013). In a recent study of over 5 million VHA patients (Yoon *et al.* 2014), researchers found that nearly one-third of veterans had ≥ 3 chronic conditions, with the most common triad being diabetes, hyperlipidemia, and hypertension. The higher rates of these preventable conditions in veterans compared to nonveterans are fully accounted for by the greater burden of obesity among veterans (Fryar *et al.* 2016).

The interaction of injuries from combat exposures with lifestyle diseases further adds to the complexity of medical care for veterans. Chronic, persistent pain is highly prevalent among veterans (44%), due in large part to musculoskeletal trauma and overuse injuries sustained during service (Goulet *et al.* 2016, Higgins *et al.* 2014). The most commonly reported painful conditions in veterans are arthritis/joint pain and back pain, both of which are more common among veterans than nonveterans, and which pose barriers to regular engagement in physical activity (Buis *et al.* 2011, Dominick *et al.* 2006, Higgins *et al.* 2016, Murphy *et al.* 2014). Moreover, the physical and psychological rehabilitation from combat injuries associated with amputations, burns, spinal cord injury, and damage is lengthy, requiring specialized exercise interventions delivered at home and clinics (Johnson *et al.* 2013, Spelman *et al.* 2012).

While musculoskeletal injuries and mental health disorders are the two most common health conditions reported by recent combat veterans, conditions with nonspecific signs and symptoms make up the third most common category (Epidemiology Group *et al.* June 2015). This category may include fatigue, and somatic and cognitive complaints such as memory and concentration problems. Although these symptoms may be associated with the high prevalence of traumatic brain injuries (10% to 20%), some forms of nonspecific medical complaints are due to occupational and combat exposures to hazardous chemicals, burns, radiation, or nerve agents. The nature of such exposures is often unique to a specific conflict and/or group of service personnel. The high prevalence and complexity of these health exposures prompted VHA to develop a pocket card for community providers to elicit these risk factors based on a veteran's service era (www.va.gov.oaa/pocketcard/).

Physical activity among veterans

Large population-based studies comparing physical activity rates among veterans and nonveterans suggest that veterans are equally active or more active than the general population (Bouldin and Reiber 2012, Littman *et al.* 2013, Littman *et al.* 2009). Among Active Duty personnel, 64% to 75% meet MVPA guidelines, which is well above the 45% to 50% rates reported by nonveterans (Hoerster *et al.* 2012b, Littman *et al.* 2013, Littman *et al.* 2015). Unfortunately, few studies make the distinction between more vulnerable veterans who use VHA services versus those who do not. One study found little difference in the prevalence rates of meeting activity guidelines between veterans and nonveterans as well as between VHA users and nonusers (Littman *et al.* 2009); however, VHA users were more likely to be inactive than nonusers (21% vs. 15%, respectively), reporting rates similar to nonveterans (21%).

While Active Duty personnel are more physically active than nonveterans, these activity levels are not maintained after military service. Results from the VA/DoD Millennium Cohort Study suggest that the transition from Active Duty to veteran status is associated with a significant reduction in physical activity (Littman *et al.* 2015). The Millennium Cohort Study is a longitudinal study of over 250,000 military personnel from all services branches, including the National Guard and Reserve that started in 2001 with periodic and ongoing health assessments. Littman and colleagues found that the proportion of individuals meeting activity guidelines (U.S. Department of Health and Human Services 2008) declined drastically from an average of 64% while Active Duty to 50% shortly after discharge.

Millennium Cohort Study findings also indicate that decline in physical activity was not equal across subpopulations of veterans. Those at risk for significant declines in physical activity were Black, less than college-educated, deployed with combat exposures, current smokers, Air Force personnel, and those who had 14 to 25 years of service. A greater decline in the proportion meeting MVPA guidelines was also seen among those who were former Active Duty (24% decrease) compared to Reserve and National Guard personnel (only 5%) (Littman *et al.* 2015). That we see smaller declines in activity rates among Reserve and National Guard service members compared to Active Duty service members may reflect greater assimilation into civilian culture among Guard and Reserve personnel. Whereas Active

Duty have the benefit of a work environment in which daily exercise is incentivized to meet fitness standards, Reserve and National Guard members must develop self-regulatory skills to sustain a regular exercise routine.

There is limited research examining physical activity correlates among minority groups of veterans except for a small number of studies in women veterans. A longitudinal analysis of the Women's Health Initiative (1998) cohort of post-menopausal women ages 50–79 years examined trajectories of physical activity and sedentary time among veterans and nonveterans (Washington et al. 2016). Although veterans exhibited higher baseline MVPA than nonveterans (13.2 vs. 12.5 MET-hours/week), veterans displayed a steeper decline in MVPA over an eight-year follow-up than nonveterans. Insufficient exercise is more prevalent among women veterans and nonveterans and least common among Active Duty women (Grossbard et al. 2013, Lehavot et al. 2012). Moreover, women veterans also report lower rates of exercise participation than male veterans (Grossbard et al. 2013). To conduct culturally tailored work with veterans, exercise professionals should consider how deeper structures related to a military culture, that is, social, historical, psychological, and environment factors in military service, affect a veteran's current engagement in physical activity (Resnicow et al. 1999).

Common barriers and facilitators to physical activity for veterans

Role of individual, social, and environmental factors

Despite a dearth of research into the determinants of physical activity among veterans, new studies suggest potential targets for tailoring physical activity promotion efforts. Chronic health conditions such as diabetes, lung disease, and sleep disorders have been commonly associated with lower activity levels (Bouldin and Reiber 2012, Chasens et al. 2009, Moy et al. 2016, Talbot et al. 2014). However, psychosocial barriers including mental disorders, pain, somatic symptom severity, and low ratings of health status are also associated with reduced odds of physical activity (Chwastiak et al. 2011, Hall et al. 2015, Hoerster et al. 2012a, Millstein et al. 2015, Mori et al. 2006, Sin et al. 2016). A substantial decline in physical activity rates on the order of 20% occurs among discharged service members who were obese or who had diagnoses of PTSD or depression. However, these same individuals were able to maintain activity levels and meet MVPA guidelines while still Active Duty (Leardmann et al. 2011, Littman et al. 2015). This finding suggests that with proactive supports and resources, veterans with these conditions may be able to continue their active lifestyle post-service.

The transition from military service to civilian life poses challenges to adhering to an exercise routine. Whereas the military provided daily structure, social support, and routine to support a physically active lifestyle, many veterans lack life skills and supportive structures to manage their disabilities and health (Buis et al. 2011,

Jay *et al.* 2015b). Low importance or lack of knowledge of the benefits of exercise does not explain the post-discharge drop in MVPA (Yaffe *et al.* 2014). In formative studies, veterans express positive attitudes toward exercise and its health protective benefits while acknowledging difficulty adhering to healthy lifestyle routines (Buis *et al.* 2011, Jay *et al.* 2015b).

Veterans experience a number of barriers to engaging in facility-based exercise programming commonly offered by health providers like VHA. Common barriers to such programs include travel distance, transportation challenges, and lack of time (Arigo *et al.* 2015, Jay *et al.* 2015a, Spring *et al.* 2014). The low use of cardiac rehabilitation programs by eligible veterans exemplifies these challenges. In a recent analysis of 88,826 veterans who were hospitalized for a significant coronary event or procedure over five years, only 10% participated in one or more sessions of facility-based cardiac rehabilitation in the year following hospitalization (Schopfer *et al.* 2016). Greater participation was associated with the proximity of a veteran's home to a VA facility and presence of an onsite cardiac rehab clinic.

The preferred types and modes of physical activity change as individuals transition from Active Duty to veteran status. Running and exercising with gym equipment are the most frequently reported Active Duty physical activities among OEF/OIF veterans (Buis *et al.* 2011, Holtz *et al.* 2014). However, post-discharge, veterans' preferences shift toward more moderate-intensity activities such as walking and jogging as they cope with chronic pain or health problems. Although male veterans typically report exercising alone, they are more likely to endorse a desire to perform physical activities with their fellow veterans (Buis *et al.* 2011, Jay *et al.* 2015b). In comparison, female veterans are more likely to endorse family, friends, and medical providers as sources of social support for exercise (Hoerster *et al.* 2015, Jay *et al.* 2015b). Other than preferences for exercising with other veterans or in neighborhoods with positive aesthetics (Hoerster *et al.* 2015, Millstein *et al.* 2015), less is known about environmental predictors of exercise participation, especially among low SES and minority veterans.

Intervention strategies

Relative to the considerable support Active Duty service members receive from their service branch to be physically active, veterans have less access to culturally tailored evidence-based physical activity interventions. For the most vulnerable veterans, VHA is likely to be the provider of preventive health services (Kizer and Dudley 2009). VHA research and clinical programs have historically focused on physical activity interventions targeting older male patients with the aims of: (1) preventing the onset of disease or disability (Kinsinger *et al.* 2009), (2) self-managing chronic conditions such as diabetes or chronic pain (Damschroder *et al.* 2015, Krein *et al.* 2013), or (3) maintaining physical function (Laferrier *et al.* 2015, Morey *et al.* 2009). Actual clinical programs reflect a dichotomy between a population-based approach that emphasizes a generic message of lifestyle physical activity through psychoeducational channels (e.g., brochures, brief counseling) and a highly specialized and intensive approach delivered by specialists like physical therapists.

Based on its expertise with complex combat injuries, VHA has become an international leader in supporting adaptive exercise and sport opportunities for veterans with serious disabilities or complications from chronic disease. This includes programs for patients with multiple limb amputations, traumatic brain injuries, and spinal cord injuries (Brenner *et al.* 2012, Laferrier *et al.* 2015). VHA is at the forefront of developing technologies for those with disabilities to be physically active due to advances in prosthetics, wheelchairs, and electronic registries to monitor health and well-being of these high-risk patients. Since 1981, VA has supported large competitive events for disabled veterans including the National Veteran Wheelchair Games (NVWG) and the National Disabled Veterans Winter Sports Clinic (WSC) (Sporner *et al.* 2009). VA also supports veteran participation in other events sponsored by the International Paralympics Committee, Invictus Games Foundation, and similar organizations. Research into the health benefits of these events is growing and represents a promising area for culturally targeted interventions for an underserved population of veterans (Littman *et al.* 2014).

Although longitudinal cohort studies of veterans (Kokkinos *et al.* 2014a, Kokkinos *et al.* 2014b) show the benefits of exercise as medical therapy, programs promoting physical activity are often implemented across VHA facilities on an *ad hoc* basis, often with highly variable results. The reach of these programs, their effectiveness, and factors impacting wider implementation are less clear and require further evaluation (Kahwati *et al.* 2011). For example, program evaluations of the nationally disseminated VA MOVE! Weight Management Program have found that the program suffers from high attrition rates (74%) while yielding modest weight loss (Kahwati *et al.* 2011, Spring *et al.* 2014). While the inclusion of physical activity in MOVE! group sessions is one of strongest predictors of program success (Arigo *et al.* 2015, Jay *et al.* 2015b, Locatelli *et al.* 2012), MOVE! providers typically lack expertise in exercise prescription for complex patients like veterans, undermining program effectiveness.

Far less attention has been put on studying younger veteran cohorts, and this research consists almost entirely of pilot work, often without regard to underserved subpopulations of veterans (Widome *et al.* 2012). Formative studies suggest that many younger veterans want activity interventions of greater intensity than their older peers (Holtz *et al.* 2014, Jay *et al.* 2015b, Rogers *et al.* 2014). Additionally, while supervised physical activity programs are first-line treatment for rehabilitation or management of complex injuries or chronic pain conditions, fewer tailored interventions are available for highly burdensome health conditions in which physical activity interventions have been found effective, including for cognitive/brain disorders, depression, pre/diabetes, lung disease, psychotic disorders, smoking cessation, and substance use disorders (Brenner *et al.* 2012, Linke *et al.* 2015, Yaffe *et al.* 2014).

BOX 12.1   EVIDENCE-BASED PRACTICE: TEAM RED, WHITE & BLUE (RWB) INTEGRATES MILITARY VETERANS WITH LOCAL COMMUNITIES THROUGH PHYSICAL AND SOCIAL ACTIVITY

Increasing opportunities for physical activity can also foster healthier social ties for veterans. Team RWB is a community-based nonprofit organization founded in 2010 that aims to connect military personnel (veterans, active duty, military families) with their local communities, using physical activity as a tool to promote social engagement. Unlike other veteran service organizations (VFW, American Legion, etc.) which focus on military veterans exclusively, RWB seeks to engage both military and civilians as team members, with the goal of promoting better integration of these two groups.

The impetus for Team RWB was the recognition that the transition from active military service to civilian life is a significant disruption in a veteran's sense of social connectedness. To help veterans rebuild these social ties in civilian life, Team RWB seeks to (1) build authentic relationships with ***people*** that are reflected in teammates' sense of belonging, purpose, and community engagement; (2) offer opportunities for team members to connect through fitness, sports, and recreation to improve ***health*** and well-being; and (3) engage members in leadership and service opportunities beyond fitness activities that renew self-identity and ***purpose*** in life.

Team RWB has expanded rapidly and is represented by 181 RWB chapters across the U.S. and five international countries. In 2015, some 271,626 people (58% veterans) participated in 32,384 events, including weekly fitness activities and outings, monthly social and/or service events, and participation in local competitions. For veterans who may not live in an area with a local chapter, or who may be living or stationed abroad, Team RWB is equipped to provide outreach and support to stay connected with other veterans and community members. The organization benefits from using an evidence-based approach to continuously evaluate its efforts and guide program development.

The adjoining box features Team Red, White & Blue (RWB; (Angel and Armstrong 2016) as a powerful illustration of how physical activity programming can be effectively implemented in community settings to reach veterans in a culturally sensitive manner. Unlike a medically based program, Team RWB taps into the strong social bond veterans share for each other as a consequence of military service (Ahern *et al.* 2015). Veterans providing peer coaching has proven effective in promoting mental health treatment and suicide prevention, yet has been largely untested for promoting physical activity. Interventions mobilizing social support must be used cautiously. For example, women veterans with a service history of MST report feeling betrayed or mistreated by the military and their peers. Consequently, these women are less likely to seek social support from their peers, especially in mixed-sex settings (Ahern *et al.* 2015, Locatelli *et al.* 2012). A recent study found offering a women-only program for female veterans appears to be a successful strategy for recruiting female veterans to participate in lifestyle interventions (Moin *et al.* 2015).

Behavioral health programs in the VHA are increasingly integrating technologies into their programming (Houston *et al.* 2013). Such technologies have an advantage over traditional face-to-face models by extending the reach to veterans across diverse geographic locations, allowing greater scheduling flexibility, and offering novelty with new telehealth and wearable technologies. Evidence shows veterans are able to use wearable devices to monitor daily activity for the application to managing pain, weight, CVD risk factors, and lung disease (Krein *et al.* 2013, Moin *et al.* 2015, Moy *et al.* 2016, Richardson *et al.* 2016). Pilot studies show that younger veterans rate *e* health programs highly. Such programs employ telephone-based lifestyle coaches or computerized tailoring programs to provide personalized exercise prescriptions and messaging via smartphones, website, or individual voice recognition platforms (Damschroder *et al.* 2016, Holtz *et al.* 2014). However, income is an important consideration of these new technologies. Lower SES veterans make up a large proportion of VHA users, and these veterans currently prefer simple text modalities, websites, and print publications versus smartphone applications (Fleming *et al.* 2016, Mendoza-Vasconez *et al.* 2016).

Implications for practice

Based on the fitness requirements for military service, veterans may be a receptive audience to messages and interventions promoting exercise. Developing tailored physical activity interventions for recently discharged military service members who are struggling to adjust to a civilian lifestyle is a priority area for future work. Another rich area for consideration is the application of exercise as an adjunct medical treatment, a relatively new idea for VHA and community settings. As we have discussed in this chapter, exercise professionals need to conduct formative work to understand a specific (sub) population of veterans' cultural and behavioral expectations before implementing exercise programming. Table 12.3 summarizes basic recommendations with which to begin culturally tailored programming efforts.

Veterans are a diverse population with complex health needs from an exercise prescription point of view but also are a health population that is generally grateful and enthusiastic in embracing programs targeted for them. Many veterans are served by integrated healthcare systems like VHA which utilizes a medical home model of care delivery and electronic medical records systems. These components of coordinated care systems are well suited to keeping a veteran's healthcare provider aware of a veteran's referral to exercise programs, current exercise prescription and activity behavior with the integration of wearable technologies, and needs for follow-up such as adjustment of medications or addressing a musculoskeletal problem

TABLE 12.3 Clinical and cultural considerations for physical activity interventions to veterans

- Physical fitness is a deeply rooted value in veteran culture and identity
- Complex health conditions associated with military service and/or older age and low income can become barriers to physical activity in veterans, especially among veterans who use VHA
- Transition from active duty to civilian life is a critical life transition for veterans in which poor social integration and lack of self-regulatory skills can lead to unhealthy lifestyle behaviors
- Interventions that incorporate messaging targeted to specific aspects of military culture are more likely to be successful than generic population-level messages
- Whereas the motivation for exercise for Active Duty personnel was extrinsically tied to job requirements, veterans may need to develop intrinsic forms of motivation to adhere to a program
- Interventions must use an appropriate delivery channel such as Physical Therapy in the VHA, veteran service organizations like Team Red, White & Blue, or health insurers linking veterans to community-based physical activity programs (e.g., YMCAs)
- Individual baseline assessments for physical activity prescription should assess a veteran's service background to understand relevant influences (e.g., self-efficacy, perceived health status)
- Exercise professionals should use patient-centered communication strategies such as motivational interviewing or the 5 As to strengthen motivation via deep cultural characteristics of the veteran
- Key veteran values include structure, a mission (purpose), sense of belonging and "teamness"
- Nonveterans should avoid asking inappropriate questions such as "Did you ever kill anyone?" and instead try to understand and empathize with a veteran's current health needs and function
- Physical activity interventions in clinical settings should aim to address physical and behavioral comorbidities that can undermine physical activity adherence
- Supervised group and individual physical activity interventions should aim to build self-regulatory skills to help veterans maintain physical activity without program supports
- Veterans with a history of discrimination (e.g., women, LGBT) may be less receptive to group interventions if their peers do not share similar military experiences
- Exercise professionals should monitor veteran progression in physical activity intensity and ensure negative aspects of the warrior identity (e.g., stoicism, suppressing pain) do not contribute to injury or aggravation of a health condition
- Effective interventions should help veterans identify preferred sources of social support and mobilize those resources to support long-term maintenance of a physically active lifestyle
- Exercise prescriptions and exercise interventions should be integrated in a coordinated fashion with the veteran's primary care provider(s) to reinforce participation and overcome barriers

(Lobelo *et al.* 2014). New and innovative community-based programs like Team Red, White & Blue provide an exciting participatory model for interventionists to emulate that attains multilevel health and psychosocial outcomes through physical activity and social activities. Although further research is needed to understand the social and cultural determinants of exercise among veterans, there is a large body of social research on veterans that can be integrated into messaging and materials to increase veteran receptivity to exercise programming (e.g., VHA Office of Health Equity; **www.va.gov/healthequity/**).

Summary points

Subgroups within the veteran population are at risk for health disparities that can often be traced directly to disabilities incurred as part of military service and to difficulties adjusting to a civilian culture that lacks the structure, camaraderie, and sense of mission that the military provides. These health disparities underscore the opportunity to reintegrate physical activity into veterans' lives as well as the need for exercise professionals to develop culturally relevant marketing messages and physical activity programs which can increase the acceptance and effectiveness of these intervention efforts.

- Veterans are a diverse health population that shares a common background in physical activity shaped by military service and culture.
- The period following military discharge represents a key time for culturally appropriate exercise interventions.
- While the vulnerable veterans served by VHA have been the focus of most studies, less is known about the physical activity needs of veterans who do not use VHA services.
- A number of veteran subpopulations exist (e.g., women, LGBT, minorities) and more work is needed to understand factors that impact physical activity behavior and preferences in these groups.
- Interventions for veterans are needed in both VHA and community settings that more effectively use culturally tailored approaches to engaging veterans in exercise therapy.

Critical thinking questions

1   How would your efforts to promote and deliver evidence-based physical activity services for a targeted health condition differ between veterans served by VHA versus veterans who seek care through community-based health providers?
2   You know that recent Iraq and Afghanistan veterans are likely to become sedentary, rapidly gain weight, and are less likely to engage in preventive health services. If you were asked by the medical director at a local VHA medical center to develop an intervention program to help these veterans become physically active again, what would be the first steps you could take to understand how to best develop and implement this program?

3 How might you modify your messaging and intervention strategies in a culturally sensitive manner when promoting physical activity to the following veteran
subcultures:

a. A group of mixed-race Vietnam-era Army soldiers attempting to lose
weight at a fitness center affiliated with a hospital system in the rural
southeastern U.S.

b. LGBT servicemen and women who retired from their service unit before
the end of the Don't Ask, Don't Tell policy.

c. A 69-year-old male Marine who fought with the Marines in Vietnam
and who has peripheral artery disease, COPD, and vision and hearing
impairments.

d. A 27-year-old female Army veteran who lost an arm and a leg to an IED
in Iraq and left her badly burned.

e. A 39-year-old man who served six deployments in the Special Forces but
now suffers from insomnia, depression, and PTSD.

References

(1998) 'Design of the Women's Health Initiative clinical trial and observational study. The
Women's Health Initiative Study Group'. *Controlled Clinical Trials*, 19: 61–109.

Ahern, J., Worthen, M., Masters, J., Lippman, S. A., Ozer, E. J. and Moos, R. (2015) 'The
challenges of Afghanistan and Iraq veterans' transition from military to civilian life and
approaches to reconnection'. *PLoS One*, 10: e0128599.

Amin M, Parisi JA, Gold MS, Gold AR. (2010) 'War-related illness symptoms among
operation Iraqi freedom/operation enduring freedom returnees.' *Military Medicine*, 175:
155–157.

Angel, C. and Armstrong, N. J. (2016) *Enriching veterans' lives through an evidence based
approach: A case illustration of Team Red, White & Blue (Measurement and Evaluation
Series, Paper 1)*. Syracuse, NY: Institute for Veterans and Military Families, Syracuse
University.

Arigo, D., Hooker, S., Funderburk, J., Dundon, M., Dubbert, P., Evans-Hudnall, G., Catanese,
S., O'donohue, J., Dickinson, E. M., Demasi, C., Downey, S. and Desouza, C. (2015)
'Provider and staff perceptions of veterans' attrition from a national primary care weight
management program'. *Primary Health Care Research and Development*, 16: 147–56.

Bagalman, E. (2014) *The number of veterans that use VA health care services: A fact sheet* [Online].
Washington, DC: Congressional Research Service. Available: www.fas.org/sgp/crs/misc/
R43579.pdf (Accessed April 14 2016).

Bagnell, M. E., Leardmann, C. A., Mcmaster, H. S., Boyko, E. J., Smith, B., Granado, N. S. and
Smith, T. C. (2013) 'The association of predeployment and deployment-related factors
on dimensions of postdeployment wellness in U.S. military service members'. *American
Journal of Health Promotion*, 28: e56–66.

Barth, S. K., Kimerling, R. E., Pavao, J., McCutcheon, S. J., Batten, S. V., Dursa, E., Peterson,
M. R. and Schneiderman, A. I. (2016) 'Military sexual trauma among recent veterans:
Correlates of sexual assault and sexual harassment'. *American Journal of Preventive Medicine*,
50: 77–86.

Bouldin, E. D. and Reiber, G. E. (2012) 'Physical activity among veterans and nonveterans
with diabetes'. *Journal of Aging Research*, 2012: 135192.

Boyd, M. A., Bradshaw, W. and Robinson, M. (2013) 'Mental health issues of women deployed to Iraq and Afghanistan'. *Archives of Psychiatric Nursing*, 27: 10–22.

Brenner, L. A., Braden, C. A., Bates, M., Chase, T., Hancock, C., Harrison-Felix, C., Hawley, L., Morey, C., Newman, J., Pretz, C. and Staniszewski, K. (2012) 'A health and wellness intervention for those with moderate to severe traumatic brain injury: A randomized controlled trial'. *Journal of Head Trauma and Rehabilitation*, 27: E57–E68.

Buis, L. R., Kotagal, L. V., Porcari, C. E., Rauch, S. A., Krein, S. L. and Richardson, C. R. (2011) 'Physical activity in postdeployment Operation Iraqi Freedom/Operation Enduring Freedom veterans using Department of Veterans Affairs services'. *Journal of Rehabilitation Research and Development*, 48: 901–11.

Burks, D. J. (2011) 'Lesbian, gay, and bisexual victimization in the military: An unintended consequence of "Don't Ask, Don't Tell"?'. *American Psychologist*, 66: 604–13.

Center for Behavioral and Health Statistics and Quality. (2015) *Behavioral health trends in the United States: Results from the 2014 National Survey on Drug Use and Health (HHS Publication No. SMA 15–4927, NSDUH Series H-50)* [Online]. Washington, DC: Center for Behavioral Health Statistics and Quality, Substance Abuse and Mental Health Services Administration. Available: www.samhsa.gov/data/sites/default/files/NSDUH-FRR1-2014/NSDUH-FRR1-2014.htm (Accessed July 16 2016).

Centers for Disease Control and Prevention. (2011) 'Quitting smoking among adults – United States, 2001–2010'. *MMWR Morbidity and Mortality Weekly Reports*, 60: 1513–9.

Chasens, E. R., Umlauf, M. G. and Weaver, T. E. (2009) 'Sleepiness, physical activity, and functional outcomes in veterans with type 2 diabetes'. *Applied Nursing Research*, 22: 176–82.

Chwastiak, L. A., Rosenheck, R. A. and Kazis, L. E. (2011) 'Association of psychiatric illness and obesity, physical inactivity, and smoking among a national sample of veterans'. *Psychosomatics*, 52: 230–6.

Conard, P. L. and Armstrong, M. L. (2015) 'Deployed women veterans: Important culturally sensitive care'. *Nursing Forum*, June 10.

Damschroder, L. J., Moin, T., Datta, S. K., Reardon, C. M., Steinle, N., Weinreb, J., Billington, C. J., Maciejewski, M. L., Yancy, W. S., Jr., Hughes, M., Makki, F. and Richardson, C. R. (2015) 'Implementation and evaluation of the VA DPP clinical demonstration: Protocol for a multi-site non-randomized hybrid effectiveness-implementation type III trial'. *Implementation Science*, 10: 68.

Damschroder, L. J., Reardon, C. M., Sperber, N., Robinson, C. H., Fickel, J. J. and Oddone, E. Z. (2016) 'Implementation evaluation of the Telephone Lifestyle Counseling (TLC) Program: Organizational factors associated with successful implementation'. *Translational Behavioral Medicine*, September.

Department of Veterans Affairs and Department of Defense. (2014) *VA/DoD clinical practice guideline for screening and management of overweight and obesity Version 2.0* [Online]. Washington, DC: VA Office of Quality, Safety and Value and Clinical Performance Assurance Directorate, United States Army MEDCOM. Available: www.healthquality.va.gov/guidelines/CD/obesity/CPGManagementOfOverweightAndObesityFINAL041315.pdf (Accessed March 1 2016).

Department of Veterans Affairs and Department of Defense. (2015) *VA/DoD clinical practice guideline for the management of substance use disorders* [Online]. Washington, DC: VA Office of Quality, Safety, and Value and U.S. Army Medical Command Office of Evidence-based Practice. Available: www.healthquality.va.gov/guidelines/MH/sud/VADoDSUD-CPGRevised22216.pdf (Accessed July 15 2016).

Dominick, K. L., Golightly, Y. M. and Jackson, G. L. (2006) 'Arthritis prevalence and symptoms among US non-veterans, veterans, and veterans receiving Department of Veterans Affairs Healthcare'. *Journal of Rheumatology*, 33: 348–54.

Epidemiology Group, Post-Deployment Health Group, Office of Public Healthand Veterans Health Administration. (June 2015) *Analysis of VA health care utilization among Operation Enduring Freedom (OEF), Operation Iraqi Freedom (OIF), and Operation New Dawn (OND) veterans: Cumulative from 1st Qtr FY 2002 through 1st Qtr FY 2015 (October 1, 2001 – December 31, 2014)* [Online]. Washington, DC: Department of Veterans Affairs. Available: www.publichealth.va.gov/docs/epidemiology/healthcare-utilization-report-fy2015-qtr1.pdf (Accessed July 15 2016).

Fleming, E., Crawford, E. F., Calhoun, P. S., Kudler, H. and Straits-Troster, K. A. (2016) 'Veterans' preferences for receiving information about VA services: Is getting the information you want related to increased health care utilization?'. *Military Medicine*, 181: 106–10.

Fryar, C. D., Herrick, K., Afful, J. and Ogden, C. L. (2016) 'Cardiovascular disease risk factors among male veterans, U.S., 2009–2012'. *American Journal of Preventive Medicine*, 50: 101–5.

Gawande, A. (2004) 'Casualties of war – military care for the wounded from Iraq and Afghanistan'. *New England Journal of Medicine*, 351: 2471–5.

Geiling, J., Rosen, J. M. and Edwards, R. D. (2012) 'Medical costs of war in 2035: Long-term care challenges for veterans of Iraq and Afghanistan'. *Military Medicine*, 177: 1235–44.

Goulet, J. L., Kerns, R. D., Bair, M., Becker, W., Brennan, P., Burgess, D. J., Carroll, C., Dobscha, S., Driscoll, M., Fenton, B. T., Fraenkel, L., Haskell, S., Heapy, A., Higgins, D., Hoff, R. A., Hwang, U., Justice, A. C., Piette, J., Sinnott, P., Wandner, L., Womack, J. and Brandt, C. A. (2016) 'The musculoskeletal diagnosis cohort: Examining pain and pain care among veterans'. *Pain*, 158(8): 1696–703.

Grossbard, J. R., Lehavot, K., Hoerster, K. D., Jakupcak, M., Seal, K. H. and Simpson, T. L. (2013) 'Relationships among veteran status, gender, and key health indicators in a national young adult sample'. *Psychiatric Services*, 64: 547–53.

Haibach, J. P., Glotfelter, M. A., Hall, K. S., Masheb, R. M., Little, M. A., Shephardson, R. L., Dobmeyer, A. C., Funderburk, J. S., Hunter, C. L., Dundon, M., Hausmann, L. R. M., Trynosky, S. K., Goodrich, D. E., Kilbourne, A. M., Knight, S. J., Talcott, G. W. and Goldstein, M. G. (2016) 'Military and veteran health behavior research and practice: Challenges and opportunities'. *Journal of Behavioral Medicine*, 40(1): 175–93.

Hall, K. S., Hoerster, K. D. and Yancy, W. S., Jr. (2015) 'Post-traumatic stress disorder, physical activity, and eating behaviors'. *Epidemiology Reviews*, 37: 103–15.

Harada, N. D., Damron-Rodriguez, J., Villa, V. M., Washington, D. L., Dhanani, S., Shon, H., Chattopadhyay, M., Fishbein, H., Lee, M., Makinodan, T. and Andersen, R. (2002) 'Veteran identity and race/ethnicity: Influences on VA outpatient care utilization'. *Medical Care*, 40: 1117–28.

Higgins, D. M., Buta, E., Dorflinger, L., Masheb, R. M., Ruser, C. B., Goulet, J. L. and Heapy, A. A. (2016) 'Prevalence and correlates of painful conditions and multimorbidity in national sample of overweight/obese veterans'. *Journal of Rehabilitation Research and Development*, 53: 71–82.

Higgins, D. M., Dorflinger, L., Macgregor, K. L., Heapy, A. A., Goulet, J. L. and Ruser, C. (2013) 'Binge eating behavior among a national sample of overweight and obese veterans'. *Obesity (Silver Spring)*, 21: 900–3.

Higgins, D. M., Kerns, R. D., Brandt, C. A., Haskell, S. G., Bathulapalli, H., Gilliam, W. and Goulet, J. L. (2014) 'Persistent pain and comorbidity among Operation Enduring Freedom/Operation Iraqi Freedom/operation New Dawn veterans'. *Pain Medicine*, 15: 782–90.

Hoerster, K. D., Jakupcak, M., Mcfall, M., Unutzer, J. and Nelson, K. M. (2012a) 'Mental health and somatic symptom severity are associated with reduced physical activity among US Iraq and Afghanistan veterans'. *Preventive Medicine*, 55: 450–2.

Hoerster, K. D., Lehavot, K., Simpson, T., Mcfall, M., Reiber, G. and Nelson, K. M. (2012b) 'Health and health behavior differences: U.S. Military, veteran, and civilian men'. *American Journal of Preventive Medicine*, 43: 483–9.

Hoerster, K. D., Millstein, R. A., Hall, K. S., Gray, K. E., Reiber, G. E., Nelson, K. M. and Saelens, B. E. (2015) 'Individual and contextual correlates of physical activity among a clinical sample of United States veterans'. *Social Science Medicine*, 142: 100–8.

Holtz, B., Krein, S. L., Bentley, D. R., Hughes, M. E., Giardino, N. D. and Richardson, C. R. (2014) 'Comparison of veteran experiences of low-cost, home-based diet and exercise interventions'. *Journal of Rehabilitation Research and Development*, 51: 149–60.

Houston, T. K., Volkman, J. E., Feng, H., Nazi, K. M., Shimada, S. L. and Fox, S. (2013) 'Veteran internet use and engagement with health information online'. *Milatary Medicine*, 178: 394–400.

Institute of Medicine (IOM). (2009) *Combatting tobacco use in military and veteran populations.* Washington, DC: The National Academies Press.

Jay, M., Chintapalli, S., Squires, A., Mateo, K. F., Sherman, S. E. and Kalet, A. L. (2015a) 'Barriers and facilitators to providing primary care-based weight management services in a patient centered medical home for Veterans: A qualitative study'. *BMC Family Practice*, 16: 167.

Jay, M., Mateo, K. F., Squires, A. P., Kalet, A. L. and Sherman, S. E. (2015b) 'Military service and other socioecological factors influencing weight and health behavior change in overweight and obese veterans: A qualitative study to inform intervention development within primary care at the United States Veterans Health Administration'. *BMC Obesity*, 3: 5.

Johnson, B. S., Boudiab, L. D., Freundl, M., Anthony, M., Gmerek, G. B. and Carter, J. (2013) 'Enhancing veteran-centered care: A guide for nurses in non-VA settings'. *American Journal of Nursing*, 113: 24–39; quiz 54, 40.

Kahwati, L. C., Lance, T. X., Jones, K. R. and Kinsinger, L. S. (2011) 'RE-AIM evaluation of the Veterans Health Administration's MOVE! Weight Management Program'. *Translational Behavioral Medicine*, 1: 551–60.

Kelly, M. M., Sido, H. and Rosenheck, R. (2016) 'Rates and correlates of tobacco cessation service use nationally in the Veterans Health Administration'. *Psychological Services*, 13: 183–92.

Kemp, J. and Bossarte, R. (2012) *Suicide Data Report, 2012* [Online]. Washington, DC: Department of Veterans Affairs, Mental Health Services, Suicide Prevention Program. Available: www.va.gov/opa/docs/suicide-data-report-2012-final.pdf (Accessed May 4 2016).

Kinsinger, L. S., Jones, K. R., Kahwati, L., Harvey, R., Burdick, M., Zele, V. and Yevich, S. J. (2009) 'Design and dissemination of the MOVE! Weight-Management Program for veterans'. *Preventing Chronic Disease*, 6: A98.

Kizer, K. W. and Dudley, R. A. (2009) 'Extreme makeover: Transformation of the veterans health care system'. *Annual Reviews in Public Health*, 30: 313–39.

Kokkinos, P., Faselis, C., Myers, J., Kokkinos, J. P., Doumas, M., Pittaras, A., Kheirbek, R., Manolis, A., Panagiotakos, D., Papademetriou, V. and Fletcher, R. (2014a) 'Statin therapy, fitness, and mortality risk in middle-aged hypertensive male veterans'. *American Journal of Hypertension*, 27: 422–30.

Kokkinos, P., Faselis, C., Myers, J., Sui, X., Zhang, J. and Blair, S. N. (2014b) 'Age-specific exercise capacity threshold for mortality risk assessment in male veterans'. *Circulation*, 130: 653–8.

Krein, S. L., Kadri, R., Hughes, M., Kerr, E. A., Piette, J. D., Holleman, R., Kim, H. M. and Richardson, C. R. (2013) 'Pedometer-based internet-mediated intervention for adults with chronic low back pain: Randomized controlled trial'. *Journal of Medical Internet Research*, 15: e181.

Laferrier, J. Z., Teodorski, E. and Cooper, R. A. (2015) 'Investigation of the impact of sports, exercise, and recreation participation on psychosocial outcomes in a population of veterans with disabilities: A cross-sectional study'. *American Journal of Physical Medicine Rehabilitation*, 94: 1026–34. Rehabiltion.

Lan, C. W., Fiellin, D. A., Barry, D. T., Bryant, K. J., Gordon, A. J., Edelman, E. J., Gaither, J. R., Maisto, S. A. and Marshall, B. D. (2016) 'The epidemiology of substance use disorders in US veterans: A systematic review and analysis of assessment methods'. *American Journal of Addiction*, 25: 7–24.

Leardmann, C. A., Kelton, M. L., Smith, B., Littman, A. J., Boyko, E. J., Wells, T. S., Smith, T. C. and Millennium Cohort Study, T. (2011) 'Prospectively assessed posttraumatic stress disorder and associated physical activity'. *Public Health Reports*, 126: 371–83.

Lehavot, K., Hoerster, K. D., Nelson, K. M., Jakupcak, M. and Simpson, T. L. (2012) 'Health indicators for military, veteran, and civilian women'. *American Journal of Preventive Medicine*, 42: 473–80.

Linke, S. E., Noble, M., Hurst, S., Strong, D. R., Redwine, L., Norman, S. B. and Lindamer, L. A. (2015) 'An exercise-based program for veterans with substance use disorders: Formative research'. *Journal of Psychoactive Drugs*, 47: 248–57.

Littman, A. J., Boyko, E. J., Thompson, M. L., Haselkorn, J. K., Sangeorzan, B. J. and Arterburn, D. E. (2014) 'Physical activity barriers and enablers in older veterans with lower-limb amputation'. *Journal of Rehabilitation Research and Development*, 51: 895–906.

Littman, A. J., Forsberg, C. W. and Boyko, E. J. (2013) 'Associations between compulsory physical activity during military service and activity in later adulthood among male veterans compared with nonveterans'. *Journal of Physical Activity and Health*, 10: 784–91.

Littman, A. J., Forsberg, C. W. and Koepsell, T. D. (2009) 'Physical activity in a national sample of veterans'. *Medicine and Science in Sports and Exercise*, 41: 1006–13.

Littman, A. J., Jacobson, I. G., Boyko, E. J. and Smith, T. C. (2015) 'Changes in meeting physical activity guidelines after discharge from the military'. *Journal of Physical Activity and Health*, 12: 666–74.

Litwack, S. D., Mitchell, K. S., Sloan, D. M., Reardon, A. F. and Miller, M. W. (2014) 'Eating disorder symptoms and comorbid psychopathology among male and female veterans'. *General Hospital Psychiatry*, 36: 406–10.

Lobelo, F., Stoutenberg, M. and Hutber, A. (2014) 'The exercise is medicine global health initiative: A 2014 update'. *British Journal of Sports Medicine*, 48: 1627–33.

Locatelli, S. M., Sohn, M. W., Spring, B., Hadi, S. and Weaver, F. M. (2012) 'Participant retention in the Veterans Health Administration's MOVE! Weight management program, 2010'. *Preventing Chronic Disease*, 9: E129.

Maguen, S., Cohen, B., Cohen, G., Madden, E., Bertenthal, D. and Seal, K. (2012) 'Eating disorders and psychiatric comorbidity among Iraq and Afghanistan veterans'. *Womens Health Issues*, 22: e403–6.

Maguen, S., Madden, E., Cohen, B., Bertenthal, D., Neylan, T., Talbot, L., Grunfeld, C. and Seal, K. (2013) 'The relationship between body mass index and mental health among Iraq and Afghanistan veterans'. *Journal of General Internal Medicine*, 28 Suppl 2: S563–70.

Mattocks, K. M., Sullivan, J. C., Bertrand, C., Kinney, R. L., Sherman, M. D. and Gustason, C. (2015) 'Perceived stigma, discrimination, and disclosure of sexual orientation among a sample of lesbian veterans receiving care in the department of veterans affairs'. *LGBT Health*, 2: 147–53.

Mendoza-Vasconez, A. S., Linke, S., Munoz, M., Pekmezi, D., Ainsworth, C., Cano, M., Williams, V., Marcus, B. H. and Larsen, B. A. (2016) 'Promoting physical activity among underserved populations'. *Current Sports Medicine Reports*, 15: 290–7.

Millstein, R. A., Hoerster, K. D., Rosenberg, D. E., Nelson, K. M., Reiber, G. and Saelens, B. E. (2015) 'Individual, social, and neighborhood associations with sitting time among veterans'. *Journal of Physical Activity and Health*, 13(1): 30–5.

Moin, T., Ertl, K., Schneider, J., Vasti, E., Makki, F., Richardson, C., Havens, K. and Damschroder, L. (2015) 'Women veterans' experience with a web-based diabetes prevention program: A qualitative study to inform future practice'. *Journal of Medical Internet Research*, 17: e127.

Monahan, P., Hu, Z. and Rohrbeck, P. (2013) 'Mental disorders and mental health problems among recruit trainees, U.S. Armed Forces, 2000–2012'. *MSMR*, 20: 13–8; discussion 16–8.

Morey, M. C., Peterson, M. J., Pieper, C. F., Sloane, R., Crowley, G. M., Cowper, P. A., McConnell, E. S., Bosworth, H. B., Ekelund, C. C. and Pearson, M. P. (2009) 'The veterans learning to improve fitness and function in elders study: A randomized trial of primary care-based physical activity counseling for older men'. *Journal of the American Geriatric Society*, 57: 1166–74.

Mori, D. L., Sogg, S., Guarino, P., Skinner, J., Williams, D., Barkhuizen, A., Engel, C., Clauw, D., Donta, S. and Peduzzi, P. (2006) 'Predictors of exercise compliance in individuals with Gulf War veterans illnesses: Department of veterans affairs cooperative study 470'. *Military Medicine*, 171: 917–23.

Moss, J. A., Moore, R. L. and Selleck, C. S. (2015) 'Veteran competencies for undergraduate nursing education'. *ANS Advances in Nursing Science*, 38: 306–16.

Moy, M. L., Martinez, C. H., Kadri, R., Roman, P., Holleman, R. G., Kim, H. M., Nguyen, H. Q., Cohen, M. D., Goodrich, D. E., Giardino, N. D. and Richardson, C. R. (2016) 'Long-term effects of an internet-mediated pedometer-based walking program for chronic obstructive pulmonary disease: A randomized controlled trial'. *Journal of Medical Internet Research*, 18: e215.

Murphy, L. B., Helmick, C. G., Allen, K. D., Theis, K. A., Baker, N. A., Murray, G. R., Qin, J., Hootman, J. M., Brady, T. J., Barbour, K. E., Centers for Disease Control and Prevention. (2014) 'Arthritis among veterans – United States, 2011–2013'. *MMWR Morbidity and Mortality Weekly Report*, 63: 999–1003.

National Center for Veterans Analysis and Statistics. (2016) *Profile of women veterans: 2014* [Online]. Washington, DC: United States Department of Veterans Affairs. Available: www.va.gov/vetdata/docs/SpecialReports/Women_Veterans_2016.pdf (Accessed May 4 2016).

National Center for Veterans Analysis and Statistics. (March 2016) *Profile of veterans: 2014: Data from the American Community Survey* [Online]. Washington, DC: United States Department of Veterans Affairs. Available: www.va.gov/vetdata/docs/SpecialReports/Profile_of_Veterans_2014.pdf (Accessed May 4 2016).

Nelson, K. M., Starkebaum, G. A. and Reiber, G. E. (2007) 'Veterans using and uninsured veterans not using Veterans Affairs (VA) health care'. *Public Health Reports*, 122: 93–100.

Office of the Surgeon General U.S. Army Medical Command, Office of the Command Surgeon Headquarters U.S. Army Central Command and Afghanistan, O. O. T. C. S. U. S. F. (2013) *Mental Health Advisory Team 9 (MHAT 9) Operation Enduring Freedom (OEF) 2013, Afghanistan* [Online]. Available: http://armymedicine.mil/Documents/MHAT_9_OEF_Report.pdf (Accessed July 10 2016).

Ogden, C. L., Carroll, M. D., Kit, B. K. and Flegal, K. M. (2014) 'Prevalence of childhood and adult obesity in the United States, 2011–2012'. *JAMA*, 311: 806–14.

Olenick, M., Flowers, M. and Diaz, V. J. (2015) 'US veterans and their unique issues: Enhancing health care professional awareness'. *Advances in Medical Education Practices*, 6: 635–9.

Park, S. Y., Zhu, K., Potter, J. F. and Kolonel, L. N. (2011) 'Health-related characteristics and dietary intakes of male veterans and non-veterans in the Multiethnic Cohort Study (United States)'. *Journal of Military and Veterans Health*, 19: 4–9.

Ramsey, C. B., Hostetler, C. and Andrews, A. (2013) 'Evaluating the nutrition intake of U.S. military service members in garrison'. *Military Medicine*, 178: 1285–90.

Rand Health. (2016) *Balancing demand and supply for veteran's health care: A summary of three RAND Assessments conducted under the Veterans Choice Act* [Online]. Santa Monica, CA: RAND Corporation. Available: www.rand.org/content/dam/rand/pubs/research_reports/RR1100/RR1165z4/RAND_RR1165z4.pdf (Accessed July 19 2016).

Resnicow, K., Baranowski, T., Ahluwalia, J. S. and Braithwaite, R. L. (1999) 'Cultural sensitivity in public health: Defined and demystified'. *Ethnicity & Disease*, 9: 10–21.

Richardson, C. R., Goodrich, D. E., Larkin, A. R., Ronis, D., Holleman, R. G., Damschroder, L. J. and Lowery, J. C. (2016) 'A comparative effectiveness trial of three walking self-monitoring strategies'. *Translational Journal of the American College of Sports Medicine*, 15: 133–42.

Rogers, C. M., Mallinson, T. and Peppers, D. (2014) 'High-intensity sports for posttraumatic stress disorder and depression: Feasibility study of ocean therapy with veterans of Operation Enduring Freedom and Operation Iraqi Freedom'. *Amercian Journal of Occupational Therapy*, 68: 395–404.

Rosenberger, P. H., Ning, Y., Brandt, C., Allore, H. and Haskell, S. (2011) 'BMI trajectory groups in veterans of the Iraq and Afghanistan wars'. *Preventive Medicine*, 53: 149–54.

Rush, T., Leardmann, C. A. and Crum-Cianflone, N. F. (2016) 'Obesity and associated adverse health outcomes among US military members and veterans: Findings from the millennium cohort study'. *Obesity (Silver Spring)*, 24: 1582–9.

Schopfer, D. W., Takemoto, S., Allsup, K., Helfrich, C. D., Ho, P. M., Forman, D. E. and Whooley, M. A. (2016) 'Notice of retraction and replacement. Schopfer D.W., et al. Cardiac Rehabilitation Use among Veterans with Ischemic Heart Disease. *JAMA Internal Medicine*, 174(10): 1687–9.

Sin, N. L., Kumar, A. D., Gehi, A. K. and Whooley, M. A. (2016) 'Direction of association between depressive symptoms and lifestyle behaviors in patients with coronary heart disease: The heart and soul study'. *Annals of Behavioral Medicine*, 50: 523–32.

Smith, C., Klosterbuer, A. and Levine, A. S. (2009) 'Military experience strongly influences post-service eating behavior and BMI status in American veterans'. *Appetite*, 52: 280–9.

Spelman, J. F., Hunt, S. C., Seal, K. H. and Burgo-Black, A. L. (2012) 'Post deployment care for returning combat veterans'. *Journal of General Internal Medicine*, 27: 1200–9.

Sporner, M. L., Fitzgerald, S. G., Dicianno, B. E., Collins, D., Teodorski, E., Pasquina, P. F. and Cooper, R. A. (2009) 'Psychosocial impact of participation in the National Veterans Wheelchair Games and Winter Sports Clinic'. *Disability & Rehabilitation*, 31: 410–8.

Spring, B., Sohn, M. W., Locatelli, S. M., Hadi, S., Kahwati, L. and Weaver, F. M. (2014) 'Individual, facility, and program factors affecting retention in a national weight management program'. *BMC Public Health*, 14: 363.

Street, A. E., Vogt, D. and Dutra, L. (2009) 'A new generation of women veterans: Stressors faced by women deployed to Iraq and Afghanistan'. *Clinical Psychology Reviews*, 29: 685–94.

Talbot, L. S., Neylan, T. C., Metzler, T. J. and Cohen, B. E. (2014) 'The mediating effect of sleep quality on the relationship between PTSD and physical activity'. *Journal of Clinical Sleep Medicine*, 10: 795–801.

Trivedi, R. B., Post, E. P., Sun, H., Pomerantz, A., Saxon, A. J., Piette, J. D., Maynard, C., Arnow, B., Curtis, I., Fihn, S. D. and Nelson, K. (2015) 'Prevalence, comorbidity, and prognosis of mental health among US veterans'. *American Journal of Public Health*, 105(12): e1–e6.

United States Census Bureau. (2014) *Definitions and concepts: Who are veterans?* [Online]. Available: www.census.gov/hhes/veterans/about/definitions.html (Accessed May 1 2016).

U.S. Department of Health and Human Services. (2008) *2008 physical activity guidelines for Americans* [Online]. Washington, DC. Available: https://health.gov/paguidelines/pdf/paguide.pdf (Accessed January 30 2010).

Vimalananda, V. G., Miller, D. R., Christiansen, C. L., Wang, W., Tremblay, P. and Fincke, B. G. (2013) 'Cardiovascular disease risk factors among women veterans at VA medical facilities'. *Journal of General Internal Medicine*, 28 Suppl 2: S517–23.

Washington, D. L., Gray, K., Hoerster, K. D., Katon, J. G., Cochrane, B. B., Lamonte, M. J., Weitlauf, J. C., Groessl, E., Bastian, L., Vitolins, M. Z. and Tinker, L. (2016) 'Trajectories in physical activity and sedentary time among women veterans in the women's health initiative'. *Gerontologist*, 56 Suppl 1: S27–39.

Widome, R., Jensen, A., Bangerter, A. and Fu, S. S. (2014) 'Food insecurity among veterans of the US wars in Iraq and Afghanistan'. *Public Health Nutrition* 18(5): 844–9.

Widome, R., Littman, A. J., Laska, M. N. and Fu, S. S. (2012) 'Preventing chronic illness in young veterans by promoting healthful behaviors'. *Preventing Chronic Disease*, 9: E19.

Yaffe, K., Hoang, T. D., Byers, A. L., Barnes, D. E. and Friedl, K. E. (2014) 'Lifestyle and health-related risk factors and risk of cognitive aging among older veterans'. *Alzheimers & Dementia*, 10: S111–21.

Yoon, J., Zulman, D., Scott, J. Y. and Maciejewski, M. L. (2014) 'Costs associated with multimorbidity among VA patients'. *Medical Care*, 52 Suppl 3: S31–6.

Zivin, K., Yosef, M., Miller, E. M., Valenstein, M., Duffy, S., Kales, H. C., Vijan, S. and Kim, H. M. (2015) 'Associations between depression and all-cause and cause-specific risk of death: A retrospective cohort study in the Veterans Health Administration'. *Journal of Psychosomatic Research*, 78: 324–31.

13

PHYSICAL ACTIVITY AMONG PHYSICALLY DISABLED POPULATIONS

Robert B. Shaw and Kathleen A. Martin Ginis

Understanding physically disabled populations

The term 'disability' refers to a complex interaction between aspects of a person's body and aspects of the society in which the person lives. A disability is not simply a health problem. Rather, people with impairments in their body function (e.g., inability to hear) or body structure (e.g., a missing limb) become 'disabled' when they encounter attitudinal, social, or physical barriers that undermine their ability to fully participate in society (World Health Organization n.d.).

Consider, for instance, a woman with a condition that causes dwarfism (defined as short stature [147 cm or less] resulting from a genetic or medical condition). On the one hand, modifications may have been made to her physical and social environments to accommodate her stature. For example, counters, appliances, and furniture in her home and in her workplace might have been lowered so that she can live and work independently; ramps and lifts may be widely available for her to use on public transportation and in other places in her community where stairs would be too high to climb; her gym might have purchased adapted equipment to accommodate her small body; and she may be surrounded by supportive friends and coworkers who include her in all aspects of life. Under such circumstances, the woman might not be considered disabled because supports are in place to ensure that she is able to fully participate in society despite her condition. On the other hand, if the woman did not have the environmental and social supports required for her to live independently, and to participate in work, recreation, and other important aspects of life, she would be disabled.

Demographic characteristics

The World Health Organization estimates that, worldwide, over 1 billion people experience disability – that is, some form of impairment that interferes with their ability to fully participate in daily activities and community life. In Canada, 13.7% of working-aged adults and 4.6% of children aged 5–14 report some form of disability (Statistics Canada 2013). Similarly, in the United States, 11.6% of adults (Carroll *et al.* 2014) and 7.4% of children aged 5–17 (Stoddard 2014) report a disability. Among adults living in these countries, the most common form of disabilities are physical disabilities (Carroll *et al.* 2014; Statistics Canada 2015) – impairments that limit pain, mobility, and flexibility. Among children, disabilities related to learning and speaking, and chronic health conditions that limit activity participation (e.g., asthma, heart conditions) are the most common (National Center for Education Statistics 2016.; Statistics Canada n.d.). Given the preponderance of people living with physical disabilities, and the expectation that this number will increase with the aging North American population, the focus of the present chapter is on people with physical disabilities.

Health disparities and inequities among physically disabled populations

People living with physical disabilities are at increased risk for a wide range of physical and psychological health problems. For instance, compared to Americans without a disability, adults with physical disabilities are more likely to report having been diagnosed with diabetes, cancer, stroke, or heart disease (Carroll *et al.* 2014). Furthermore, adults with physical disabilities are more likely to have risk factors for chronic conditions such as high blood pressure and high cholesterol, and are less likely to receive forms of health care that can detect or prevent illness, such as cancer screening tests or flu shots (Reichard *et al.* 2011). People with physical disabilities are also at increased risk for psychological health problems, particularly depression. It is estimated that the overall rate of depressive disorders among people with physical disabilities is between 25–50%. This estimate is nearly four times higher than the rate in nondisabled populations (Kemp 2006).

Physical activity among the physically disabled

The United Nations Convention on the Rights of Persons with Disabilities protects the rights of people with disabilities to participate, on an equal basis with others, in sport, exercise, and other recreational physical activities (United Nations General Assembly 2006). Despite this protection, disabled populations are less likely to participate in leisure-time physical activity than able-bodied populations. For instance, data collected from nearly 84,000 Americans who participated in the National Health Interview Study revealed that only 21% of adults with a mobility limitation reported doing enough physical activity to meet national and international physical activity guidelines (i.e., > 150 min/wk of moderate-heavy aerobic activity). In contrast, 54% of adults without a disability reported meeting the guidelines (Carroll *et al.* 2014). Although population-level data from children and youth with disabilities are scarce, data collected from adolescents with cerebral palsy suggest young people with disabilities also participate in significantly less physical activity compared to their typically developing peers (Carlon *et al.* 2013). Likewise, parallel-ing trends seen in the able-bodied population, women with physical disabilities tend to participate in less leisure-time physical activity than men with physical disabilities (Martin Ginis *et al.* 2010). These statistics are not particularly surprising given the numerous barriers that prevent people with disabilities from leading a physically active lifestyle.

Common barriers and facilitators to physical activity

Researchers have conducted dozens of studies in which they have asked people with physical disabilities to list the factors that serve as barriers and facilitators to their participation in sport and exercise. A group of researchers compiled all of these factors into a comprehensive list (Martin Ginis *et al.* 2016). The list consisted of over 200 barriers and facilitators which were subsequently organized into five different themes: *Intrapersonal Factors, Interpersonal Processes, Institutional/Organiza-tional Factors, Community Factors,* and *Public Policy Factors* as outlined in the social ecological model in Chapter 1. Unfortunately, given that few studies focused on children or youth with disabilities, or distinguished between salient barriers and facilitators for women versus men, it is not possible to draw conclusions regarding the relative importance of specific barriers and facilitators across these various sub-groups of people with disabilities.

Intrapersonal factors

Intrapersonal factors refer to a person's individual characteristics. In general, two types of individual characteristics have been linked with physical activity participation among persons with physical disabilities: *psychological factors* and *physical factors.* Of the *psychological* factors, elevated levels of depression and anxiety, and fears about getting hurt or embarrassing oneself are often-reported barriers to participation. In contrast, holding positive attitudes and beliefs about being active (e.g., believing that sport provides opportunities to meet others, or that exercise can improve physi-cal function) and having confidence in one's capabilities to be active are important facilitators of sport and exercise participation. Among the *physical* factors, pain, fatigue, poor health, and a lack of energy and strength have been consistently identi-fied as significant barriers. It is not surprising that people with physical disabilities report so many physical barriers to participation given that they tend to experience more health problems and greater physical deconditioning than able-bodied people (Carroll *et al.* 2014).

Interpersonal processes

Interpersonal processes refer to aspects of how people interact and engage with one another. Within the disability literature, the provision of social support is one interpersonal process that has been consistently identified as facilitating participation in sport and exercise. In study after study, people with physical disabilities have cited the importance of receiving social support from a wide variety of sources including family members, friends, neighbors, peers, and healthcare professionals. People with disabilities have also indicated the importance of receiving different types of support, such as information, instruction, encouragement, and assistance obtaining access to equipment and facilities. In addition, both being a role model and having a role model have been identified as facilitating sport and exercise participation.

Conversely, when other people hold negative attitudes toward sport and exercise for persons with disabilities, this can be a profound impediment to participation. For instance, when gym employees make people with disabilities feel like they are a burden or an inconvenience, or when others talk disparagingly about adapted forms of popular sports (e.g., wheelchair basketball, sledge hockey), such negative interpersonal encounters can be highly discouraging for a person with a disability who wants to be active. Unfortunately, negative attitudes in gyms and other recreational facilities are often reflective of negative societal attitudes toward people with disabilities and their right to be physically active. Indeed, it is highly unusual for people with disabilities to be featured in campaigns promoting physical activity, and many campaigns are downright exclusionary, if not offensive, to people who rely on wheelchairs or other mobility devices, such as the currently popular "Sitting Kills" and "Move More Sit Less" campaigns.

Institutional factors

Institutional factors are characteristics of formal and informal institutions or settings (e.g., hospitals, schools, recreation centers, gyms) including their rules and regulations of operation. Understandably, the location and accessibility of places to be active have a profound influence on sport and exercise participation. If people cannot get to a recreation facility (e.g., because the approaching sidewalks are too badly damaged for wheelchair and other mobility-device users to navigate) or cannot move freely about the facility once they are inside (e.g., because there are too many stairs), participation will be hindered. In addition, the types and availability of programs offered by institutions are important. Program factors that facilitate participation include the delivery of fun, enjoyable activities, and the provision of individualized instruction and assistance. Program factors that hinder participation include inadequate staffing, an over-emphasis on competition, and restrictions on the types of mobility devices that people may use while participating (e.g., power wheelchairs). In addition, the level of knowledge displayed by the people working in institutions is important. Healthcare providers, teachers, coaches, and fitness professionals become key participation facilitators when they understand how to modify sports and exercises so that people with disabilities can participate safely.

Community factors

Broadly conceptualized, 'community' encompasses the structures and groups to which people belong (e.g., teams, neighborhoods) within a politically or geographically defined area. The availability of accessible sport and exercise equipment within one's community is one of the most potent influences on participation. Adapted fitness equipment is costly and if people are not able to access it, they are unlikely to participate. For instance, sit skis, hockey sledges, hand bikes, and sport wheelchairs can each cost in the thousands of dollars, while accessible exercise equipment typically costs more than generic equipment. When communities are able to provide adapted equipment at recreation and fitness centers or through equipment loaning programs, a significant barrier to participation is alleviated. Spreading and sharing information on how and where to be active in one's community is also important, as people with disabilities often cite a lack of access to such information to be a significant barrier.

Yet, whereas access to equipment and information are potentially modifiable community influences on participation, one key factor is not: weather. Many people with physical disabilities face tremendous challenges moving about their communities when weather conditions are not ideal. For instance, during winter months, people who use mobility devices (walkers, wheelchairs) are often unable to use icy or snow-covered sidewalks and paths. In hot summer months, individuals with certain disabling conditions (e.g., tetraplegia, multiple sclerosis) may face health risks associated with an increased risk for over-heating. Thus, unpleasant weather can be a significant barrier to sport and exercise participation.

Policy factors

Government and organizational decision-making and policies can function as barriers or facilitators to physical activity participation. At the *government* level, two types of policies have been repeatedly identified as having a positive effect on participation: policies that provide funding for programs, and transportation polices. Program funding is important to alleviate cost barriers such as those associated with specialized equipment and staff training. Transportation policies are important for supporting accessible services and systems so that people with disabilities can move freely about their communities and get to sport and exercise facilities. At the *organizational* level, policies related to the pricing of programs and equipment can be profound barriers if people cannot afford to participate. In addition, if organizations do not have policies requiring their staff to be trained on how to facilitate participation for people with disabilities, then staff lack of knowledge may also be a significant barrier to participation.

Intervention strategies

As previously reported in this chapter, physical inactivity rates for people living with physical disabilities are alarmingly high. This is a very serious public health issue as physical inactivity can lead to reduced strength, flexibility, bone density, and physical independence, while increasing the risk of developing chronic diseases such as heart disease and type 2 diabetes. A sedentary lifestyle is also linked to a greater risk of developing mental health problems such as depression and anxiety, as well as reduced participation in various aspects of family and community life. Given the negative impact of physical inactivity on the physical, psychological, and social well-being of people with physical disabilities, it should come as no surprise that an increasing number of approaches are being used to facilitate physical activity participation in these populations.

The goal of physical activity interventions is to modify one or more physical activity determinants that will then lead to increases in physical activity. As such, it is important to consider what strategies or approaches are effective at facilitating change in these determinants. In this section, we will briefly describe four general types of physical activity interventions. Although most of the research on these interventions has been conducted in samples of able-bodied individuals (Kahn *et al.* 2002), some studies have demonstrated the utility of these interventions to promote physical activity in people with physical disabilities. To facilitate deeper understanding, we will illustrate each of the four approaches by providing examples drawn from the research involving people with physical disabilities (see Table 13.1).

TABLE 13.1 Types of interventions and the determinants of physical activity they influence

Intervention Approaches	Examples of Interventions	Modifiable Determinants of Physical Activity	Real-world Intervention Examples
Informational	• Telephone-based physical activity education • Physiotherapist-delivered education on the importance of physical activity delivered to patients in rehabilitation hospitals	• Knowledge about the unique benefits of physical activity for people with disabilities • Knowledge on where and how to be active with a disability • Other people's attitudes toward the importance of physical activity for people with disability	• Get in Motion is a free physical activity telephone-based counselling service for people with physical disabilities. Counselling is performed by trained peers who have a physical disability. Peers provide users with information and support for how to start and maintain a physical activity program.

(Continued)

TABLE 13.1 (Continued)

Intervention Approaches	Examples of Interventions	Modifiable Determinants of Physical Activity	Real-world Intervention Examples
Behavioural	• Online modules that teach behaviour change techniques • Group behaviour change education classes that teach the most effective techniques for people with disabilities	• Behavioral management skills for successfully initiating and maintaining physical activity if you have a disability (e.g., goal-setting, self-monitoring)	• MacWheelers is an adapted exercise program for people with spinal cord injuries, based at McMaster University. In addition to providing an exercise facility, the program teaches users how to set goals and how to self-monitor their progress.
Social	• Organized exercise groups with inclusive programming and modified equipment • Telephone peer support programs for people to connect with others with disabilities • Peer-assisted programming and/or physical activity buddy systems	• Social influences and social environments that facilitate physical activity (e.g., socially supportive peers with disabilities, inclusive group exercise classes)	• The Disabled Sailing Association of Kelowna offers a weekly sailing program for people with disabilities. New users are paired with experienced sailors, and equipment is provided.
Environmental/ Policy	• Modifying the physical environment to improve accessibility (e.g., curb cuts) • Developing community-wide policies that address specific barriers for people with disabilities	• Physical environments to support physical activity (e.g., accessible pathways) • Policies that reduce barriers and support physical activity for people with disabilities (e.g., free transportation)	• The city of Dundas, Ontario, modified its local tennis courts to allow easier access for people with disabilities. The city paved over the crushed stone path leading to the courts and the members built a removable ramp to allow access to the clubhouse.

Source: Adapted from Lox et al. (2014)

Informational approaches

Informational approaches are designed to motivate people to become physically active by providing them with information about why they should be active, how to get started, or how to maintain their participation over time. Interventions for people with physical disabilities using this approach have concentrated mainly on providing educational information about the benefits of physical activity, how to overcome barriers restricting participation, the risk factors associated with being inactive, as well as specific information regarding physical activity guidelines. This would constitute surface-level strategies, most notably evidential approaches. While few studies have tested the effectiveness of informational approaches that are delivered at the community- or population-level to people with disabilities (e.g., point-of-decision prompts, mass media campaigns), several studies have tested the effectiveness of individualized educational interventions for people with disabilities. The rationale behind individualized education is that teaching people where, why, and how to engage in physical activity targets determinants of motivation (e.g., perceived health benefits of activity, control over one's ability to participate) which can spur them on to become more active (Lox *et al.* 2014).

Individualized educational interventions

These types of interventions are usually conducted in-person or over the telephone, and involve a counselor or some other knowledgeable person providing individuals with physical activity information. An illustrative study from the disability literature involved sedentary older adults with osteoarthritis (Halbert *et al.* 2001). In that study, participants who were provided with personalized physical activity information (e.g., what type of physical activity to perform, how frequently to participate, and participation intensity) from an exercise physiologist reported significant increases in the frequency and duration of walking and vigorous exercise compared to individuals who received no information. Furthermore, those who received physical activity information reported stronger intentions to continue exercising 12 months later. Another study showed that individualized interventions can also be effective when delivered in the form of a printed sheet of information. Adults with a spinal cord injury increased their time spent participating in physical activity after they received individualized information indicating their own personal level of risk for developing heart disease, diabetes, and obesity (Bassett and Martin Ginis 2011).

Behavioral approaches

Behavioral approaches involve teaching people specific behavioral techniques (e.g., self-monitoring, goal setting, action planning, etc.) to help facilitate physical activity participation and promote long-term adherence to a sport or exercise program. Often taught through Internet-based, telephone-based, or face-to-face counselling sessions, behavioral interventions have been readily used to promote physical activity in populations with physical disabilities. Behavioral approaches are effective because they have the potential to influence theoretical determinants of physical activity (e.g., self-efficacy) known to influence participation.

Internet-based interventions

Internet-based programs that teach behavioral techniques have become increasingly popular because they alleviate barriers that may impede one's ability to participate in a face-to-face intervention (e.g., lack of transportation to the intervention site). Support for the utility of this type of intervention is indicated in a study involving people with multiple sclerosis (Dlugonski *et al.* 2012). Through the web-based delivery of text- and video-based information, participants were taught behavioral techniques such as how to overcome barriers, set goals, monitor activity, and prevent relapse. Physical activity was measured for 12 weeks prior to the intervention using both self-report measures and pedometer step count measures. Physical activity was found to have increased over the 12-week intervention, thus providing support for the utility of Internet-based behavior change interventions. This type of intervention also appears to be suitable and effective for children with physical disabilities. Children with cerebral palsy who engaged in a 20-week web-based therapy program that involved tracking their progress online (a form of self-monitoring) displayed improved motor skills for activities of daily living compared to a control group who only engaged in standard care activities prescribed by their health professional (James *et al.* 2015).

Face-to-face interventions

While the use of Internet-delivered interventions is increasing, some people may not have access to the Internet, or they may prefer to learn behavior change techniques through face-to-face consultation with a trained professional. The effectiveness of group-based, face-to-face interventions was demonstrated in a study of people with spinal cord injury. Participants significantly increased their weekly self-managed physical activity levels after being taught a variety of self-regulatory skills (e.g., planning, self-monitoring) by a trained exercise interventionist (Brawley *et al.* 2013). In a similar vein, the benefits of individualized face-to-face interventions were demonstrated in a study of adults with multiple sclerosis (Carter *et al.* 2014). Participants who were taught goal-setting techniques and how to utilize their social support networks by a physical therapist reported increases in their exercise behavior as well as their daily step counts.

Social approaches

Social approaches aim to influence people's physical activity behavior by structuring their social environment to be more supportive toward engaging in and adhering to physical activity. This may involve modifying one's existing social network or creating completely new social networks that provide supportive relationships for behavior change. Creating exercise groups, telephone support systems, and having peer-assisted programs are three social approaches that have been used to positively influence physical activity behavior for people with physical disabilities. These approaches are hypothesized to influence physical activity behavior by providing people with the support they need (e.g., encouragement, companionship, practical assistance, information) from support networks they consider to be important (e.g., family, peers, health professionals).

Exercise groups

Organized exercise groups are one of the most basic social approaches to influencing physical activity behavior. Bringing a group of individuals together to work out, or to play a sport, has the potential to create a socially supportive environment that can increase participants' motivation toward achieving their activity goals. For instance, in a study involving adults with multiple sclerosis, participants who completed a 12-week *group-based* exercise program significantly improved their balance and functional status compared to a control condition who exercised alone, at home (Tarakci *et al.* 2013). Exercise groups also have been shown effective for children with cerebral palsy who demonstrated improvements in aerobic and anaerobic capacity, strength, agility, and participation when participating in a group exercise program in addition to their standard care (Verschuren *et al.* 2007).

Telephone support systems

Regularly scheduled telephone calls from a counsellor, mentor, peer, or interventionist can provide individuals with emotional and informational support that can help facilitate and promote physical activity participation. For example, *Get in Motion*, a free physical activity counselling service, has proven effective at promoting and increasing intentions to participate in leisure-time physical activity for people with spinal cord injury living in the community (Arbour-Nicitopoulos *et al.* 2014). Similarly, for people recovering from amputations, stroke, and other disabilities, telephone counselling has also been shown to positively influence physical activity and sport participation during the first year after rehabilitation (Ploeg *et al.* 2007).

Peer-assisted programs

Instruction, encouragement, and praise from peers have been identified as facilitators of physical activity participation for people with disabilities (Shields *et al.* 2012). Peers with a disability can be powerful role models, instilling the beginner athlete or exerciser with a sense of self-efficacy and belief that "if s/he can do it, then I can do it." For instance, Latimer-Cheung *et al.* (2010) found that adults with paraplegia nearly tripled the amount of time they spent each week on strength-training, after a single session of exercise training and counseling from a peer with paraplegia and a fitness trainer. Ongoing peer-assisted physical activity programs also allow people to monitor one another's behavior and motivate each other. This type of social intervention approach has been shown effective at influencing physical activity behaviors of children with disabilities. For example, participating alongside a trained peer (a classmate trained to interact with students who have disabilities) resulted in deaf children increasing their physical activity levels by nearly 20% during physical education classes (Lieberman *et al.* 2000). Similar results were found for visually impaired children who increased their time spent actively involved in physical education classes by 21% when they attended classes with a trained peer (Wiskochil *et al.* 2007).

Environmental and policy approaches

Environmental and policy approaches are designed to provide environmental opportunities, support, and cues to help people engage in physical activity. Unlike the approaches previously discussed in this section, environmental and policy approaches target the physical and organizational structures that impede participation rather than affecting change in the individual. Given that people with physical disabilities continuously indicate characteristics of the environment as barriers to participation (e.g., sidewalk access, access to facilities, transportation), this type of approach has the potential to impact large segments of disabled populations. Reducing the prevalence of modifiable barriers (e.g., inaccessible doorways) is one example of how environmental and policy approaches can positively contribute to physical activity behavior change for people with physical disabilities.

Environmental approaches

Despite the breadth of research implicating the built environment as a barrier to participation for people with physical disabilities (Martin Ginis *et al.* 2016), very little has been done to address this barrier. However, a recent observational study provides some insight on how the built environment can be modified to promote physical activity (Spivock *et al.* 2008). In that study, a greater presence of environmental buoys (e.g., access ramps, curb cuts, accessible pathways) within a neighborhood was associated with greater leisure-time physical activity in a sample of 205 individuals with varying physical disabilities. These findings suggest that even minor modifications to the built environment can facilitate physical activity participation. Additional research is needed to determine which environmental buoys have the greatest impact on physical activity.

Policy approaches

Although an increasing number of policies to promote physical activity are being implemented (e.g., mandatory physical education in schools, wheelchair accessible public transportation), there is limited information on the most effective policies to guide population-wide interventions for people with physical disabilities. In the able-bodied literature, community- and street-scale urban design and land use policies have been shown as effective policy approaches for promoting physical activity (Heath *et al.* 2006). These policies aim to promote physical activity by improving the livability of communities and their streets (e.g., improved street lighting, street crossings, sidewalk availability, proximity of facilities, landscaping, etc.). For example, in the recent Surgeon General's Call to Action to Promote Walking and Walkable Communities, having well-maintained sidewalks, pedestrian-friendly streets, access to public transit, and adequate lighting were highlighted as methods to improve the walkability of communities (United States Department of Health and Human Services 2015). Ongoing data collection is needed to determine the impact of these policies on the activity levels of people with disabilities. Additionally, because a lack of transportation is such a prevalent barrier to sport and exercise participation (Martin Ginis *et al.* 2016), collaborative efforts are needed across policy makers and agencies (e.g., city councils, transportation boards) to improve transportation access. An example of agencies working together to fix transportation problems comes from the small rural town of Peterborough, Ontario. The city council worked with the city bus service to extend the final bus stop by 1 km, on Monday nights, so that passengers could get to an adapted curling program. As a result of this policy, the program had a substantial increase in the number of participants with disabilities.

All four types of approaches have the potential to positively influence physical activity participation for people with different types of physical disabilities. It is important to keep in mind, however, that because people with different physical disabilities experience different limitations and have varying functional impairments, an approach that is effective for people with one type of disability may not be appropriate or effective for people with another type. Furthermore, although research on physical activity–enhancing interventions for people with disability is growing, there is not yet enough evidence to indicate which type, or combination of intervention approaches, are most effective. Nevertheless, we cautiously suggest that because accessibility is such a common and significant barrier, environmental and policy interventions could be maximally effective when combined with behavioral interventions. By combining these approaches, people with disabilities would have the behavioral skills needed to take advantage of accessible opportunities to be physically active. As intervention research grows, so will our understanding of what approach, or combination of approaches, are best suited to influence physical activity behavior for people with physical disabilities.

BOX 13.1   EVIDENCE-BASED PRACTICE: ACTIVE ACCESSIBLE LIVING IN CANADA'S OKANAGAN VALLEY

Accessible Okanagan is a community-based organization in Kelowna, British Columbia, Canada, that offers programming to help encourage and facilitate physical activity participation for people with physical disabilities. Utilizing various **social approaches** (e.g., peer-assisted programs, exercise groups), the organization offers weekly accessible recreational opportunities (e.g., hand cycling, wheelchair tennis, seated yoga) that are led by experienced community members who have a disability. By providing specialized adaptive equipment, and not charging program admission fees, these programs are tailored to people with disabilities who often report a lack of resources/equipment and financial restrictions as limitations to participation. The organization also utilizes **environmental/policy approaches** to facilitate participation by networking with city councils to ensure recreational facilities are meeting accessibility requirements. For example, the city of Kelowna installed a fully accessible portable restroom adjacent to the public tennis courts after being notified by Accessible Okanagan that the current restrooms were inaccessible. The tennis courts now play host to a weekly wheelchair tennis program. Lastly, Accessible Okanagan has an interactive social media webpage whereby people can ask questions and gain access to resources by networking with other people in the community who have a disability. This informal peer-to-peer connection service is one example of how Accessible Okanagan utilizes **informational approaches** to promote, encourage, and facilitate participation for people living in the community.

Implications for practice

Based on the low physical activity participation rates coupled with the risks of inactivity, interventions to facilitate physical activity for people with physical disabilities are imperative. Although scientists have a good understanding of the barriers that impede participation and the facilitators that encourage it (Martin Ginis et al. 2016), there is still much that needs to be investigated and considered when designing effective interventions to influence physical activity in these populations. Given the limited number of published studies, few conclusions can be made regarding which intervention approaches are most appropriate or effective. However, based on the able-bodied literature, we suggest that at a minimum, interventions should be tailored for the target population, grounded in theory (e.g., self-determination theory, social cognitive theory, social ecological model, theoretical domains framework), and use evidence-based strategies that target specific, theory-based physical activity determinants that have the potential to cause behavior change. By incorporating theoretical determinants of change into the design of an intervention, the intervention can be designed to have an impact on those determinants, thus maximizing the likelihood of changing people's behavior.

People working in the recreation sector should attempt to create inclusive interventions or environments within existing community programs. Truly inclusive environments are those that consider the full range of human diversity with respect to ability language, culture, gender, age, ability, and any other form of human difference (Inclusive Design Research Centre 2016). With this in mind, program developers need to go beyond creating environments that meet the minimum architectural accessibility recommendations (e.g., wide doors for wheelchairs to pass through, wheelchair-accessible washroom) and ensure that programs are inclusive from all perspectives (e.g., instructors trained to work with people with disabilities, modified equipment, appropriate education material). Adapting *existing* community programs to be inclusive would also reduce the financial burden of developing *new* disability-specific programming.

Creating socially supportive environments should also be considered when developing inclusive programming for people with physical disabilities. Offering incentives (e.g., free admission) that encourage family and friends to participate in programming could help encourage people with disabilities to build and utilize their social support networks. Furthermore, programming could be designed to facilitate peer support, peer mentoring, and the use of role models to foster a sense of community and relatedness. Involving peer mentors could help alleviate informational/knowledge barriers (e.g., where to purchase adapted equipment) experienced by people with physical disabilities and allow people with disabilities to reap the social benefits of participating in physical activity.

Another practical consideration to help facilitate participation is to create stronger relationships between researchers, community-based physical activity programs, and disability organizations, in order to encourage information sharing (Martin Ginis *et al.* 2016), as has been mentioned in several of the other chapters. Researchers need to ensure that their findings are translated into usable information that is readily available to, and understood by, individuals responsible for creating and administering programming for people with physical disabilities. Furthermore, disability organizations should also share information regarding the needs of people with particular physical disabilities so that community-based physical activity programs can determine what programming is currently available for these populations and how these programs can be tailored to improve their effectiveness. Improving the spread of information would also ensure that staff at physical activity programs are educated and up to date with specific information that may help improve the quality and specificity of their programming (e.g., new physical activity guidelines, new exercise modalities, etc.).

Existing and new physical activity programs need to be tailored to address individual needs. People with disabilities are not a homogeneous population, just as the other populations discussed in this text are diverse. A "one-size-fits-all" mentality to recreation programming ignores the fact that physical activity preferences, desires, and abilities vary drastically between individuals. Communities should attempt to offer a variety of different program settings (e.g., inclusive, disability-specific) to address this reality. In addition, ensuring that exercise programs have a range of equipment (e.g., arm ergometers, wheelchair treadmills, hand bikes) will allow people to have greater autonomy over the type of physical activity they perform, potentially leading to increased enjoyment and adherence. Continuing to tailor interventions, services, and programs, based on the specific characteristics and needs of people with physical disabilities, will help create impactful initiatives that are meaningful and sustainable.

Although good quality research has been conducted to promote and facilitate physical activity participation among people with physical disabilities, overall there remains a dearth of information on how best to increase participation. As the number of adults living with a disability is expected to increase as the North American population ages, greater resources must be devoted toward creating and improving physical activity programming for these populations. The creation of policies, and tailored programs/services, to alleviate transportation, financial, environmental, and other systemic barriers must be a priority; these barriers must be removed if people with disabilities are to reap the maximal benefits of informational, behavioral, and social physical activity–enhancing interventions.

Summary points

- The concept of disability reflects an interaction between characteristics of the individual's body and aspects of the physical and social environments.
- Extensive research has been conducted on barriers and facilitators to sport and exercise participation among people with disabilities. Barriers and facilitators can be categorized as interpersonal, intrapersonal, community, institutional, and policy-related factors.
- Physical inactivity is associated with reduced physical, social, and psychological well-being among people with disabilities.
- Informational, social, behavioral, and environmental/policy approaches are all appropriate intervention strategies to promote and facilitate physical activity participation for people with physical disabilities. Continued research is needed to determine if certain types of intervention approaches are more effective than others and if combining intervention types results in added effectiveness.
- Ongoing communication between researchers, disability organizations, community members, and people with physical disabilities may help to develop truly inclusive and socially supportive physical activity programs that are tailored to the needs of people with physical disabilities.

Critical thinking questions

1   Environmental approaches to promote and facilitate physical activity participation for people with physical disabilities are lacking. Imagine you are working for a public health agency with unlimited access to resources and participants. Design an intervention that focuses on modifying one or several aspects of the environment that you believe would help facilitate participation. Your intervention should include how you plan to facilitate physical activity, how you will measure participation levels, how long your intervention will last, and the proposed impact the intervention would have on society.

2   James, a 20-year-old college student, recently incurred a spinal cord injury as a result of a motor vehicle accident. The severity of his injury has left him with paralysis in his legs resulting in him being reliant on a manual wheelchair. Prior to his injury, James was very athletic and enjoyed the outdoors. Now that he uses a manual wheelchair, James doesn't know how he's going to be active like he was before. Using what you've learned in this chapter, discuss what you believe to be the most significant factors facilitating or restricting James from being active.

References

Arbour-Nicitopoulos, K.P., Tomasone, J.R., Latimer-Cheung, A.E. and Martin Ginis, K.A. (2014). 'Get in motion: An evaluation of the reach and effectiveness of a physical activity telephone counseling service for Canadians living with spinal cord injury.' *PM&R*, 6: 1088–1096.

Bassett, R.L. and Martin Ginis, K.A. (2011). 'Risky business: The effects of an individualized health information intervention on health risk perceptions and leisure time physical activity among people with spinal cord injury.' *Disability and Health Journal*, 4: 165–176.

Brawley, L.R., Arbour-Nicitopoulos, K.P. and Martin Ginis, K.A. (2013). 'Developing physical activity interventions for adults with spinal cord injury: Part 3: A pilot feasibility study of an intervention to increase self-managed physical activity.' *Rehabilitation Psychology*, 58: 316–321.

Carlon, S., Shields, N., Dodd, K. and Taylor, N. (2013). 'Differences in habitual physical activity levels of young people with cerebral palsy and their typically developing peers: A systematic review.' *Disability Rehabilitation*, 35: 647–655.

Carroll, D., Courtney-Long, E.A., Stevens, A.C., Sloan, M.L., Lullo, C., Visser, S.N., Fox, M.H., Armour, B.S., Campbell, V.A., Brown, D.R., Dorn, J.M. and Centers for Disease Control and Prevention. (2014). 'Vital signs: Disability and physical activity – United States, 2009–2012.' *Morbidity and Mortality Weekly Report (MMWR)*, 63: 407–413.

Carter, A., Daley, A., Humphreys, L., Snowdon, N., Woodroofe, N., Petty, J., Roalfe, A., Tosh, J., Sharrack, B. and Saxton, J. (2014). 'Pragmatic intervention for increasing self-directed exercise behavior and improving important health outcomes in people with multiple sclerosis: A randomised controlled trial.' *Multiple Sclerosis Journal*, 20: 1112–1122.

Dlugonski, D., Motl, R.W., Mohr, D.C. and Sandroff, B.M. (2012). 'Internet-delivered behavioral intervention to increase physical activity in persons with multiple sclerosis: Sustainability and secondary outcomes.' *Psychology, Health and Medicine*, 17: 636–651.

Halbert, J., Crotty, M., Weller, D., Ahern, M. and Silagy, C. (2001). 'Primary care-based physical activity programs: Effectiveness in sedentary older patients with osteoarthritis symptoms.' *Arthritis and Rheumatism*, 45: 228–234.

Heath, G.W., Brownson, R.C., Kruger, J., Miles, R., Powell, K.E., Ramsey, L.T. and Task Force on Community Preventive Services. (2006). 'The effectiveness of urban design and land use and transport policies and practices to increase physical activity: A systematic review.' *Journal of Physical Activity and Health*, 3: S55–S76.

Inclusive Design Research Centre. (2016). '*About the IRDC: What is inclusive design*.' Available: http://Idrc.ocadu.ca/ (Accessed April 20 2016).

James, S., Ziviani, J., Ware, R.S. and Boyd, R.N. (2015). 'Randomized controlled trial of web-based multimodal therapy for unilateral cerebral palsy to improve occupational performance.' *Developmental Medicine and Child Neurology*, 57: 530–538.

Kahn, E.B., Ramsey, L.T., Brownson, R.C., Heath, G.W., Howze, E.H., Powell, K.E., Stone, E.J., Rajab, M.W. and Corso, P. (2002). 'The effectiveness of interventions to increase physical activity: A systematic review.' *American Journal of Preventive Medicine*, 22: 73–107.

Kemp, B. (2006). 'Depression as a secondary condition in people with disabilities.' In M.J. Field, A.M. Jette and L. Martin (eds.) *Workshop on disability in America: A new look-summary and background papers.* Washington, DC: National Academies Press.

Latimer-Cheung, A.E., Brawley, L.R., Ginis, K.M., Prapavessis, H. and Tomasone, J.R. (2010). 'Active homes: A preliminary evaluation of a peer-mediated, home-based strength training session for people with paraplegia.' *Journal of Exercise, Movement, and Sport*, 42(1): 123.

Lieberman, L.J., Dunn, J.M., Mars, H. van der and McCubbin, J. (2000). 'Peer tutors' effects on activity levels of deaf students in inclusive elementary physical education.' *Adapted Physical Activity Quarterly*, 17: 20–39.

Lox, C.L., Martin Ginis, K.A. and Petruzzello, S.J. (2014). *The psychology of exercise: Integrating theory and practice.* 4th ed. Scottsdale, AZ: Holcomb Hathaway Publishers.

Martin Ginis, K.A., Latimer, A.E., Arbour-Nicitopoulos, K.P., Buchholz, A., Bray, S.R., Craven, B., Hayes, K.C., Hicks, A.L., McColl, M., Potter, P.J., Smith, K. and Wolfe, D.L. (2010). 'Leisure-time physical activity in a population-based sample of people with spinal cord injury part I: Demographic and injury-related correlates.' *Archives of Physical Medicine and Rehabilitation*, 91, 722–728.

Martin Ginis, K.A., Ma, J.K., Latimer-Cheung, A.E. and Rimmer, J.W. (2016). 'A systematic review of review articles addressing factors related to physical activity participation among children and adults with physical disabilities.' *Health Psychology Review*, 10(4): 478–494.

National Center for Education Statistics. (2016). '*Fast facts: Students with disabilities* [Online].' Available: https://nces.ed.gov/fastfacts/display.asp?id=64 (Accessed April 4 2016).

Ploeg, H.P. van der, Streppel, K.R.M., Beek, A.J. van der, Woude, L.H.V. van der, Vollenbroek-Hutten, M.M.R., Harten, W.H. van and Mechelen, W. van. (2007). 'Successfully improving physical activity behavior after rehabilitation.' *American Journal of Health Promotion*, 21: 153–159.

Reichard, A., Stolzle, H. and Fox, M.H. (2011). 'Health disparities among adults with physical disabilities or cognitive limitations compared to individuals with no disabilities in the United States.' *Disability and Health Journal*, 4, 59–67.

Shields, N., Synnot, A.J. and Barr, M. (2012). 'Perceived barriers and facilitators to physical activity for children with disability: A systematic review.' *British Journal of Sports Medicine*, 46: 989–997.

Spivock, M., Gauvin, L., Riva, M. and Brodeur, J.-M. (2008). 'Promoting active living among people with physical disabilities.' *American Journal of Preventive Medicine*, 34: 291–298.

Statistics Canada. (2013). '*Disability in Canada: Initial findings from the Canadian survey on disability* [Online].' Available: www.statcan.gc.ca/pub/89-654-x/89-654-x2013002-eng. htm (Accessed April 4 2016).

Statistics Canada. (2015). '*A profile of persons with disabilities among Canadians aged 15 years or older, 2012.*' Available: www.statcan.gc.ca/pub/89-654-x/89-654-x2015001-eng. htm#a2 (Accessed April 4 2016).

Statistics Canada. (n.d.). '*Profile of disability for children* [Online].' Available: www.statcan.gc.ca/ pub/89-628-x/2007002/4125020-eng.htm (Accessed April 4 2016).

Stoddard, S. (2014). *Disability statistics annual report.* New Hampshire: University of New Hampshire.

Tarakci, E., Yeldan, I., Huseyinsinoglu, B.E., Zenginler, Y. and Eraksoy, M. (2013). 'Group exercise training for balance, functional status, spasticity, fatigue and quality of life in multiple sclerosis: A randomized controlled trial.' *Clinical Rehabilitation*, 27: 813–822.

United Nations General Assembly. (2006). '*Convention of the rights of persons with disabilities* [Online].' Available: www.un.org/disabilities/convention/conventionfull.shtml (Accessed December 29 2015).

United States Department of Health and Human Services (USDHHS). (2015). '*Step it up! The surgeon general's call to action to promote walking and walkable communities* [Online].' Available: www.surgeongeneral.gov/library/calls/walking-and-walkable-communities/call-to-action-walking-and-walkable-communites.pdf (Accessed September 12 2016).

Verschuren, O., Ketelaar, M., Gorter, J.W., Helders, P.J.M., Uiterwaal, C.S.P.M. and Takken, T. (2007). 'Exercise training program in children and adolescents with cerebral palsy: A randomized controlled trial.' *Archives of Pediatrics and Adolescent Medicine*, 161: 1075–1081.

Wiskochil, B., Lieberman, L.J., Houston-Wilson, C. and Petersen, S. (2007). 'The effects of trained peer tutors on the physical education of children who are visually impaired.' *Journal of Visual Impairment and Blindness*, 101: 339–350.

World Health Organization. (n.d.). '*Health topics: Disabilities* [Online].' Available: www.who.int/topics/disabilities/en/ (Accessed April 4 2016).

14

PHYSICAL ACTIVITY AMONG DIVERSE POPULATIONS INTERNATIONALLY

Justin Richards, Adewale Oyeyemi and Adrian Bauman

Understanding international populations

In 2016, there were 194 member states recognized by the World Health Organization (WHO). The World Bank classifies these countries into high income (*n* = 55), upper-middle income (*n* = 55), lower-middle income (*n* = 50) and low income (*n* = 34). However, the distribution of the world's population is heavily skewed towards low- and middle-income countries. World Bank data from 2014 indicate that approximately 81% of the estimated 7.3 billion people living on earth were in either low- or middle-income countries. Furthermore, The Worldometer Report (2016) indicates that there are also geographical differences with approximately 76% of the global population living in either Asia or Africa.

Despite the concentration of the world's population in Asian and African low- and middle-income countries, the majority of health research comes from high-income countries in Europe, North America and Australasia (Siron *et al.* 2015). Although this includes diverse populations within the local contexts, the evidence generated is not always globally transferrable. Specifically, low-income populations within high-income countries have inherently different socioecological characteristics (as noted in Chapter 9) to the norms observed in low-income countries and may benefit from different health promotion strategies (Siron *et al.* 2015). Similarly, the report of the WHO Global Health Observatory (2016) indicates that there are geographical differences in health priorities that may not be captured by examining culturally and environmentally diverse populations in countries with large research outputs. Consequently, there is a relative lack of data that accurately represents the health of the majority of the world's population.

However, the WHO STEPS global surveillance system for non-communicable diseases (e.g. cardiovascular disease, type II diabetes) and associated risk factors (e.g. smoking, physical inactivity) in adults has been widely implemented in low- and middle-income countries globally. This has made a substantial contribution to adult physical activity surveillance data being available for a total of 146 countries representing 93.3% of the global population (Sallis *et al.* 2016). Similarly, data primarily from the Global School-Based Health Survey and Health Behavior in School-Age Children Study provide an indication of adolescent physical activity levels in 120 countries representing 76.3% of the global population (Sallis *et al.* 2016).

Despite progress in global physical activity surveillance and the development of the Global Observatory for Physical Activity (2016), the recently established Country Report Cards indicate that high-income countries continue to produce the majority of physical activity research publications (83.5%) and researchers (82.0%). Although there are several established research groups rapidly expanding the physical activity evidence base in Latin America, there continues to be a lack of physical activity research conducted in Africa and Asia (Pratt *et al.* 2015). Consequently, it is important to understand what health and physical activity evidence has global utility and what may be unique to different settings.

Notable global disparities and inequities in health

Existing data indicate disparities in the distribution of the overall disease burden experienced by different countries and regions globally. According to the WHO Global Health Observatory (2016) there is a marked deficit in life expectancy when comparing countries at varying levels of development. This is largely driven by factors associated with poor sanitation and hygiene affecting child and maternal health in low-income settings. Furthermore, the fractured health systems and barriers to accessing quality health care that are common in low-income countries contribute to the persistence of communicable diarrheal and mosquito-borne diseases as well as tuberculosis and HIV/AIDS.

Despite ongoing conjecture, it is widely accepted that as a country develops an epidemiological transition occurs as the prevalence of deaths caused by communicable disease decreases relative to those caused by non-communicable disease (McKeown 2009). However, this should not be misinterpreted as an absence of non-communicable disease burden in lower-income settings. On the contrary, according to the latest WHO Global Status Report on Non-communicable Diseases (World Health Organization 2014) it is estimated that globally 74% of deaths from non-communicable diseases occur in low- and middle-income countries. It is also important to note that non-communicable diseases are responsible for more deaths than communicable diseases in low- and middle-income countries. Furthermore, the onset of non-communicable diseases in lower-income settings tends to be at a younger age, which further exacerbates health disparities when comparing morbidity and premature mortality. Consequently, lower-income countries experience the greatest burden of both non-communicable and communicable diseases – a phenomenon recognized as the double burden of disease (Boutayeb 2006).

Physical activity in global populations

Although it is widely accepted that physical inactivity is a leading risk factor for many non-communicable diseases, there is significant variation in its global prevalence. In 2016, it was estimated that 23.3% of adults and 81.4% of adolescents did not meet the WHO Global Recommendations for Physical Activity (Sallis *et al.* 2016). As noted in Chapter 1, for adults this was defined as not completing at least 150 minutes of moderate-intensity or 75 minutes of vigorous-intensity physical activity per week, or an equivalent combination. For adolescents, insufficiently active was defined as not completing at least 60 minutes of moderate- to vigorous-intensity physical activity daily. This ranged from 4.1% (Nepal) to 65.0% (Cook Islands) in adults and from 70.5% (India) to 94.8% (Republic of Korea) in adolescents (Sallis *et al.* 2016). The prevalence and distribution of insufficiently active adults and adolescents at the country level is summarized in Figure 14.1.

Despite wide variation in physical activity levels at the country level, there appear to be common trends that occur according to level of socioeconomic development and geographical location. This may have implications for the relative contribution of physical inactivity to the burden on non-communicable diseases in different income groups and WHO regions. For example, the contribution of physical inactivity to the total disease burden may be different when comparing high-income versus low-income countries or Africa versus Europe. These patterns may provide important insights into the potential transferability of public health policy and interventions across settings.

Differences in prevalence of overall physical inactivity according to income

When considering adult physical activity prevalence according to country income, there are data available from the majority of countries at all levels (high = 82%; upper-middle = 75%; lower-middle = 69%; low = 77%) (Sallis *et al.* 2016). According to data from the WHO Global Status Report on Non-communicable Diseases (World Health Organization 2014), there is a larger prevalence of insufficient activity in high (28.0%) and upper-middle (27.5%) countries than in lower-middle (17.9%) and low- (18.2%) income countries.

By contrast, the representativeness of the adolescent data according to income level was more disparate (high = 82%; upper-middle = 71%; lower-middle = 60%; low = 20%) (Sallis *et al.* 2016). Data presented in the WHO Global Status Report on Non-communicable Diseases (2014) suggest that there is no clear pattern across income groups in adolescents – the prevalence of insufficient physical activity was lowest in lower-middle income countries (77.6%) and highest in upper-middle income countries (84.2%). The prevalence of insufficient physical activity for both adults and adolescents according World Bank income status is summarized in Figure 14.2.

The distribution of these data suggests that as a country undergoes socioeconomic development the transition from lower-middle to upper-middle income levels may

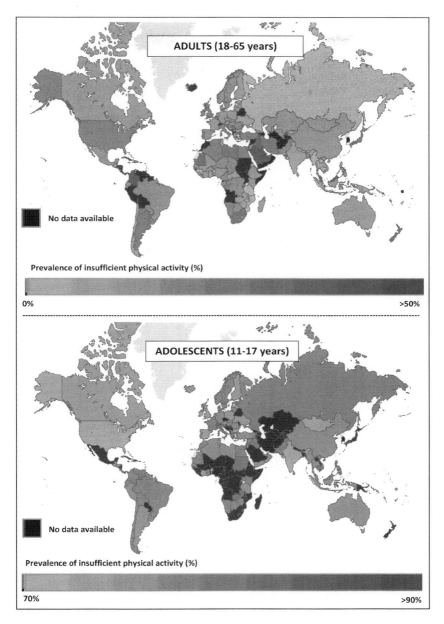

FIGURE 14.1 Prevalence of people insufficiently active by country
Source: Data from Global Observatory for Physical Activity (2016).

be the most critical point for physical activity behavior change. This appears to be particularly the case in adults, but may also be important during adolescence. It is likely that this is partly explained by the increasing proportion of people living in urban settings as a country develops from low (30%) to lower-middle (39%) to

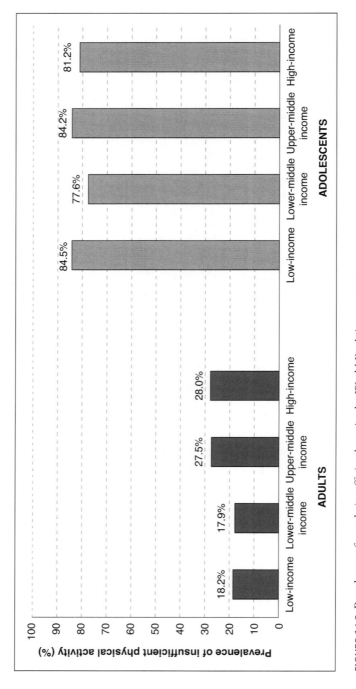

FIGURE 14.2 Prevalence of people insufficiently active by World Bank income status

Source: Data from Global Observatory for Physical Activity (2016).

upper-middle (62%) to high (81%) income (World Bank 2016). Of particular note is that there is a relatively large increase in urbanization as a country shifts from lower-middle to upper-middle income. Despite a lack of data, it appears that this manifests as significant decreases in incidental activity in the transport and vocation domains as motorized vehicle ownership increases and more people undertake sedentary employment (Bauman *et al.* 2011). This is not offset by progressive public health policy and infrastructure more common in high-income countries that promotes intentional physical activity participation, particularly during leisure time (Sallis *et al.* 2106).

Differences in prevalence of overall physical inactivity according to region

When considering adult physical activity prevalence according to WHO regions, there are data available from the majority of countries in all regions (Africa = 87%; Americas = 57%; Eastern Mediterranean = 57%; Europe = 75%; South-East Asia = 82%; Western Pacific = 89%) (Sallis *et al.* 2016). There are notable regional differences in the proportion of adults not meeting the physical activity guidelines. According to data from the WHO Global Status Report on Non-communicable Diseases (2014), South-East Asia (15.9%) performed markedly better than Africa (21.8%), Europe (22.8%) and the Western Pacific (24.9%), which were notably better than the Americas (31.4%) and the Eastern Mediterranean (33.1%).

Similar to the income-stratified data described previously, the representativeness of adolescent data across WHO regions was more disparate (Africa = 30%; Americas = 77%; Eastern Mediterranean = 76%; Europe = 68%; South-East Asia = 55%; Western Pacific = 78%) (Sallis *et al.* 2016). Calculations using data presented in the WHO Global Status Report on Non-communicable Diseases (2014) indicates that the relative differences among regions for adolescents meeting the physical activity recommendations is broadly similar to the patterns observed for adults. Specifically, the prevalence of adolescents not meeting physical activity recommendations was lowest in South-East Asia (73.7%) and highest in the Eastern Mediterranean (87.3%). Similarly, there was little difference when comparing adolescents from Europe (83.4%), Africa (84.7%) and the Western Pacific (84.8%). However, it appears that the performance of adolescents in the Americas (80.4%) relative to other regions was better than in adults. Despite these trends, as noted throughout this text, there is tremendous variability in physical activity participation based on the social determinants of health (race, ethnicity, income, etc.), even among the most active regions. The prevalence of insufficient physical activity for both adults and adolescents according WHO region is summarized in Figure 14.3.

These data suggest that the greatest burden of physical inactivity is experienced by countries in the Eastern Mediterranean region and people living in South-East Asia are the most active at the population level. It also appears that countries in the Americas may be relatively better at facilitating physical activity for adolescents than adults when compared to other WHO regions. The variation in physical activity

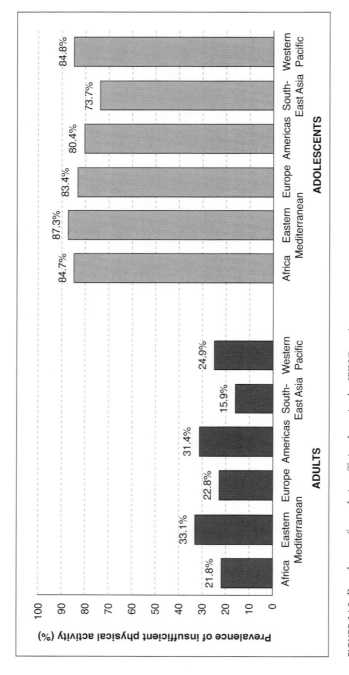

FIGURE 14.3 Prevalence of people insufficiently active by WHO region

Source: Data from Global Observatory for Physical Activity (2016).

prevalence according to region is likely to be partly explained by climatic differences. For example, several countries in the Eastern Mediterranean experience extreme heat that may be prohibitive of various outdoor physical activities readily accessible to people living in more temperate climates. Previous studies have shown that extreme temperatures can adversely affect physical activity in the transport, vocation and leisure domains (Chan and Ryan 2009). Finally, it is also important to recognize that relative differences in physical activity according to region may be a function of broader diversity in sociocultural and legislative norms that influence known correlates of physical activity behavior.

Common barriers and facilitators to physical activity globally

As previously described increasing participation in regular physical activity in the population is a national health priority in low-, middle- and high-income countries. However, interventions to promote physical activity are most effective when they address the underlying factors that influence physical activity behaviors (Heath *et al.* 2012; Sallis and Owen 2015). When considering factors that influence physical activity participation, we understand that they are referred to as 'correlates' if they have been identified in cross-sectional studies or 'determinants' if there is evidence from prospective or longitudinal studies. There are numerous correlates and determinants of physical activity that are consistent across settings and have global utility when planning potential interventions to change behavior. However, more recent research has begun to elucidate the relative importance of various correlates and determinants in various settings.

Common correlates and determinants of physical activity globally

The global correlates and determinants of physical activity are broad and could include demographic and biological factors, behavioral factors, psychosocial factors, sociocultural factors and environmental and policy factors (Sallis and Owen 2015). The common physical activity correlates or determinants that are of global utility for adults and young people are highlighted in Table 14.1.

Younger age and male gender are the most consistent positive demographic correlates for physical activity globally. However, the physical activity patterns of youth are different from that of adults (Caspersen *et al.* 2000; Troiano *et al.* 2008). Furthermore, the strength of the association between physical activity and many of its correlates and determinants varies across age groups. Review-level evidence indicates that psychosocial and environmental factors are the most consistent correlates and determinants of adult physical activity, while sociocultural and behavioral factors are the most consistent correlates and determinants of youth physical activity. Consequently, the physical activity of young people is often associated with external sociocultural factors such as parental rules, role modelling and peer support and/or behavioral factors like physical education class participation, school sports engagements and spending time outdoors (Dollman *et al.* 2005). In contrast, adult

TABLE 14.1 Common physical activity correlates and determinants globally

Adult Physical Activity	Youth Physical Activity
Demographic and Biological Correlates	**Demographic and Biological Correlates**
Age	Age
Gender	Gender
Income/socioeconomic status (SES)	Family income/SES
Education	Parental education
Occupation	Marital status of parent
Marital status	Race/ethnic origin
Parity	Body-mass index or anthropometry
Race/ethnic origin	Maternal body-mass index
Health status or perceived fitness	**Psychosocial Correlates**
Overweight/obesity	Self-esteem
Hereditary	External locus of control
Psychosocial Correlates	Attitude
Attitudes	Physical activity intention
Enjoyment of exercise	Perceived competence
Expected benefits	Sport/athletic competence
Barriers to exercise	Self-perception
Lack of time	Fun/enjoyment/preference of physical activity
Perceived behavioral control	Dislike physical education
Intention to exercise	Self-motivation/goal orientation
Action planning	Perceived behavioral control
Self-efficacy	Perceived benefits
Self-motivation	Value of health and status
Stage of change	Barriers to physical activity
Process of change	Lack of time
Normative belief	Stress
Personality variables	Depression
Psychological health	**Behavioral Correlates**
Openness to experience	PE/school sports/school sports team
Agreeableness	Organized competitive sports
Conscientiousness	Community sport
Knowledge of health/exercise	Watching TV/sedentary time/screen time
Stress	Time outdoors
High job strain	Previous physical activity
Susceptibility to/seriousness of illness	Healthy diet
(Fear of) symptoms	Caloric intake

Adult Physical Activity	Youth Physical Activity
Mood disturbance, mental health	Smoking
Psychological health, well-being	Chewing tobacco
PA characteristics, perceived effort	Alcohol use
Perceived benefits	Sensation seeking
Value of exercise outcomes	Fighting
Behavioral Correlates	**Sociocultural Correlates**
Activity history during childhood/youth	Parental involvement (PA with youth)
Activity history during adulthood	Perceived parental role model
Dietary habits (quality)	Parental activity
Alcohol	Sibling physical activity
Contemporary exercise program	Support for physical activity
Past exercise program	Parental/family support
Skills for coping with barriers	Direct parental help
Smoking	Parental encouragement, persuasion
Sports media use	Parental discouragement
Type A behavior pattern	Parent transports child
Decisional balance sheet	Parent pays physical activity fees
Sociocultural Correlates	Teacher support or modelling
Social support	Peer modelling
Social support from friends/peers	Friend/significant other support
Social support from spouse/family	Subjective norms
Physician influence	Parental attitudes
Social norms	Parent benefits of physical activity
Class size	Parent barriers to physical activity
Exercise models	**Environmental Correlates**
Group cohesion	Residential density
Past family influence	Access to destinations (land use mix)
Social isolation	Street connectivity
Environmental Correlates	Walkability (composite)
Residential density	Access/proximity to recreational facilities/areas
Access to destinations (land use mix)	Traffic speed/volume
Street connectivity	Safety from crime
Walkability (composite)	Neighbourhood incivilities/disorders
Access/proximity to recreational facilities/areas	Aesthetics/enjoyable scenery
Walking/biking infrastructures (e.g., sidewalks, cycle lane, trails or paths)	Walking/biking infrastructures (e.g., sidewalks, cycle lane, trails or paths)
Heavy traffic	

(Continued)

TABLE 14.1 (Continued)

Adult Physical Activity	Youth Physical Activity
Safety from crime	
Aesthetics/enjoyable scenery	
Adequate lighting	
Neighbourhood safety	
Frequently observe others exercising	
Hilly terrain	
Home equipment	
Satisfaction with facilities	
Unattended dogs	
Urbanization	

Source: Adapted from Bauman *et al.* (2012), Ding *et al.* (2011), Sallis *et al.* (2016), and Trost *et al.* (2002)

physical activity is more closely associated with internal psychosocial factors like self-efficacy, perceived benefits and physical self-concept and/or environmental factors such as access to recreational facilities and community walkability.

Unique correlates and determinants of physical activity according to income

There are subtle differences in correlates and determinants of physical activity between populations in low-, middle- and high-income countries. However, there is currently a lack of evidence that specifically stratifies low-income from middle-income countries and they are commonly grouped together in research assessing the correlates and determinants of physical activity. The unique correlates and determinants of youth and adult physical activity according to country income are highlighted in Table 14.2.

Socioeconomic status (SES) is a global demographic correlate of physical activity, but its association is different when comparing high-income countries to low- and middle-income countries. While high SES is a positive correlate for adult physical activity unique to high-income countries, low SES is a specific correlate of adult physical activity in low- and middle-income countries. For young people, family SES is not a consistent correlate of youth physical activity in high-income countries, but low family SES is a unique positive correlate in low- and middle-income countries. Differences in SES correlates of physical activity between high-income countries and low- and middle-income countries could be a reflection of the social patterns of physical activity in these diverse settings. For example, walking for transportation and manual high energy–dependent occupation are dominant physical activity patterns among the majority of low SES individuals in low- and

TABLE 14.2 Unique physical activity correlates and determinants according to country income

	High-income Countries		Low- and Middle-income Countries	
Correlates/Determinants*	Adult Physical Activity	Youth Physical Activity	Adult Physical Activity	Youth Physical Activity
Demographic and Biological Factors				
Age	Younger age		Younger age	
Gender	Male	Male^	Male	Male
SES/family income	High SES		Low SES	Low SES
Education				
Parental education		High education		
Race/ethnic origin		White		
Health status or fitness	Good health^			
Psychosocial Factors				
Self-efficacy	High self-efficacy^	High self-efficacy^	High self-efficacy	High self-efficacy
Perceived competent		High competence		
Perceived behavioral control		High ability		
Perceived/expected benefits	Benefit		Benefit	
Intention to exercise	Intent			
Barrier to exercise	Less barrier			
Stage of change	Positive change^			
Stress	Less stress^			
Perceived health/fitness			Healthy/high fitness	
Behavioral Factors				
Activity during childhood	Activity^			
Previous physical activity		Participation^	Participation	

(Continued)

TABLE 14.2 (Continued)

Correlates/Determinants*	High-income Countries		Low- and Middle-income Countries	
	Adult Physical Activity	Youth Physical Activity	Adult Physical Activity	Youth Physical Activity
Present physical activity			Participation	
Time outdoors		More time (HICs)		
Risk behavior/other risk factors			Low risk	
Sociocultural Factors				
Parental/family support		Support		
Friend/significant other support	Support	Support	Support	Support
General support for physical activity		Support^		
Environmental Factors				
Residential density	High density	High density		
Land use mix and access to destinations	Good access	Good access	Good access	Good access
Street connectivity	High connectivity			
Walkability (composite)	Walkable	Walkable		
Access/proximity to recreational facilities/areas	Good/proximal access	Good/proximal access	Good/proximal access	Good/proximal access
Traffic speed/volume		Low volume		
Walking/biking infrastructures (sidewalks, cycle lane, trails or paths)	Presence			
Aesthetics	Good			
Urbanization			Rural location	

* Factors listed in the table are those that have been reported as consistent positive correlates and determinants in at least 3 systematic reviews.

^ Factors that have been found as determinants of physical activity in longitudinal studies.

Note: Blank spaces indicate variables with inconclusive evidence for their role as correlates/determinants of physical activity.

middle-income countries (Atkinson *et al.* 2016; Guthold *et al.* 2011). In contrast, leisure-time physical activity, including sports participation, predominantly occurs in high-income countries and is associated with populations with a high SES in these settings (Finger *et al.* 2012; Juneau and Potvin 2010; Knuth and Hallal 2009; Stamatakis *et al.* 2008).

Self-efficacy is a global psychosocial determinant of physical activity across the lifespan in low-, middle- and high-income countries. Self-efficacy has consistently been documented as a strong psychosocial factor that can exert direct and indirect effects on the initiation and maintenance of physical activity (Craggs *et al.* 2011; Stralen *et al.* 2009). Other psychosocial correlates of physical activity common to adults in countries of all income levels include perceived and expected benefits of the behavior. There are several psychosocial correlates of physical activity for which there is only evidence from adults in high-income countries. In contrast, there are currently no unique psychosocial correlates or determinants of physical activity specific to low- and middle-income countries documented in the published literature. However, it is important to recognize that the relative lack of correlates and determinants in low- and middle-income countries may be an artifact of fewer studies in these settings rather than fewer factors associated with physical activity.

Of behavioral factors, activity during childhood and previous physical activity are positive determinants of physical activity unique to adults and youth, respectively, in high-income countries. Also, more time outdoors is a unique correlate of youth's physical activity in high-income countries. In contrast, previous and present physical activity and low-risk behavior are consistent positive behavioral correlates unique to adult physical activity in low- and middle-income countries. There is no evidence for any unique behavioral correlates or determinants for youth physical activity in low- and middle-income countries. However, it is again important to recognize that this may only reflect a lack of research rather than a lack of correlates and determinants in low- and middle-income countries.

Of sociocultural factors, support from friends and significant others to participate in physical activity are the most consistent correlates across the lifespan in low-, middle- and high-income countries. Parental and family support is a correlate and general support for physical activity is a determinant of youth physical activity specific to high-income countries. It appears that sociocultural correlates of physical activity are more prevalent in high-income countries when compared to low- and middle-income countries, particularly in youth. This may be explained by differences in sociocultural values and expectations regarding physical activity for youth and adult women that are relatively unique to low- and middle-income countries. Though difficult to examine, investigating cultural differences in correlates and determinants of physical activity could be an important research direction that may help explain discrepancies in physical activity levels observed in different regions throughout the world.

Although research investigating the influence of the environment on physical activity is relatively new, some important correlates of physical activity have emerged and few distinct patterns exist when comparing high-income to low- and middle-income countries. There is evidence to suggest that environmental factors such as access to destinations (i.e. mixed land use) and access to recreational facilities are global correlates of physical activity. However, there are several positive environmental correlates of physical activity that appear to be specific to high-income countries, which include high residential density, high street connectivity, high walkable neighborhood, presence of active transport infrastructures and aesthetically appealing surroundings. In contrast, rural living is a consistent positive environmental correlate of physical activity unique to low- and middle-income countries.

Unique correlates and determinants of physical activity according to region

There is currently limited research that discerns the correlates and determinants of physical activity according to WHO region. This is particularly the case for countries located in Africa, South-East Asia and the Eastern Mediterranean. Consequently, we can only make generalizations based on the location of countries that have made the most predominant contributions to existing relevant physical activity research.

Most of the physical activity correlates and determinants evidence described previously for high-income countries has come from Western Europe, North America and Australia. This evidence is remarkably consistent across these diverse geographical locations. Consequently, it appears that being a high-income country may supersede the influence of a specific WHO region when considering physical activity correlates and determinants.

Similarly, the correlates and determinants of physical activity identified for low- and middle-income countries were primarily derived from studies conducted in middle-income countries in South America (i.e. Brazil, Colombia), the Eastern Mediterranean (i.e. Iran) and the Western Pacific (i.e. China, Malaysia). However, emerging evidence from low-income countries supported some demographic (i.e. age, gender, SES, education) and environmental (i.e. rural location, crime safety) factors as important correlates of physical activity. In many African and South-East Asian nations, physical activity decreases with increasing SES, education and urban living as the population's primary source of physical activity shifts away from active transportation and manual occupation (Guthold et al. 2011; Muthuri et al. 2014; Ranasinghe et al. 2013; Sullivan et al. 2011).

Current evidence for physical activity interventions globally

In the past 15 years, there has been an increase in the number of peer-reviewed publications specifically about physical activity interventions from 40–50 papers in the year 2000 to approximately 500 papers per year in 2014–2016. Although this is still only a small proportion of all physical activity papers, it has increased from 8% in 2000 to approximately 16–17% in 2014–2016. Of these intervention papers, most are reporting research conducted in high-income countries with only 1–2%

being completed in low- and middle-income countries in 2014–2016. The majority of the studies conducted in low- and middle-income countries were in Latin America or China, with only very few conducted elsewhere in the world. Even a specific review of physical activity programs in Latin America concluded that there was limited evidence to guide policy (Hoehner *et al.* 2008).

The lack of evidence for interventions in low- and middle-income countries parallels the overall physical activity publication trends described previously. Furthermore, the existing evidence focuses on increasing physical activity at the individual and community level (Baker *et al.* 2011; Bock *et al.* 2014). Consequently, there is limited information on the implementation and effectiveness of strategies to promote physical activity at the population level for the majority of countries globally and where the need for intervention continues to increase. This is likely to result in insufficient policy attention focused on physical activity in many countries, which in turn will limit the implementation and evaluation of interventions at scale. The WHO Global Strategy on Diet, Physical Activity and Health identified the translation and generation of evidence across countries at varying levels of development and in different regions as a critical next step for delivering effective interventions in low- and middle-income settings (World Health Organization 2004).

Principles for developing physical activity interventions across different settings

When considering public health interventions to promote physical activity, it is important to differentiate between broad population-wide initiatives and smaller community-based programs. Population-wide approaches are inherently complex and involve numerous stakeholders across multiple disciplines. In contrast, the complexity of community-based programs varies and the extent of stakeholder engagement varies accordingly. Despite these differences, there are several common principles that underlie the effective development and delivery of both population-wide and community-based interventions for promoting physical activity.

Population-wide approaches to physical activity promotion require policy commitment that includes a clearly defined plan of action with adequate funding and robust monitoring and evaluation. Cross-agency partnerships that enable the implementation of multiple actions are integral. Specifically, health-centric approaches to physical activity promotion only influence information dissemination and structured exercise delivery by professionals in healthcare settings. This fails to recognize the potential to promote physical activity at a population level by engaging the education, parks and recreation, transport, urban planning and sport sectors in a diverse range of accessible community programs and infrastructure development (World Health Organization 2007). However, the logistical and financial challenges of genuine cross-sectoral and cross-agency interventions means that implementation is often compromised. Common pitfalls include organizational restructuring, under-resourcing, changing stakeholder priorities, competing policy interests and/ or poor governance (Evenson and Satinsky 2014; Eyler *et al.* 2014, Kohl *et al.* 2013;

Seguin *et al.* 2008). Consequently, population-wide plans to promote physical activity require genuine commitment from all relevant stakeholders to a well-defined logic model, pre-specified deliverables and a detailed work plan that clearly allocates organizational responsibilities.

Furthermore, it is important that physical activity plans are socially inclusive and have strategies targeting the groups identified as the least active in population-level surveys. This may vary according to country or region, but often constitutes older adults, socioeconomically disadvantaged groups, ethnic minorities and people with special needs or disabilities. Effectively communicating the potential benefit of physical activity to those who are least active is critical to the successful implementation of physical activity plans. There are cultural, language, religious, gender and age differences in the meaning of physical activity and appropriate adaptation is often required in diverse populations. This may include varying communication methods and marketing strategies for physical activity promotion according to different social norms and local contexts, as noted in several other chapters in this text (Keller *et al.* 2014).

Similar principles can be applied to the development and implementation of a community-based program, albeit on a smaller scale. Although community-based programs can be delivered in isolation, ideally they are targeted interventions for specific settings that are embedded in a broader population-wide action plan. This enables adaptation of population-wide initiatives to the 'local realities' and contextual differences of specified target groups, which may differ according to resources, staff capacity, physical infrastructure, social norms and built environments. Successful implementation and adaptation of national programs to different communities is enhanced by engaging with professionals and community members (e.g. constituent-involving strategies) and using grass-roots experiences of implementing programs in specific settings. This process, known as community-based participatory planning, engages stakeholders in contributing to the development of locally acceptable programs (Hogan *et al.* 2014, Reger-Nash *et al.* 2005; Teufel-Shone *et al.* 2014).

Adapting the "Seven Best Investments for Physical Activity" globally

The "Seven Best Investments for Physical Activity" document was based on consensus from physical activity experts across the world and developed by the International Society of Physical Activity and Health (Global Advocacy for Physical Activity 2007). This provided evidence for actions to promote physical activity that were likely to be generalizable to many countries and settings (Trost *et al.* 2014). Table 14.3 summarizes several potential actions for implementing the "Seven Best Investments for Physical Activity" and the relevance of these to community-based programs with specific reference to adaptation for delivery in low- and

TABLE 14.3 Application of the "Seven Best Investments for Physical Activity" in community settings and low- and middle-income countries

Potential Actions	Relevance for Community-based Programs	Adaptation to Low- and Middle-income Countries	Evaluation/Monitoring of Implementation
1) 'Whole of school' programs			
• Embed physical education in curriculum and develop active after-school programs • Support active travel to/from school	• Working with local schools and School Boards • Promoting active travel and after-school programs	• Mandatory physical education policies for all students • Encouraging cross-sectoral work to promote active travel for school children	• % of schools delivering physical education and active after-school programs • % of children engaging in active travel to/from school
2) Transport policies and systems that prioritize walking, cycling and public transport			
• Increase public transport options (co-benefits of less traffic and air quality) • Include active travel options as a priority in all transport policy and development	• Improving public transport usability and accessibility in conjunction with active travel options • Working on local walking and cycling routes for active travel	• Strategies to improve public transport systems to reduce traffic congestion and air pollution • Restrict car access in urban centers	• Number of people using public transport (and changes in traffic flow and air quality) • Number of users of walking and cycling infrastructure
3) Urban design regulations and infrastructure that provide for equitable and safe access for recreational physical activity, and recreational and transport-related walking and cycling across the life course			
• Plan urban environments that include parks and that enable recreational walking, running, cycling and play • Build infrastructure that enables active travel	• Working across sectors that are involved in local-level planning (e.g. local municipalities) • Promoting the inclusion of active transport options in all urban development	• Policies to reduce local traffic and increase the provision of parks and recreation areas • Inclusion of infrastructure' for walking and cycling high-use transport corridors	• Accessibility (e.g. distance) and number of people using active recreation facilities • Extent of active travel infrastructure (e.g. miles of footpaths/cycle lanes)

(Continued)

TABLE 14.3 (Continued)

Potential Actions	Relevance for Community-based Programs	Adaptation to Low- and Middle-income Countries	Evaluation/Monitoring of Implementation
4) Physical activity and non-communicable disease prevention integrated into primary healthcare systems			
• Provide advice to increase physical activity (and sit less) to all patients in healthcare settings • Distribute resources for physical activity promotion through healthcare professionals	• Training local healthcare providers to disseminate effective messages about physical activity participation • Improving the provision of physical activity resources through existing local healthcare networks	• Utilize various healthcare providers in primary health centers to deliver culturally adapted physical activity messages and guidelines • Identify local facilities and programs for accessing key local healthcare workers	• % of all health professionals recommending physical activity to their patients • % of patients receiving promotional material for physical activity
5) Public education, including mass media to raise awareness and change social norms on physical activity			
• Improve awareness of the physical activity recommendations • Highlight the benefits of being physically active and opportunities to increase participation	• Developing community campaigns delivered through local media, printed materials, online resources and advocates • Identifying physical activity opportunities and benefits of particular relevance locally	• Utilize locally accessible media to deliver campaigns as an initial part of a national strategy (e.g. local radio) • Mobilize local luminaries who may inspire broader changes in physical activity behavior	• % of the population aware of the physical activity recommendations • Attitudes towards physical activity and uptake of directly promoted opportunities

6) Community-wide programs involving multiple settings and sectors and that mobilize and integrate community engagement and resources

- Develop comprehensive approaches to physical activity promotion in community settings (e.g. worksites, religious centers)
- Facilitate community ownership of physical activity promotion

- Developing physical activity programs in consultation with local worksites and community centers
- Training local 'champions' who can lead physical activity advocacy in the community

- National policies targeting relevant settings and populations in the community (e.g. sedentary workplaces, religious centers)
- Community forums led by local leaders promoting physical activity opportunities

- % of community settings (e.g. worksites, religious centers) with strategies to promote physical activity
- Number of local people in governance and delivery structures of community-wide physical activity programs

7) Sports systems and programs that promote 'sport for all' and encourage participation across the lifespan

- Promote non-elite sport for all people in society
- Encourage participation in traditional sport and games

- Working with clubs/schools to foster community participation
- Promoting cultural norms that promote active games and play

- Prioritize local participation (not just elite sport)
- Maintain infrastructure for traditional games

- Number of participants in sport and traditional games
- % of total physical activity from sport and games

Source: World Health Organization (2009)

middle-income countries. In addition, evaluation indicators or metrics are suggested, indicating how progress could be monitored.

When implementing these guidelines, one key question asked in many settings is how to prioritize these 'seven areas' for population-wide action? The best approach is to identify any physical activity program that has already been effectively delivered at scale in that setting and use this as the basis for developing a broader population strategy: this recognizes that it may be difficult to implement all 'seven areas' concurrently.

There are varying levels of evidence to support the implementation of each of these seven investments in different settings. It is also important to note that interventions in each of these areas can involve various components targeted at influencing different physical activity behaviors in specific sub-populations. For example, whole-of-school programs to promote physical activity often include multiple intervention components that are seldom evaluated at scale (Centers for Disease Control and Prevention 2013), but are promising approaches for children and adolescents that are generalizable in many countries. In addition, sedentary behaviors can also be addressed through changes to in-school patterns of prolonged sitting. Better outcomes are related to effective implementation of multiple program components (Naylor et al. 2015).

There is good evidence to support transport-focused interventions and in natural experiments of building transport or trip-focused infrastructure (Brown et al. 2016, Rissel et al. 2012). An excellent example of a community-wide intervention with a strong transport component has taken place in the city of Bogota, in Colombia, where public policies have encouraged cycling and walking and discouraged car use (Díaz del Castillo et al. 2011, Torres et al. 2013).

For the built environment, the vast majority of published studies report the 'potential' for intervention based on cross-sectional associations between walkable environments and overall physical activity levels. However, very limited intervention evidence exists on changes to the built environment and its impact on community or population physical activity levels. This was recognized many years ago (Bauman 2005), and has persisted (De Rezende and Rey-López 2015), indicating that there has been limited evolution of the evidence in this area.

Efforts to promote physical activity through healthcare settings have been encapsulated in the concept of "Exercise is Medicine", which is being disseminated in high-, middle- and low-income countries (Lobelo et al. 2014). Similar efforts through general practice, family medicine and primary care provide further evidence in this area, although dissemination and uptake across healthcare providers remains low (Orrow et al. 2012).

Public education and mass media communication campaigns are a central part of a national physical activity plan, or can be operationalized to target a specific community or sub-population group. Examples of comprehensive national campaigns include the United States' VERB campaign (Huhman et al. 2005), and at the local level, social marketing campaigns have been used to target specific members of smaller communities (Eakin et al. 2007, Kamada et al. 2013). However, almost no such campaigns have been evaluated in low- or middle-income countries as part of physical activity strategies.

Community-wide programs are inherently complex and arguably require the highest level of coordination and communication among multiple stakeholders with divergent agendas. Interventions that have shown the most promise are those where legislation for changes to the built environment have occurred at the municipality level and have been integrated with other physical activity–promoting strategies specifically targeted at the least active people in the community (Reger-Nash et al. 2005). This has included physical activity advocacy through various established community settings (e.g. churches, worksites, community centers). However, generating evidence for these multi-faceted community-wide approaches is complex and limited across all income settings (Day 2016).

Finally, the "Sport for all" movement has received high-level endorsement as an important strategy to promote physical activity participation (Mountjoy et al. 2011). The premise is that sport is a potentially popular way of encouraging physical activity, for all ages, and particularly in sports-oriented low-income countries with limited resources for physical activity promotion. A related area is "sport for development" interventions, usually in low-income and sometimes post-conflict regions; this approach uses sport to contribute to social and mental health as well as to physical activity (Richards and Foster 2013). The "sport for development" field has an emerging evidence base and is likely to be applicable in low- and middle-income countries where it may garner political support at an early stage (Richards et al. 2013). The Kau Mai Tonga initiative is widely regarded as one of the most successful "sport for all" programs previously delivered in a middle-income country and is highlighted in Box 14.1.

BOX 14.1 EVIDENCE-BASED PRACTICE: KAU MAI TONGA USES NETBALL TO REDUCE THE BURDEN OF NON-COMMUNICABLE DISEASES AND ADDRESS BROADER SOCIAL INEQUITIES

Tonga has one of the highest incidences of non-communicable diseases in the world and social norms put women particularly at risk. Kau Mai Tonga is a "sport for all" initiative that was initially aimed at highlighting the risks of non-communicable diseases caused by physical inactivity and combating this by promoting participation in community-level netball. It commenced in 2012 and targeted women aged 15–45 years. The program has continued annually and evolved to include all age groups, genders and ability levels. It has catalyzed the delivery of a suite of netball programs in Tonga with a scope that has broadened to include gender equity objectives particularly focusing on leadership skill development and the inclusion of women in local community governance.

Kau Mai Tonga currently constitutes a national advocacy campaign accompanied by infrastructure development and resource mobilization to facilitate participation in netball. Specifically, a six-week mass media campaign aimed at raising awareness of the benefits of physical activity and changing social norms precedes a large-scale netball carnival that takes place across Tonga each year. This is the largest annual netball carnival in the world and has provided access to over 4,000 people for healthcare workers (i.e. nurses) to conduct non-communicable disease screening of all participants.

The success of Kau Mai Tonga is largely dependent on the effective engagement of multiple cross-sectoral stakeholders and the local communities. It is internally coordinated by the Tonga Netball Association in partnership with the Tongan Government (Ministry of Internal Affairs, Ministry of Health). Strategic and financial support is provided by Netball Australia and the Australian Government (Department of Foreign Affairs and Trade). Extensive consultation and capacity building of community stakeholders facilitates local adaptation and leadership of program delivery. Further details can be accessed at http://netball.com.au/kau-mai-tonga.

In summary, the "Seven Best Investments for Physical Activity" provide an evidence-informed framework for local community and national approaches in low-, middle- and high-income countries. These approaches are generalizable and when adapted appropriately they are likely to work in populations and sub-groups anywhere in the world where non-communicable disease and physical inactivity are important public health issues.

Implications for practice

It is evident that physical inactivity is an international phenomenon that has important implications for non-communicable disease outcomes and global mortality. In practice, the variation in physical activity behavior, correlates and determinants among countries suggests that a "one-size-fits-all" approach to promoting physical activity is unlikely to be successful.

However, consistent patterns in physical activity participation and its correlates as a country undergoes socioeconomic development indicate that while some leverage points for intervention may be effective in all settings, there may also be some unique opportunities that vary according to country income level. This has practical implications when prioritizing intervention types and developing optimal intervention components in resource-limited settings. Although this process should be informed by the physical activity correlates and determinants unique to different settings, it is important to recognize that there is a relative paucity of evidence from low- and middle-income countries. Consequently, an absence of published literature for several potential physical activity correlates in low- and middle-income countries may be explained by an absence of evidence and should not be misconstrued as contradicting evidence.

The practical application of the "Seven Best Investments for Physical Activity" recognizes this limitation by providing evidence-based general principles for promoting physical activity at the population level. A key principle for low- and middle-income countries is to move beyond strategic plans for physical activity and actually implement wide-reaching prevention programs targeting inactivity at the population level. The "Seven Best Investments" effectively addresses the global need for physical activity interventions by providing a range of options, of which at least one is intended to be accessible to any country as a starting point for implementation and delivery across the population. This approach embraces the organic nature in which various physical activity promotion strategies have developed in different countries. After countries have effectively harnessed physical activity interventions that "come naturally", selecting which of the "Seven Best Investments" to pursue next should be informed by identifying successes in similar settings and thoroughly evaluating its transferability to the new context. This inherently requires understanding critical program processes when translating evidence across diverse international populations.

Summary points

- Physical inactivity is a global phenomenon, but its relative health burden varies according to country income and geographical location in both adults and adolescents.
- There are several common demographic, psychosocial, behavioral, sociocultural and environmental correlates and determinants for physical activity participation that appear to have global utility across diverse populations.
- Although there are some physical activity correlates that appear to be unique to high-income countries, it is important to recognize that this may be an artifact of the relative lack of research conducted in low- and middle-income countries.
- Across all settings, increasing physical activity at a population level requires coordinated action that engages a diverse range of relevant stakeholders and is adapted to the local context and the needs of specific target groups.
- The "Seven Best Investments for Physical Activity" include actions in healthcare settings, built environments, transport systems, school programs, community-based approaches, public education and "sport for all" programs.
- Countries and jurisdictions aiming to increase physical activity levels at the population level or in targeted sub-groups should first focus on scaling up existing actions and then consider implementing programs that have evidence of success in similar contexts.

Critical thinking questions

1   What factors may confound the observed differences in physical activity prevalence according to country income and geographical location? How might other contextual factors be responsible for these variations?

2   What emerging issues in the global sociopolitical and physical environment may be important determinants of physical activity behavior? How might this differ according to country income and geographical location?

3   What should be included if the WHO decided to increase to the "Twelve Best Investments for Physical Activity"? How would this be justified to countries with limited resources to invest in physical activity interventions?

4   What should be prioritized with the limited physical activity research resources available in low- and middle-income countries? How might a shift from further research into physical activity correlates to focusing on intervention evaluation be beneficial and/or problematic?

Acknowledgments

The authors acknowledge Andrea Ramirez for her contribution to preparing Figure 14.1.

References

Atkinson K., Lowe S., and Moore S. (2016). 'Human development, occupational structure and physical inactivity among 47 low and middle income countries.' *Preventive Medicine Reports*, 3:40–45.

Baker P.R.A., Francis D.P., Soares J., Weightman A.L., and Foster C. (2011). 'Community wide interventions for increasing physical activity.' *Sao Paulo Medical Journal*, 129:436–437.

Bauman A.E. (2005). 'The physical environment and physical activity: Moving from ecological associations to intervention evidence.' *Journal of Epidemiology and Community Health*, 59:535–536.

Bauman A.E., Ma G., Cuevas F., Omar Z., Waqanivalu T., Phongsavan P., Keke K., and Bhushan A. (2011). 'Cross-national comparisons of socioeconomic differences in the prevalence of leisure-time and occupational physical activity, and active commuting in six Asia-Pacific countries.' *Journal of Epidemiology Community Health*, 65:35–43.

Bauman A.E., Reis R.S., Sallis J.F., Wells J.C., Loos R.J.F., and Martins B.W. (2012). 'Correlates of physical activity: Why are some people physically active and others are not?' *Lancet*, 380:257–271.

Bock C., Jarczok M.N., and Litaker D. (2014). 'Community-based efforts to promote physical activity: A systematic review of interventions considering mode of delivery, study quality and population subgroups.' *Journal of Science and Medicine in Sport*, 17:276–282.

Boutayeb A. (2006). 'The double burden of communicable and non-communicable diseases in developing countries.' *Transactions of the Royal Society of Tropical Medicine & Hygiene*, 100:191–199.

Brown V., Diomedi B.Z., Moodie M., Veerman J.L., and Carter R. (2016). 'A systematic review of economic analyses of active transport interventions that include physical activity benefits.' *Transport Policy*, 45:190–208.

Caspersen C.J., Pereira M.A., and Curran K.M. (2000). 'Changes in physical activity patterns in the United States, by age and cross-sectional age.' *Medicine and Science in Sports and Exercise*, 32:1601–1609.

Centers for Disease Control and Prevention (CDC). (2013). '*Comprehensive School Physical Activity Programs: A Guide for Schools* [Online].' Available: www.cdc.gov/healthyschools/physicalactivity/cspap.htm (Accessed June 2016).

Chan C., and Ryan D. (2009). 'Assessing the effects of weather conditions on physical activity participation using objective measures.' *International Journal of Environmental Research in Public Health*, 6(10):2639–2654.

Craggs C., Corder K., Sluijs E.M.F. van, and Griffin S.J. (2011). 'Determinants of change in physical activity in children and adolescents: A systematic review.' *American Journal of Preventive Medicine*, 40:645–658.

Day K. (2016). 'Built environmental correlates of physical activity in China: A review.' *Preventive Medicine Reports*, 3:303–316.

De Rezende L.F.M., and Rey-López J.P. (2015). 'Environmental interventions are needed to provide sustained physical activity changes.' *Exercise and Sport Sciences Reviews*, 43:238.

Díaz del Castillo A., Sarmiento O.L., Reis R.S., and Brownson R.C. (2011). 'Translating evidence to policy: Urban interventions and physical activity promotion in Bogotá, Colombia and Curitiba, Brazil.' *Translational Behavioral Medicine*, 1:350–360.

Ding D., Sallis J.F., Kerr J., Lee S., and Rosenberg D.E. (2011). 'Neighborhood environment and physical activity among youth: A review.' *American Journal of Preventive Medicine*, 41:442–455.

Dollman J., Norton K., and Norton L. (2005). 'Evidence for secular trends in children's physical activity behavior.' *British Journal of Sports Medicine*, 39:892–897.

Eakin E.G., Mummery K., Reeves M.M., Lawler S.P., Schofield G., Marshall A.J., and Brown W.J. (2007). 'Correlates of pedometer use: Results from a community-based physical activity intervention trial (10,000 Steps Rockhampton).' *International Journal of Behavioral Nutrition and Physical Activity*, 4:31.

Evenson K.R., and Satinsky S.B. (2014). 'Sector activities and lessons learned around initial implementation of the United States national physical activity plan.' *Journal of Physical Activity and Health*, 11:1120–1128.

Eyler A., Chriqui J., Maddock J., Cradock A., Evenson K.R., Gustat J., Hooker S., Lyn R., Segar M., O'Hara Tompkins N., and Zieff S.G. (2014). 'Opportunity meets planning: An assessment of the physical activity emphasis in state obesity-related plans.' *Journal of Physical Activity and Health*, 11:45–50.

Finger J.D., Tylleskar T., and Lampert T.T. (2012). 'Physical activity patterns and socioeconomic position: The German National Health Interview and Examination Survey, 1998 (GNHIES98).' *BMC Public Health*, 12:1079.

Global Advocacy for Physical Activity (GAPA), and the Advocacy Council of the International Society for Physical Activity and Health (ISPAH). (2007). 'NCD prevention: Investments that work for physical activity.' *Reproduced in: British Journal of Sports Medicine*, 46:709–712.

Global Observatory for Physical Activity. (2016). '*Country Cards* [Online].' Available: www.globalphysicalactivityobservatory.com/ (accessed June 2016).

Guthold R., Louazani S.A., Riley L.M., Cowan M.J., Bovet P., Damasceno A., Sambo B.H., Tesfaye F., and Armstrong T.P. (2011). 'Physical activity in 22 African countries: Results from the World Health Organization STEPwise approach to chronic diseases risk factor surveillance.' *American Journal of Preventive Medicine*, 41:52–60.

Heath G.W., Parra-Perez D., Sarmiento O.L., Andersen L.B., Owen N., Goenka S., Montes F., and Brownson R.C. (2012). 'Evidence-based physical activity interventions: Lessons from around the world.' *Lancet*, 380:272–281.

Hoehner C.M., Soares J., Perez D.P., Ribeiro I.C., Joshu C.E., Pratt M., Legetic B.D., Malta D.C., Matsudo V.R., Ramos L.R., and Simões E.J. (2008). 'Physical activity interventions in Latin America: A systematic review.' *American Journal of Preventive Medicine*, 31;34(3):224–233.

Hogan L., Bengoechea E.G., Salsberg J., Jacobs J., King M., and Macaulay A.C. (2014). 'Using a participatory approach to the development of a school-based physical activity policy in an indigenous community.' *Journal of School Health*, 84(12):786–792.

Huhman M., Potter L.D., Wong F.L., Banspach S.W., Duke J.C., and Heitzler C.D. (2005). 'Effects of a mass media campaign to increase physical activity among children: Year-1 results of the VERB campaign.' *Pediatrics*, 116:e277–e284.

Kamada M., Kitayuguchi J., Inoue S., Ishikawa Y., Nishiuchi H., Okada S., Harada K., Kamioka H., and Shiwaku K. (2013). 'A community-wide campaign to promote physical activity in middle-aged and elderly people: A cluster randomized controlled trial.' *International Journal of Behavioral Nutrition and Physical Activity*, 10:44.

Keller C., Vega-López S., Ainsworth B., Nagle-Williams A., Records K., Permana P., and Conrod D. (2014). 'Social marketing: Approach to cultural and contextual relevance in a community-based physical activity intervention.' *Health Promotion International*, 29:130–140.

Knuth A.G., and Hallal P.C. (2009). 'Temporal trends in physical activity: A systematic review.' *Journal of Physical Activity and Health*, 6:548–559.

Kohl H.W., Satinsky S.B., Whitfield G.P., and Evenson K.R. (2013). 'All health is local: State and local planning for physical activity promotion.' *Journal of Public Health Management and Practice*, 19:S17–S22.

Juneau C.E., and Potvin L. (2010). 'Trends in leisure-, transport-, and work-related physical activity in Canada 1994–2005.' *Preventive Medicine*, 51:384–386.

Lobelo F., Stoutenberg M., and Hutber A. (2014). 'The "exercise is medicine" global health initiative: A 2014 update.' *British Journal of Sports Medicine*, 48:1627–1633.

McKeown R. (2009). 'The epidemiologic transition: Changing patterns of mortality and population dynamics.' *American Journal Lifestyle Medicine*, 3:19S–26S.

Mountjoy M., Andersen L.B., Armstrong N., Biddle S., Boreham C., Bedenbeck H.P., Ekelund U., Engebretsen L., Hardman K., Hills A.P., Kahlmeier S., Kriemler S., Lambert E., Ljungqvist A., Matsudo V., McKay H., Micheli L., Pate R., Riddoch C., Schamasch P., Sundberg C.J., Tomkinson G., Sluijs E. van, and Mechelen W. van. (2011). 'International Olympic Committee consensus statement on the health and fitness of young people through physical activity and sport.' *British Journal of Sports Medicine*, 45:839–848.

Muthuri S.K., Wachira L.J.M., Leblanc A.G., Francis C.E., Sampson M., Onywera V.O., and Tremblay M.S. (2014). 'Temporal trends and correlates of physical activity, sedentary behavior, and physical fitness among school-aged children in Sub-Saharan Africa: A systematic review.' *International Journal of Environmental Research in Public Health*, 11:3327–3359.

Naylor P.J., Nettlefold L., Race D., Hoy C., Ashe M.C., Wharf Higgins J., and McKay H.A. (2015). 'Implementation of school based physical activity interventions: A systematic review.' *Preventive Medicine*, 72:95–115.

Orrow G., Kinmonth A.L., Sanderson S., and Sutton S. (2012). 'Effectiveness of physical activity promotion based in primary care: Systematic review and meta-analysis of randomised controlled trials.' *BMJ*, 344:e1389.

Pratt M., Ramirez A., Martins R., Bauman A., Heath G., Kohl H.W. 3rd, Lee I.M., Powell K., and Hallal P. (2015). '127 steps toward a more active world.' *Journal of Physical Activity and Health*, 12:1193–1194.

Ranasinghe C.D., Ranasinghe P., Jayawardena R., and Misra A. (2013). 'Physical activity patterns among South-Asian adults: A systematic review.' *International Journal of Behavioral Nutrition and Physical Activity*, 10:116.

Reger-Nash B., Bauman A., Butterfield-Booth S., Smith H., Chey T., and Simon K. (2005). 'Wheeling walks – long term evaluation.' *Family and Community Health*, 28:64–78.

Richards J., and Foster C. (2013). 'Sport-for-development interventions: Whom do they reach and what is their potential for impact on physical and mental health in low-income countries?' *Journal of Physical Activity and Health*, 10:929–931.

Richards J., Kaufman Z.A., Schulenkorf N., Wolff E., Gannett K., Siefken K., and Rodriguez G. (2013). 'Advancing the evidence base of sport for development: A new open-access, peer-reviewed journal.' *The Journal of Sport for Development*, 1:1–3.

Rissel C., Curac N., Greenaway M., and Bauman A. (2012). 'Physical activity associated with public transport use-a review and modelling of potential benefits.' *International Journal of Environmental Research and Public Health*, 9(7):2454–2478.

Sallis J.F., Bull F., Guthold R., Heath G., Inoue S., Kelly P., Oyeyemi A., Perez L.C., Richards J., and Hallal P. (2016). 'Progress in physical activity over the Olympic quadrennium.' *Lancet*, 388:1325–1336.

Sallis J.F., and Owen N. (2015). 'Ecological models of health behavior.' In Glanz K., Rimer B., and Viswanath V. (eds.) *Health behavior: Theory, research & practice*. 5th ed., San Francisco: Jossey-Bass.

Seguin R.A., Palombo R., Economos C.D., Hyatt R., Kuder J., and Nelson M.E. (2008). 'Factors related to leader implementation of a nationally disseminated community-based exercise program: A cross-sectional study.' *International Journal of Behavioral Nutrition and Physical Activity*, 5:62.

Siron S., Dagenais C., and Ridde V. (2015). 'What research tells us about knowledge transfer strategies to improve public health in low-income countries: A scoping review.' *International Journal of Public Health*, 60:849–863.

Stamatakis E., and Chaudhury M. (2008). 'Temporal trends in adults' sports participation patterns in England between 1997 and 2006: The health survey for England.' *British Journal of Sports Medicine*, 42:901–908.

Stralen M.M. van, De Vries H., Mudde A.N., Bolman C., and Lechner L. (2009). 'Determinants of initiation and maintenance of physical activity among older adults: A literature review.' *Health Psychology Review*, 3:147–207.

Sullivan R., Kinra S., Ekelund U., Bharathi A.V., Vaz M., Kurpad A., Collier T., Reddy K.S., Prabhakaran D., Ben-Shlomo Y., Davet Smith G., Ebrahim S., and Kuper H. (2011). 'Socio-demographic patterning of physical activity across migrant groups in India: Results from the Indian migration study.' *PLoS One*, 6:e24898.

Teufel-Shone N.I., Gamber M., Watahomigie H., Siyuja T.J. Jr., Crozier L., and Irwin S.L. (2014). 'Using a participatory research approach in a school-based physical activity intervention to prevent diabetes in the Hualapai Indian community, Arizona, 2002–2006.' *Preventing Chronic Disease*, 11.

Torres A., Sarmiento O.L., Stauber C., and Zarama R. (2013). 'The ciclovia and cicloruta programs: Promising interventions to promote physical activity and social capital in Bogotá, Colombia.' *American Journal of Public Health*, 13:103.

Troiano R.P., Berrigan D., Dodd K.W., Mâsse L.C., Tilert T., and McDowell M. (2008). 'Physical activity in the United States measured by accelerometer.' *Medicine and Science in Sports and Exercise*, 40:181–188.

Trost S.G., Blair S.N., and Khan K.M. (2014). 'Physical inactivity remains the greatest public health problem of the 21st century: Evidence, improved methods and solutions using the '7 investments that work' as a framework.' *British Journal of Sports Medicine*, 48:169–170.

Trost S.G., Owen N., Bauman A.E., Sallis J.F., and Brown W. (2002). 'Correlates of adults' participation in physical activity: Review and update.' *Medicine and Science in Sports and Exercise*, 34:1996–2001.

World Bank. (2016). 'World Development Indicators [Online].' Available: http://data.worldbank.org/ (accessed June 2016).

World Health Organization. (2004). *Global strategy on diet, physical activity and health.* Geneva: World Health Organisation.

World Health Organization. (2007). *A guide for population-based approaches to increasing levels of physical activity: Implementation of the WHO global strategy on diet, physical activity and health.* Geneva: World Health Organization.

World Health Organization. (2009). *Interventions on diet and physical activity: What works? Summary report.* Geneva: World Health Organization.

World Health Organization. (2010). *Global recommendations on physical activity for health.* Geneva: World Health Organization.

World Health Organization. (2014). *Global action plan for the prevention and control of noncommunicable diseases.* Geneva: World Health Organization.

World Health Organization Global Health Observatory. (2016). *World Health Statistics 2016: Monitoring health for the SDGs.* Geneva: World Health Organization.

Worldometers. (2016). '*World Population* [Online].' Available: www.worldometers.info/world-population/ (accessed June 2016).

15

FUTURE DIRECTIONS FOR ADDRESSING PHYSICAL ACTIVITY IN DIVERSE POPULATIONS

Melissa Bopp

The main goal of this text was to provide you with an overview of how the social determinants of health can impact physical activity participation, examine the current status of the evidence, and provide some implications for practice. Throughout the chapters we have examined how race, ethnicity, socioeconomic status, residence location, sexual orientation, veterans status, and level of disability are related to individuals' health and physical activity behavior. These factors create the health disparities related to physical inactivity and inactivity-related chronic disease found in the United States and around the world. In order to address these inequities, initiatives need to be developed at multiple levels, targeting along a spectrum of individual approaches up to policy implementation. The World Health Organization's Global Strategy for Diet and Physical Activity has also stressed the importance of considering social and cultural norms, religions, values, gender issues, political support, and local-level capacity for promoting physical activity (World Health Organization 2010).

Social ecological approaches to health disparities

Within a social ecological framework, there is extensive evidence for intervening at all levels of the model. There are a number of national and international position stands, reviews, and programs that have highlighted the importance of multi-level approaches to drive programming, policies, and initiatives (Heath *et al.* 2012, National Physical Activity Plan 2016, Reis *et al.* 2016, U.S. Department of Health and Human Services (USDHHS) 2012, World Health Organization 2004). Throughout the chapters in this book we have highlighted effective strategies for addressing inactivity across all levels for many different populations.

Individual-level approaches

At an individual level there is extensive research that has evaluated the best approaches to increasing physical activity behavior. These strategies have included education, behavior change techniques, health-risk appraisals, and other approaches to increase the adoption and improve the maintenance of physical activity (Dishman and Buckworth 1996). Though there is a significant body of knowledge in this area, limited research has been conducted with many of the underserved populations included in this text. An intervention featured in Chapter 13 outlined an individually based strategy for individuals with disability. This Internet-based intervention provided education and encouragement along with behavior change techniques (self-monitoring) among disabled youth, resulting in improved behavioral and health outcomes (James *et al.* 2015). Though not wide-reaching, many individual-level approaches have significant potential to improve physical activity and health outcomes in a targeted population.

Social/interpersonal approaches

The social environment for physical activity has been shown to be very important for physical activity in a variety of populations and settings. Social support has been noted repeatedly throughout this text as an important influence for women, older adults, and racial/ethnic minorities. Interventions grounded in a social environmental approach have tremendous versatility and can be delivered in a variety of settings. In Chapter 5, a study by Arredondo and colleagues (2014) was highlighted. This program included Latina mothers and daughters and used educational sessions and encouraged the women to walk together. This approach was an excellent way to create a supportive social environment for physical activity and was culturally tailored at both surface and deep levels (Arredondo *et al.* 2014). Chapter 11 also featured a group-based intervention for lesbian women that included group exercise along with discussion sessions about barriers and coping strategies, using deep cultural tailoring (Fogel *et al.* 2016).

Setting-based approaches

Throughout this text the benefits of setting-based approaches were highlighted for many different populations. The additional benefit of targeting settings is the potential to target the physical and/or social environment of the setting along with the individuals, thus providing a potential for a longer-lasting intervention. Among youth, pre-school, school, and after-school programs have served as an effective partner for changing behavior and were all notable locations for a number of the populations highlighted in this book. Worksites and faith-based organizations were all noted as potential locations for changing physical activity in adult populations and healthcare organizations have the potential for reaching older adults and clinical populations. This text provided a number of examples of setting-based approaches effectively targeting underserved populations. In Chapter 8 we discussed a program that used traditional hula dancing to increase activity levels among Native Hawaiians.

This program was based in a healthcare setting, a cardiac rehabilitation clinic, and provides participants with the benefits of working within an established institution. Inclusion of both surface and deep structure elements, like hula dancing and elements of spiritual health, allowed for a very tailored approach within a setting.

Community-based approaches

Among the more broad-brush approaches, community-based approaches often employ strategies at the individual, social, and setting levels along with other initiatives to target physical activity participation for the general population.

Chapter 7 outlined how community-level strategies could be used to target inactivity among Native Americans through reducing barriers to access facilities, engaging youth through coaches and participation in traditional Native American activities (Findlay and Kohen 2007). These types of approaches allow for extensive reach throughout the community, targeting males and females of all ages using culturally tailored strategies and increasing the likelihood that the intervention will be well received and effective. Chapter 12 also highlighted a study that used community-based approaches to encourage physical activity among veterans. This study included outreach and support through different community organizations and was culturally tailored based on military identity (Angel and Armstrong 2016). These community-level strategies that were effectively tailored to meet the needs of the population have great potential for effectiveness and long-term sustainability by partnering with existing community organizations.

Policy approaches

Perhaps the most far-reaching approaches are those that focus on policy. In terms of addressing health inequities and disparities, policy approaches can be effective when considering issues associated with resources or access that have the potential to reach a particular population. Effective policies have included increasing opportunities or access to places for people to be active through physical education, walkable or bikeable communities, or other places for access. These types of policies to promote physical activity have the potential to encourage behavior change regardless of race, ethnicity, gender, sexual orientation, income level, ability level, veterans' status, or location. In Chapter 10, the authors outlined the importance of supportive policies for physical activity, especially among youth. A number of school-based policies were implemented to increase opportunities for extracurricular physical activity among rural youth with many positive outcomes (Umstattd Meyer et al. 2016).

Environmental approaches

Approaches grounded in environmental change have the capacity to work across multiple levels of the social ecological framework. Environmental changes could take place in a setting (e.g., a workplace installing locker rooms to allow employees to clean up after a mid-day workout), at a community level (e.g., walking trails installed throughout a neighborhood), or work in conjunction with policy (e.g., policies put in place to enhance an environment's walkability). Chapter 9 outlined how the physical activity friendliness of the environment of neighborhoods was different among low-, middle-, and high-income areas (Taylor *et al.* 2012).

Among all of the levels of the social ecological model, the approaches with the greatest potential public health impact on health disparities are those which have the broadest reach. These would be strategies focused on settings, communities, policies, and the environment. Given the extensive health disparities noted in this text, broad-based approaches that have the potential to reach across races, ethnicities, income levels, location, sexual orientation, disability level, or veterans' status have a greater likelihood of impacting health and physical activity outcomes.

A foundation for moving forward

The extensive inequities outlined in this text highlight the importance of an organized strategy moving forward in any attempt to address these problems. The U.S. Department of Health and Human Services' Healthy People 2020 initiative goals and objectives for physical activity stress not only individual-level behavior goals (e.g., changes in participation in leisure-time physical activity), but also goals for environments, settings, and policies across multiple sectors that can support individual-level behavior change (e.g., recess offerings in elementary schools). Two documents that outline strategies and tactics for moving forward are the United States' National Physical Activity Plan (National Physical Activity Plan Alliance 2016) and the World Health Organization Non-communicable Disease Action Plan (World Health Organization 2013).

National Physical Activity Plan

As noted in Chapter 1, the National Physical Activity Plan (NPAP) envisions a future where all individuals are active and live, work, and play in environments that support physical activity (National Physical Activity Plan Alliance 2016). The NPAP is also grounded in a social ecological approach and emphasizes the importance of working within established sectors:

- Business and Industry
- Community, Recreation, Fitness and Parks
- Education
- Faith-based Settings
- Healthcare
- Mass Media
- Public Health
- Sport
- Transportation, Land Use, and Community Design

with recommended strategies and tactics to improve physical activity participation. This comprehensive approach is well suited to impact many of the health disparities outlined in this text. Similar to our evidence-based practice focus in this text, the NPAP draws from initiatives supported by the evidence of effectiveness. The strategies outlined within the sectors provide a foundation to help address the disparities in activity levels outlined throughout the chapters. For example, in the Community Recreation, Fitness and Parks Sector, strategy 2 indicates that communities should improve availability and access to places to support physical activity for all residents. Among disabled populations, this would mean that facilities adhere to guidelines for allowing access for a wide range of physical abilities, including equipment and physical spaces and programming that is adaptable. In the Business Sector, strategy 1 indicates that businesses should provide employees opportunities and incentives to be active. Rural workplaces could use this tactic to provide a space for employees to engage in exercise before, during, or after work where adults in rural communities may not have access otherwise to places to be active. If approached strategically these sectors may have the potential to impact many of the health disparities associated with physical inactivity noted throughout this text.

WHO Global Action Plan for the Prevention and Control of Non-communicable Diseases

As noted in Chapter 14, the World Health Organization's approach to non-communicable diseases focuses on policy, capacity building, leadership, and partnerships to address the risk factors associated with non-communicable diseases (World Health Organization 2013). The WHO Plan has a strong focus on equity and health for all global citizens, aiming to reduce disparities through multisectoral action and evidence-based strategies across the life course. Specific to physical activity, the WHO Plan aims to target underlying social determinants through creation of health-promoting environments. As noted previously, policy approaches can be effective for combating health disparities. For example, urban planning policy approaches to improve pedestrian and bicyclist safety in low-income neighborhoods could increase active travel and contribute to overall physical activity for residents. Policies aimed to improve access to and quality of physical education can impact the health of children of all racial or ethnic backgrounds, income levels, or residence locations. This comprehensive plan provides a foundation for addressing many of the disparities outlined through the chapters in this book.

Healthy People 2020 and beyond

More than midway through the timeframe for Healthy People 2020, progress has been made in a number of physical activity topics and objectives (U.S. Department of Health and Human Services (USDHHS) 2012). National Snapshot data have indicated that the proportion of adults getting no leisure-time physical activity has decreased, and the 2020 target goal of 32.6% has been met. However, upon examining trends by race/ethnicity and education level, there are still a number of population groups that are not meeting the target as noted in Figure 15.1 by the dashed line. The trends for youth are less promising; overall progress toward increasing the percent of youth meeting current aerobic physical activity guidelines is not progressing at similar rates to adults. Among adolescents, only males have achieved the target goal of 31.6% (noted in Figure 15.2 by the dashed line). Differences are noted by grade level and racial/ethnic group.

Other objectives for 2020 have included creating healthier and more supportive environments for physical activity through schools, worksites, healthcare

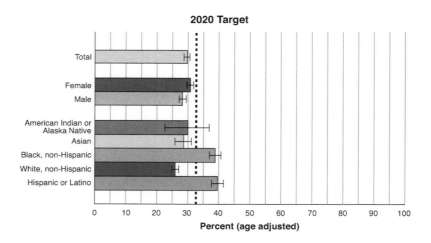

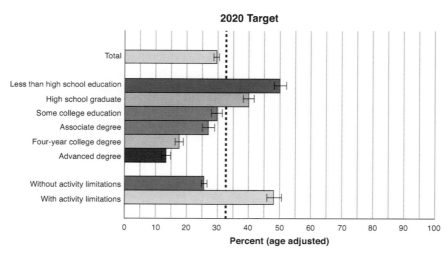

FIGURE 15.1 Prevalence of no leisure-time physical activity among adults by race/ethnicity, education level, and disability status, 2012

Source: U.S. Department of Health and Human Services (2016).

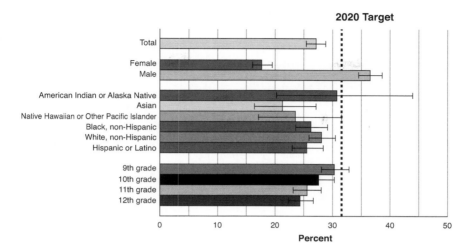

FIGURE 15.2 Prevalence of meeting guidelines for aerobic physical activity among adolescents, 2011

Source: U.S. Department of Health and Human Services (2016).

organizations, and legislative policies. The inclusion of these types of objectives can enhance the likelihood that individual-level outcomes will be achieved by making being physically active the easier choice. These objectives are also very much in line with the NPAP and WHO's Plan and can target the social determinants of health more comprehensively.

Implications for practice

Throughout this text we have outlined how the current body of knowledge can influence public health practice to improve physical activity participation among multiple population groups. A number of overarching themes emerged to address physical inactivity across a variety of different population groups.

Surveillance and measurement

One of the more consistent issues noted throughout the chapters is the lack of population-level data about health outcomes and physical activity for several of the population groups included in this text. For example, in the United States, national data collected through the Behavioral Risk Factor Surveillance System (BRFSS), Youth Risk Behavior Survey (YRBS), National Health Interview Survey (NHIS), or National Nutrition and Health Examination Survey (NHANES) does not consistently or not at all assess sexual orientation, presenting a significant gap in knowledge for the prevalence of physical inactivity and related chronic disease for LGBT youth and adults. The BRFSS, which is administered in each state with slightly different modules covering different topics, may not adequately sample in rural areas to get a representative sample for the region. All of the national data collection systems are also limited in their findings by their recruitment methods and response bias. Many rely on phones to recruit, which may not be effective for low-income populations, those who work shift-work with incompatible hours, or those who aren't comfortable speaking English. Other countries' surveillance systems struggle with similar issues, indicating the importance of creating data collection methods that adequately cover all the diversity of the population.

Another concern with measurement is the method of assessment of physical activity. Aside from NHANES, there is limited national-level data using objective measures of physical activity. This indicates a significant portion of our current information on physical activity comes from a self-report, which comes with some limitations in terms of reliability and accuracy. This is of concern for many population groups considering the tremendous variability in domains of activity (occupational, transportation, household, leisure-time) and specific types of activity (e.g., sport, dance, gardening, aerobics) that could be assessed. It is difficult for measurement tools to be designed to work well for all sexes, ages, ethnicities, social classes, ability levels, and so forth. Further investigation is needed on the most effective methods for determining physical activity participation across diverse populations.

Evidence-based practice

The Task Force on Community Preventive Services' Community Guide is a resource for interpreting the current evidence for changing physical activity participation and determining the most effective strategy (Task Force on Community Preventive Services 2002). For physical activity, the three main areas which have been systematically reviewed for evidence are: (1) behavioral and social approaches, (2) campaigns and informational approaches, and (3) environmental and policy approaches. The Community Guide provides practitioners with a summary of "best practices" and recommended strategies and, where available, an indication of which population groups the strategies have been tested for. This tool can be helpful for communities to determine the best place to invest resources for trying to promote physical activity.

Increasing awareness

This book serves as a foundation for students, healthcare providers, and practitioners to increase their competence in dealing with diverse population groups. The importance of cultural competency for twenty-first-century health and wellness professionals cannot be stressed enough. With changing demographics, it is important for professionals and practitioners to be capable and confident in helping a multitude of populations address their activity levels. Developing an awareness of the health inequities outlined in this book and translating that information to daily practice will enhance the likelihood that we can reduce health disparities related to inactivity in the future.

Summary points

- The social determinants of health discussed in this text – race, ethnicity, socio-economic status, residence location, sexual orientation, veterans' status, and level of disability –are related to individuals' health and physical activity behavior.
- These factors create the health disparities related in physical inactivity and inactivity-related chronic disease found in the United States and around the world.
- In order to address these inequities, initiatives need to be developed at multiple levels, targeting along a spectrum of individual approaches up to policy implementation.
- The consideration of social and cultural norms, religions, values, gender issues, political support, and local-level capacity for promoting physical activity is essential for developing tailored and effective programs promoting physical activity.
- With changing demographics, it is important for health and wellness professionals and practitioners to be capable and confident in helping a multitude of populations address their activity levels.

Critical thinking questions

1 Consider a population of your choice. How could strategies at each level of the social ecological model be effective to promote physical activity?
2 Why are national and international plans for promoting physical activity necessary and useful?
3 Describe how measurement can result in limitations with understanding physical activity participation in different population groups.
4 Why is it important to use evidence-based strategies to promote physical activity?

References

Angel, C. and Armstrong, N. J. (2016). *Enriching veterans' lives through an evidence based approach: A case illustration of Team Red, White & Blue (Measurement and Evaluation Series, Paper 1).* Syracuse, NY: Institute for Veterans and Military Families, Syracuse University.

Arredondo, E. M., Morello, M., Holub, C. and Haughton, J. (2014). Feasibility and preliminary findings of a church-based mother-daughter pilot study promoting physical activity among young Latinas. *Family & Community Health,* 37: 6–18.

Dishman, R. K. and Buckworth, J. (1996). Increasing physical activity: A quantitative synthesis. *Medicine and Science in Sports and Exercise,* 28: 706–719.

Findlay, L. C. and Kohen, D. E. (2007). Aboriginal children's sport participation in Canada. *Pimatisiwin: A Journal of Aboriginal and Indigenous Community Health,* 5: 185–206.

Fogel, S. C., Mcelroy, J. A., Garbers, S., Mcdonnell, C., Brooks, J., Eliason, M. J., Ingraham, N., Osborn, A., Rayyes, N., Redman, S. D., Wood, S. F. and Haynes, S. G. (2016). Program design for healthy weight in lesbian and bisexual women: A ten-city prevention initiative. *Womens Health Issues,* 26 Suppl 1: S7–S17.

Heath, G. W., Parra, D. C., Sarmiento, O. L., Andersen, L. B., Owen, N., Goenka, S., Montes, F. and Brownson, R. C. (2012). Evidence-based intervention in physical activity: Lessons from around the world. *Lancet,* 380: 272–281.

James, S., Ziviani, J., Ware, R. S. and Boyd, R. N. (2015). Randomized controlled trial of web-based multimodal therapy for unilateral cerebral palsy to improve occupational performance. *Developmental Medicine & Child Neurology*, 57: 530–538.

National Physical Activity Plan Alliance. (2016). *National Physical Activity Plan* [Online]. Available: www.physicalactivityplan.org/index.php (Accessed August 8 2016).

Reis, R. S., Salvo, D., Ogilvie, D., Lambert, E. V., Goenka, S., Brownson, R. C. and Lancet Physical Activity Series 2 Executive Committe. (2016). Scaling up physical activity interventions worldwide: Stepping up to larger and smarter approaches to get people moving. *Lancet*, 388: 1337–1348.

Task Force on Community Preventive Services. (2002). Recommendations to increase physical activity in communities. *American Journal of Preventive Medicine*, 22: 67–72.

Taylor, W. C., Franzini, L., Olvera, N., Carlos Poston, W. S. and Lin, G. (2012). Environmental audits of friendliness toward physical activity in three income levels. *Journal of Urban Health*, 89: 296–307.

Umstattd Meyer, M. R., Perry, C. K., Sumrall, J. C., Patterson, M. S., Walsh, S. M., Clendennen, S. C., Hooker, S. P., Evenson, K. R., Goins, K. V., Heinrich, K. M., O'hara Tompkins, N., Eyler, A. A., Jones, S., Tabak, R. and Valko, C. (2016). Physical activity-related policy and environmental strategies to prevent obesity in rural communities: A systematic review of the literature, 2002–2013. *Preventing Chronic Disease*, 13: E03.

U.S. Department of Health and Human Services. (2012). *Healthy People 2020* [Online]. Available: www.healthypeople.gov/2020/default.aspx (Accessed June 20 2016).

U.S. Department of Health and Human Services. (2016). *Physical Activity* [Online]. Available: www.healthypeople.gov/2020/topics-objectives/topic/physical-activity (Accessed June 20 2016).

World Health Organization. (2004). *Global strategy on diet, physical activity & health*. Geneva: World Health Organization.

World Health Organization. (2010). *Global recommendations on physical activity for health*. Switzerland: World Health Organization.

World Health Organization. (2013). Global Action Plan for the Prevention and Control of Noncommunicable Diseases. *In:* Non-communicable Disease and Mental Health (ed.). Switzerland: WHO Document Production.

INDEX

Note: Page numbers in italics indicate figures and tables.

Aboriginal Coaching Modules 116
Aboriginal RunWalk Program 115–16
Aboriginal Sport, Recreation and Physical
   Activity Partners Council (ASRPAPC)
   115–16
accelerometers *3*, 46–7, *72*, 130, 191
Accessible Okanagan 237–8
action, as stage of change 17, *18*
Active Duty service members 201, 202,
   206, 208–9, 210, 211, 212, *216*
Active Living by Design (ALbD) 173
*Active Transportation Beyond Urban
   Centers* 170–1
activity monitors *4*, 95, 193, 215
adults: Asian Americans *86*, 86–9, 87–9, *88*;
   Latinos 70; LGBT populations 185–6;
   rural adults 168–71; 2020 target goal
   for aerobic physical activity among
   277–8, *278*
aerobics 111, 113, 114, 280
African American Collaborative Obesity
   Research Network (AACORN) 48,
   48, 55
African Americans: chronic diseases among
   64; common barriers and facilitators to
   physical activity for 48–56; community
   involvement and social support 49;
   cultural and psychosocial processes
   49–50; demographic characteristics 45–6;
   evidence-based practice 53–4; family
   responsibilities 50; health disparities
   and inequities among 46; heart disease

among 64–5; historical and social
   contexts 49–50; implications for practice
   54–5; *Instant Recess*® 53–4; intervention
   strategies for 51–5; limitations of studies
   focused on 52–3; metabolic health among
   64–5; personal demographic variables 50;
   physical activity among 46–8; physical
   and economic environments 50–1;
   poor health conditions 50; sociocultural
   knowledge and beliefs 49; studies focused
   on promoting physical activity among
   52–3; understanding 45; women, unique
   influences among 49–50; youth, unique
   influences among 50
alcohol use: among diverse populations
   internationally *253*; among LGBT
   populations 183, 190, 192; among military
   veterans 208; among Native Americans
   109; among rural populations 172
Alzheimer's disease 65, 70
American Heart Association 4
American Indian Games 113
ANGELO (Analysis Grid for
   Environments/Elements Linked to
   Obesity) model 136
appraisal support *72*
arthritis: among LGBT populations 183;
   among military veterans 209; among
   Native Americans 103, *104*; among
   physically disabled populations 233
Asian Americans: barriers to physical
   activity for 85–97; community health

workers among 93–4; community participatory methods 93–4; culturally competent/sensitive interventions 92–3; demographic characteristics 84–5; evidence-based practice 94; healthcare settings 95; health disparities and inequities among 85; implications for practice 96; intervention strategies for 92–6; middle-aged adults, unique influences among 87–9, *88*; mode of physical activity 94–5; neighborhood and built environment *90*, 90–2; physical activity among 85; seniors, unique influences among 87–9, *88*; technology-based intervention 95; understanding 84; women, unique influences among 89–90; youth and younger adults, unique influences among *86*, 86–7
Asian and Pacific Islander Obesity Prevention Alliance (APIOPA) 94
asthma: among LGBT populations 183; among Native Americans 103, *104*; among physically disabled populations 227
awareness, increasing 280

barrier, defined 10
Barriers to Engaging in Physical Activity Among Lesbians (BE-PALS) 191
barriers to physical activity: for African Americans 48–56; for Asian Americans 85–97; cultural 26–41; for diverse populations internationally 251–68; Ecologic Model of Physical Activity and 15–16; for Latinos 66–78, *67*; for LGBT populations 187–95, *188–9*; for low-income populations 147–55; for military veterans 211–18; for Native Americans 108–17; for NHPI population 131–7; for physically disabled populations 228–41; for rural populations 165–75; time 15
behavioral approaches to intervention *232*, 233–4; face-to-face interventions 234; Internet-based interventions 234; for rural adults 169
behavioral capabilities 19
behavioral economics 150–1
Behavioral Risk Factor Surveillance System (BRFSS) 46, 47–8, 103, 126, 127–9, *128*, 182, 186, 279–80
behavioral theories of health disparities 17–19
"Bike to China" program 94
biological theories of health disparities 14–15

blood pressure: among Asian Americans 95; among Latinos 65, 77; among Native Americans 114, 115; among NHPI population 135; among physically disabled populations 227
body mass index (BMI): among African Americans 48, 50; among Asian Americans 84, 95; among LGBT populations 192; among low-income populations 151; among NHPI populations 125, 126, 129; among rural populations 165

California Health Interview Study 103
cancer: among Asian Americans 85, 93–4; among LGBT populations 183; among military veterans *207*; among Native Americans 103, *104*; among NHPI population 126–7; among physically disabled populations 227; epigenetic modifications and 14–15; LHW nutrition and physical activity intervention 93–4; outcome expectancies 1
cardiovascular disease (CVD) *see* heart disease (HD)
categories of difference 21–3, 161
Centers for Disease Control and Prevention (CDC) 37, 166; MET recommendations 133–4; obesity-related policy and environmental change recommendations 168; *Partnerships to Improve Community Health* 162–3
Chamorros 123, 126, 130
change, stages of 17, *18*
change theories 13
Cherokee Choices 113
Children's Healthy Living Project 136
chronic diseases: among African Americans 45, 46, 51, 53, 54; among Asian Americans 84, 85, 89, 95, 96; among Latinos 64, 66, 73, 78; among LGBT populations 279; among military veterans 206, 209, 212, 213; among Native Americans 103, 109; among NHPI population 125, 127; among physically disabled populations 227, 231; among rural populations 159, 161, 162–3, 169; outcome expectancies 1; physical inactivity/sedentary behavior and 4, 7
chronic pain 70, *205*, 207, 212, 213
church-based intervention *see* faith-based intervention
Coaching Association of Canada 116

cognitive health: among Latinos 65, 73; among military veterans *205,* 206, 209–10, 213
collectivism 29, 50
community-based participatory approaches 20, 153–4
community-based participatory planning 260
Community Based Participatory Research (CBPR) *14,* 20–1, 75, 134, 135, 153–4, 192, 195
community-based strategies: for Native Americans 114; for rural adults 170–1; for rural youth 172–3
Community Energy Balance Framework 154
community factors for physical activity: for African Americans 48, 49; for Asian Americans 85–6, 90, 93; in evidence-based practice 9; in future directions 275; for Latinos 74, 75–6, 77; for LGBT populations *189;* for Native Americans 109, 110, 112, 113, 114, 115; for NHPI population 131; overview of 8, *8;* for physically disabled populations 230; in theories of health disparities related to physical activity *14,* 20–1
community health workers (CHWs): among Asian Americans 93–4; among Latinos 73–4
community-level interventions, conceptual frameworks for 20–1
community participatory methods 93–4
community partnerships for rural populations 167–8
community readiness, determining 36–7
Community Readiness Model 21, 167
computer use 4, 75, 86
constituent-involving strategies 32, *33*
contemplation, as stage of change 17, *18*
Country Report Cards 245
cultural barriers: community readiness, determining 36–7; culturally competent/sensitive interventions 34–6, *35–6,* 38–40; culturally targeting and tailoring 29; deep structure strategies 29–30, *30–2,* 33; developing or adapting intervention, deciding between 33–4; family responsibilities 33; goals of intervention, identifying 37; intervention strategies for 28, *31–2;* method of delivery 36–7; to physical activity 26–41; physical activity measurement considerations 37–8; racial/ethnic backgrounds 27; social class 27–8;

surface structure strategies 29–33, *30–2, 33;* target group, identifying and characterizing 36–7; for women 27
cultural competency, defined 10
culturally appropriate strategies for promoting physical activity 26–41; *see also* culturally competent/sensitive interventions; cultural targeting and tailoring 29; culture and health, understanding 26–8; deep structure strategies 29–30, *30–2,* 33, 38; developing or adapting an intervention, deciding between 33–4; health and, understanding 26–8; physical activity and 26–8; surface structure strategies 29–33, *30–2, 33*
culturally competent/sensitive interventions: for Asian Americans 92–3; community readiness, determining 36–7; for cultural barriers 28, 34–6, *35–6,* 38–40; goals of 37; integrating 38–9; method of delivery 36–7; overview of 28; physical activity measurement considerations 37–8; pilot testing and refining 39–40; promotion strategies 38–9; steps to develop or adapt 34–6, *35–6;* target group, identifying 36–7
cultural targeting and tailoring 29

dance: Bollywood 95; hula 132–5; Latin 38, 73, 74
deep structure strategies 29–30, *30–2,* 33, 38; among Asian Americans 94; among Latinos 74, 76; among LGBT populations 195; among military veterans *203–4;* among Native Americans 112–13, 114; among NHPI population 133, 134
diabetes: among African Americans 14, 45, 46; among Asian Americans 84, 85, 93, 94, 95; among diverse populations internationally 244–5; among Latinos 65, 70, 77; among military veterans 207, *207,* 209, 211, 212, 213; among Native Americans 103, *104,* 108, 113, 114, 115; among NHPI population 125, 126, 135, 136; among physically disabled populations 227, 231, 233; among rural populations 159, 161; outcome expectancies 1; physical inactivity/sedentary behavior and 5; racial differences to insulin secretion and disparities in 14
Diabetes Prevention Program 135
diaries/logs *3*
Diffusion of Innovation Theory *14,* 20, 21

diverse populations internationally: common barriers and facilitators to physical activity for 251–68; common correlates and determinants of physical activity globally 251–8, *252–4, 255–6*; current evidence for physical activity interventions globally 258–9; evidence-based practice 265–6; global correlates and determinants 251–4, *252–4*; implications for practice 266–7; income, physical inactivity according to 246–9, *247, 248*, 254–8, *255–6*; intervention strategies for 258–68; notable global disparities and inequities in health 245; physical activity in 246; principles for developing interventions across different settings 259–60; region, physical inactivity according to 249–51, *250*, 258; "Seven Best Investments for Physical Activity" 260–6, *261–3*; understanding 244–5

Doing It For Ourselves (DIFO) 192

"Don't Ask Don't Tell" (DADT) policy 201

drug use: among military veterans 208; among Native Americans 109

Ecologic Model of Physical Activity (EMPA) 14, 15–16

economic barriers to physical activity for African Americans 50–1

economic stability as social determinant of health 6, *6,* 7

educational attainment: among African Americans 46, 50, 51, 53, 55; among Asian Americans 85, 87, 89, 92; among diverse populations internationally *255,* 258; among Latinos 63, 65, *67;* among LGBT populations 182; among low-income populations 145, 146, 147, 153; among military veterans 202; among Native Americans 103, 104, *104,* 111, 113; among rural populations 160, 161, 173; culture and 27; Healthy People 2020 objectives and 278, *278*; as social determinant of health *6,* 7, 7

emotional support *72,* 76, 235

employment: African Americans and 48, 50; Asian Americans and 87, 90; diverse populations internationally and 249; Latinos and 75; military veterans and *204, 205*; Native Americans and 103, 104, *104*; rural populations and 170; as social determinant of health 7

environmental approaches to intervention: for NHPI population 135–6; for

physically disabled populations *232,* 236, 238; for rural populations 168

environmental issues as barriers to physical activity: for Asian Americans *90,* 90–2; barriers to physical activity for Latinos *67,* 68–9; for Latinos *67,* 68–9; for low-income populations 147–50; for military veterans 211–12; for NHPI population 131–2; for rural populations 165–6

ethnicity, defined 10

evidence-based practice: Aboriginal RunWalk Program 115–16; active accessible living in Okanagan Valley 237–8; for African Americans 53–4; APIOPA 94; for Asian Americans 94; community partnerships 167–8; for diverse populations internationally 265–6; in future directions for addressing physical activity 280; hula dancing 134–5; HWLB 190–1; *Instant Recess®* 53–4; Kau Mai Tonga 265–6; for Latinos 76–7; for LGBT populations 190–1; for low-income, Hispanic community parks 152–3; for military veterans 214; for Native Americans 115–16; for NHPI population 134–5; for physically disabled populations 237–8; for rural populations 167–8; RWB 214; social ecological framework in SDOH 9

evidential strategies 32, *33*

exercise groups 235

exo-environment 15–16

explanatory theories 13

face-to-face interventions 234

facilitator, defined 10

Fair Market Rent Document 143

faith-based intervention 20–1, 34, 36, 37, 38, 39–40; for African Americans 29, 51, 53; for diverse populations internationally 265; *Fe en Acción* (Faith in Action) study 30, 34, 36, 37–9, 77 *30–1*; in future directions 274, 276; for Latinos 29, 71, 75, 76–7; for LGBT populations 191, 195; in National Physical Activity Plan 276

faith-placed intervention 53

familismo 63

family responsibilities: for African Americans 50; cultural barriers to physical activity and 33; levels of 29

fatalismo 63

Federal TRIO Programs *144*

Fe en Acción (Faith in Action) study 30, 34, 36, 37–9, 77 *30–1*

females *see* women
Fitbit 95, 193
food insecurity: among military veterans
    208; among Native Americans 103, 104,
    104; economic stability and 7
four Ds 148–9
future directions for addressing physical
    activity 273–81; awareness, increasing
    280; community factors in 275;
    evidence-based practice 280; faith-based
    intervention in 274, 276; foundation for
    moving forward 276–9; Healthy People
    2020 277–9; implications for practice
    279–80; institutional factors in 274–5;
    interpersonal factors in 274; intrapersonal
    factors in 274; National Physical Activity
    Plan 276–7; public policy factors in 275;
    social ecological approaches in 273–6;
    surveillance and measurement 279–80;
    WHO Plan 277, 279

gardening 93, 129, 132, 280
gender, defined 180
gender identity, defined 180
Global Action Plan for the Prevention and
    Control of Non-communicable Diseases
    (WHO) 276, 277, 279
global correlates and determinants 251–4,
    252–4; according to income 254–8,
    255–6; according to region 258
Global Health Observatory (WHO)
    244, 245
Global Observatory for Physical
    Activity 245
Global Physical Activity Questionnaire
    (GPAQ) 37–8
Global Recommendations on Physical
    Activity for Health (WHO) 2, 246
Global School-Based Health Survey 245
Global Status Report on Non-
    communicable Diseases (WHO) 245,
    246, 249, *250*
Global Strategy on Diet, Physical Activity
    and Health (WHO) 258, 259, 273

Hālau Mōhala ʻIlima 134
Hawaiʻi, NHPIs in 129–30
Health Behavior in School-Age Children
    Study 245
healthcare settings to promote physical
    activity: for Asian Americans 95; for
    diverse populations internationally 259,
    262, 264
health equity 5–7, 16, 163, 168, 173,
    265–6, 277

*Health of Lesbian, Gay, Bisexual, and
    Transgender People: Building a Foundation
    for Better Understanding, The* (IOM) 182
Health Promotion Model and Self
    Determination Theory 152
Healthy People 2020 181, 277–9; goals for
    adults 277–8, *278*; goals for youth 278–9,
    279; Rural Healthy People 2020 160–1,
    166, 169; targeting LGBT health 181
Healthy People Initiative (USDHHS) 2, 5;
    see also Healthy People 2020
Healthy Weight Disparity Index 151
Healthy Weight in Lesbian and Bisexual
    Women: Striving for a Healthy
    Community (HWLB) 190–1, 192, 194–5
heart disease (HD): among African
    Americans 45; among Asian Americans
    84, 85, 93, 94; among international
    populations 244; among Latinos 64–5,
    75; among LGBT populations 183;
    among low-income populations 153;
    among military veterans 209; among
    Native Americans 103, *104,* 114, 115;
    among NHPI population 125–6; among
    physically disabled populations 227,
    231, 233; among rural populations 161;
    outcome expectancies 1, 19; physical
    inactivity/sedentary behavior and 4, 5
high school education: among Latinos 63;
    among Native Americans *104*
Hispanic Community Health Study/Study
    of Latinos (HCHS/SOL) 64
Hispanics *see* Latinos
HIV/AIDS 183, 245
HŌʻALA research project 136
home-based strategies to intervention for
    rural adults 169
HUD Income Limits Documentation
    System 143
hula dancing 132–5
Hula Enabling Lifestyles Adaptation
    (HELA) 134–5

implications for practice, in intervention
    strategies: for African Americans 54–5;
    for Asian Americans 96; for diverse
    populations internationally 266–7; future
    directions for addressing physical activity
    279–80; for Latinos 78; for LGBT
    populations 195–6; for low-income
    populations 153–4; for military veterans
    215–17; for Native Americans 116; for
    NHPI population 136–7; for physically
    disabled populations 238–40; for rural
    populations 173–4, *174*

informational support *72, 77, 231, 233*, 235, 238, 280
Instant Recess® 53–4
Institute of Medicine (IOM) 182
institutional factors to physical activity: for African Americans 48; for Asian Americans 92, 94–5; in evidence-based practice 9; in future directions 274–5; for LGBT populations 187, *188–9*; for Native Americans 109–10; overview of 8, *8*; for physically disabled populations 228, 229; for rural populations 169
instrumental support *72*
interlocking systems of oppression theory 22
International Paralympics Committee 213
international populations *see* diverse populations internationally
Internet-based interventions 234
interpersonal factors for physical activity: for African Americans 48, 49; for Asian Americans 85, 93, 95; in evidence-based practice 9; in future directions 274; for Latinos 77; for LGBT populations 187, *188*; for low-income populations 147; for Native Americans 109; overview of 8, *8*; for physically disabled populations 228–9; for rural populations 165; in theories of health disparities related to physical activity *14*, 18–19, 21
intervention, defined 10
intervention strategies: for African Americans 51–5; for Asian Americans 92–6; conceptual frameworks for community-level interventions 20–1; for cultural barriers 28–40, *31–2*; for diverse populations internationally 258–68; examples of, in stages of change 17, *18*; for Latinos *67*, 71–8; for LGBT populations 190–6; for low-income populations 151–5; for military veterans 212–18; for Native Americans 112–16; for NHPI population 132–7; for physically disabled populations 230–41, *231–2*; for rural populations 166–74
intrapersonal factors for physical activity: for African Americans 48, 49; for Asian Americans 85, 92, 95; in evidence-based practice 9; in future directions 274; for LGBT populations 187, *188*; for low-income populations 147; for Native Americans 109; overview of 8, *8*; for physically disabled populations 228; for rural populations 165; stages of change

17, *18*; in theories of health disparities related to physical activity *14*, 17, 22
Invictus Games Foundation 213

Kahnawake Schools Diabetes Prevention Project 113
Kalihi Valley Instructional Bike Exchange (KVIBE) 136
Kau Mai Tonga 265–6
Kitigan Zibi school program 113
Kokua Kalihi Valley Comprehensive Family Services 136
Kumu hula 134

Latinos: acculturation 66, 67–8; cognitive health among 65, 73; common barriers and facilitators to physical activity for 66–78, *67*; community health workers among 73–4; cultural beliefs 63; demographic characteristics 63; environmental issues *67*, 68–9; evidence-based practice 76–7; faith-based intervention 76–7; health disparities and inequities among 64–6; historical background 63–4; immigration status 70–1; implications for practice 78; intergenerational intervention 74–5; intervention strategies for *67*, 71–8; language 68, 74; men, unique influences among 69; mental health among 65, 70; modes of physical activity 73; older adults, unique influences among 70; physical activity among 66; physical environment *67*, 68; policy level 68–9; self-efficacy 66, *67*; social support *67*, 68, 71–2, *72*; technology 75–6; time constraints *67*, 68; understanding 62–3; women, unique influences among 69; youth, unique influences among 69–70
lay health workers (LHW) 93–4
"Let's Move" campaign 84
LGBT populations: adults 185–6, 187, 190; BE-PALS 191; college years 184–5, *185*; common barriers and facilitators to physical activity for 187–95, *188–9*; demographic characteristics 181–2; DIFO 192; evidence-based practice 190–1; gender, defined 180; gender identity, defined 180; health disparities and inequities among 182–3; HWLB interventions 190–1, 192, 194–5; implications for practice 195–6; intervention strategies for 190–6; LOLA 193; mental health among 183; MOVE

193–4; physical activity among 183–6; physical health among 183; sexual orientation, defined 181; SHE 193; understanding 180–1; WHAM 194; youth 184, *184*, 187

LHW nutrition and physical activity intervention 93–4

limited English proficiency (LEP) 92

linguistic strategies 32, *33*, 92, 112, 113

Living Out, Living Actively (LOLA) 192, 193

low-income populations: behavioral economics 150–1; built environment 147–50; CBPR 153–4; common barriers and facilitators to physical activity for 147–55; Community Based Participatory Research 153–4; Community Energy Balance Framework 154; definitions of low income 143–5; demographics of 145; evidence-based practice 152–3; health disparities and inequities among 145; Healthy Weight Disparity Index and 151; implications for practice 153–4; intervention strategies for 151–5; levels of physical activity among 145–7, *146*; physical activity among 145–51, *146*; policy and ordinance decision making 154; poverty guidelines 144, *144*; social capital 150; understanding 143–5

machismo 63

macro-environment 15–16

maintenance, as stage of change 17, *18*

Making Our Vitality Evident (MOVE) 192, 193–4

marianismo 63

measures of physical activity 2–4; frequency 2; intensity 2; methods of 3, *3–4*; objective 3, 130, 164, 280; self-reported 52; subjective 3, *3–4*; time/duration 2; type 2

mental health: among African Americans 46, 54; among diverse populations internationally *253*, 265; among Latinos 65, 70; among LGBT populations 183; among military veterans *204*, 205, *205*, 206, *207*, 208–9, 214; among Native Americans 109, 115, 116; among physically disabled populations 231

meso-environment 15–16

metabolic equivalent (MET) 4–5, 133–4, 211

metabolic health: among Latinos 64–5; among military veterans 207; among

NHPI population 125–6; among rural populations 161–2

military culture 202–6; veteran identity 203, 205, 206

military sexual trauma (MST) 205, 215

military veterans 200–18; Active Duty service members 201, 202, 206, 208–9, 210, 211, 212, *216*; behavioral health risk factors 208; chronic health conditions among 211; clinical and cultural considerations for 215–17, *216*; cognitive health among *205*, 206, 209–10, 213; common barriers and facilitators to physical activity for 211–18; deep structure strategies among *203–4*; demographic characteristics 201; deployment 202, 203, *204*, 205, 209; environmental factors 211–12; evidence-based practice 214; facility-based exercise programming 212; healthcare use and access 206–7, *207*; health disparities and inequities among 206–10; implications for practice 215–17; individual factors 211–12; intervention strategies for 212–18; mental health among *204*, 205, *205*, 206, *207*, 208–9, 214; metabolic health among 207; military culture 202–6; military service 202; physical activity among 210–11; physical health disparities among 209–10; poor nutrition among 208; role of individual, social, and environmental factors 211–12; service-related disabilities 205–6, *206*; social factors 211–12; surface structure strategies among 200, *203–4*; transition from military service to civilian life 211–12; understanding 200; veteran identity 203–6; VHA physical activity programming 212–15

Millennium Cohort Study (VA/DoD) 210–11

moderate-to-vigorous physical activity (MVPA) 77, 164–5, 171, 210, 211, 212

Molokai Heart Study 125

morbidity, defined 10

mortality, defined 10

MOVE! Weight Management Program (VA) 213

National Center for Children in Poverty 144

National Disabled Veterans Winter Sports Clinic (WSC) 213

National Health Interview Survey (NHIS) 46, 47–8, 279
National Household Travel Survey (2009) 170–1
National Nutrition and Health Examination Survey (NHANES) 46–8, 103, 279–80
National Physical Activity Plan (NPAP) 10, 166, 276–7
National Veteran Wheelchair Games (NVWG) 213
Native Americans: Aboriginal RunWalk Program 115–16; chronic disease among 103; common barriers and facilitators to physical activity for 108–17; community-based approaches 114; community factors 110; deep structure strategies 112, 113, 114; determinants of health among 103, 104–5; evidence-based practice 115–16; health disparities and inequities among 103, *104*; health-focused strategies 114–15; implications for practice 116; institutional factors 109–10; interpersonal factors 109; intervention strategies for 112–16; linguistic strategies 112, 113; peripheral strategies 112, 113; physical activity levels among 105–8, *106*; policy factors 110–11; on reservations 111; in rural and remote communities 111–12; school-based approaches 113–14; socioeconomic status among 112; understanding 102–3; youth, unique influences among 111
Native Hawaiian and Pacific Islanders (NHPIs): cancer among 126–7; cardiovascular health among 125–6; common barriers and facilitators to physical activity for 131–7; community influences 131–2; demographic characteristics *124*, 124–5; environmental change 135–6; environmental influences 131–2; evidence-based practice 134–5; in Hawai'i 129–30; health disparities and inequities among 125–7; hula dancing 132–5; implications for practice 136–7; intervention strategies for 132–7; metabolic health among 125–6; physical activity among 127–9, *128*; Tongans 130; understanding 123; youth, unique influences among 131
Native Hawaiian Health Research Project (NHHRP) 125
Non-Latino Whites (NLWs) 63, 66, 68, 71, 73, 74, 75, 76

obesity: among African Americans 45, 46, 48, *48*, 51–2; among Asian Americans 84, 87, 93, 94; among diverse populations internationally *252*; among Latinos 65; among LGBT populations 183, 190–1, 192, 195; among low-income populations 145, 146, 147, 151; among military veterans *205*, 207, 209; among Native Americans 103, *104*, 114, 115; among NHPI population 125–6, 136, 137; among physically disabled populations 233; among rural populations 159, 161–2, 163, 167, 168; health disparities/equity and 5; outcome expectancies 1
observational learning 19
Okanagan Valley, active accessible living in 237–8
older adults: Asian Americans 87–9, *88*; Latinos 70
operations Enduring Freedom, Iraqi Freedom, and New Dawn (OEF, OIF, OND) 201, *204*, 206, 207, 208, 209, 212
osteoarthritis 233
outcome expectancies 19

Partnerships to Improve Community Health (CDC) 162–3
Pathways 113
pedometers *3*, *72*, 95, 114, 193, 194, 234
peer-assisted programs 235–6
peripheral strategies 32, *33*
personalismo 63
physical activity: health disparities and equity 5–10; importance of 1–5; measures of 2–4; sedentary behavior and 4–5; social determinants of health 5–17
physical education: among diverse populations internationally 251, *252*, *261*; among LGBT populations 187, *189*; among Native Americans 116; among physically disabled populations 236; among rural populations 168, 172; in Ecologic Model of Physical Activity 16; policies aimed to improve access to and quality of 275, 277
physical inactivity 4–5
physically disabled populations: behavioral approaches *232*, 233–4; common barriers and facilitators to physical activity for 228–41, *232*, 234–6, 238; community factors 230; demographic characteristics 226–7; educational interventions, individualized 233;

environmental approaches *232, 236,* 238; evidence-based practice 237–8; exercise groups 235; face-to-face interventions 234; goal of intervention 231; health disparities and inequities among 227; implications for practice 238–40; individualized educational interventions 233; informational approaches *231,* 233, 238; institutional factors 229; Internet-based interventions 234; interpersonal processes 228–9; intervention strategies for 230–41, *231–2;* intrapersonal factors 228; Okanagan Valley, active accessible living in 237–8; peer-assisted programs 235–6; physical activity among 227–8; policy approaches *232, 236–7,* 238; policy factors 230; social approaches *232,* 234–6, 238; telephone support systems 235; understanding 226
physicians, access to 104, *104,* 148
physiological theories of health disparities 14–15
PILI 'Ohana Program 135
pilot testing 39–40
poor nutrition among military veterans 208
Post Traumatic Stress Disorder (PTSD) 207, 209, 211
poverty: among African Americans 46; among low-income populations 144, *144, 146,* 148, 149, 150; among military veterans *205;* among Native Americans 104, *104,* 109; among rural populations 160, 162, 173; economic stability and 7
precontemplation, as stage of change 17, *18*
preparation, as stage of change 17, *18*
psychosocial theories of health disparities 17–19
public policy factors for physical activity: in evidence-based practice 9; in future directions 275; for LGBT populations 187, *189;* for Native Americans 109, 110–11; for NHPI population 136; overview of 8, *8;* for physically disabled populations 228, 230

race, defined 10
Rails to Trails Conservancy 170
randomized controlled trial, defined 10
RE-AIM model 152
recall measure *3, 4*
Resource Deprivation Theory *14,* 20
Risk Exposure Theory *14,* 20
Rural Active Living Call to Action 173–4, *174*

Rural America at a Glance: 2015 Edition 173
Rural Healthy People 2020 160–1, 166, 169
rural populations: adults, interventions for 168–71; adults, unique challenges for 163–4; behavioral and home-based strategies, individually tailored 169; common barriers and facilitators to physical activity for 165–75; community-based strategies 170–1, 172–3; demographic characteristics 160; environmental approaches 168; environmental barriers 165–6; evidence-based practice 167–8; family home strategies 171; health disparities and inequities among 160–1; implications for practice 173–4, *174;* individual barriers 165; individually tailored behavioral and home-based strategies 169; intervention strategies for 166–74; metabolic health among 161–2; physical activity among 163–5; for rural adults 168–71; rural contexts, unique challenges for 162–3; school-based strategies 172; social barriers 165; understanding 159–60; worksite strategies 170; youth, interventions for 171–3; youth physical activity 164–5

Safe Routes to School programs 136
Samoans 123, 124, 130
school-based strategies: among Native Americans 113–14; among rural populations 172
sedentary behavior 4–5
self-efficacy: for African Americans 49; for diverse populations internationally *252,* 254, *255,* 257; for military veterans *204, 216;* for NHPI population 129; for physically disabled populations 234, 235; sources impacting levels of, for Latinos 66, *67;* in theories of disparities 15, 17, *18,* 19
seniors *see* older adults
"Seven Best Investments for Physical Activity" 260–6, *261–3*
sex, defined 180
sexual orientation, defined 181
Siglang Buhay 93
smoking: among diverse populations internationally 244, *253;* among Latinos 65; among LGBT populations 183, *188;* among low-income populations 145; among military veterans 205, 208, 213; among Native Americans 103, *104,* 113,

114, 115; among NHPI population 137;
among rural populations 159; cessation
113, 114, 213; health disparities/
inequities and 5
social barriers to physical activity for:
Latinos *67, 68*; low-income populations
150; military veterans 211–12; rural
populations 165
social capital 150
social class as barrier to physical activity
27–8
Social Cognitive Theory *14,* 19, 20, 151,
165–6, 191, 238
social determinants of health (SDOH) 5–17;
see also individual determinants; application
in different populations 10; community
8, *8, 9*; evidence-based practice (social
ecological framework) 9; examples of 7;
institutional 8, *8,* 9; interpersonal 8, *8, 9*;
intrapersonal 8, *8, 9*; public policy 8, *8,*
9; social ecological framework 7–10, *8*;
USDHHS model of 5–7, *6*
social ecological approaches to health
disparities 273–6; community-based
approaches 275; environmental
approaches 275–6; individual-level
approaches 274; policy approaches 275;
setting-based approaches 274–5; social/
interpersonal approaches 274
social justice, defined 22–3
social support: for African Americans 49;
for Latinos 71–2, *72*; for physically
disabled populations *232,* 234–6, 238
social systems 21–3
socioeconomic status (SES): among
African Americans 50; among diverse
populations internationally *252,* 254,
255–6, 257–8; among Latinos 64, 66,
68–9, 78; among military veterans 206,
208, 212, 215; among Native Americans
112; among rural populations 159, 169;
defined 11; indicators of 27–8
socioenvironmental theories of health
disparities 19–20
"Sport for all" movement 265
SportMedBC 115–16
Sports, Play and Active Recreation for Kids
program 113
step counters *see* pedometers
Step It Up 2015 Call to Action 16, 237
STEPS global surveillance system (WHO)
244–5
Strong, Healthy, Energized (SHE) 192, 193

suicide: among LGBT populations 183;
among military veterans 209, 214; among
Native Americans 103, *104*
surface structure strategies 29–33, *30–2, 33*;
among LGBT populations 191, 195–6;
among military veterans 200, *203–4*
Surgeon General: Report of the Surgeon
General for Physical Activity and Health
(1996) 145–6; *Step It Up* 2015 Call to
Action 16, 237

Tai Chi 92, 132
tailoring 29
target group: cultural targeting and tailoring
29; identifying and characterizing 36–7;
LGBT health 181
Task Force on Community Preventive
Services' Community Guide 280
Team Red, White, and Blue (RWB) 214
technology-based intervention strategies: for
Asian Americans 95; for Latinos 75–6
telephone support systems 235
television viewing 4, 7, 9, 70, 75, 86, 92, *104*
termination, as stage of change 17, *18*
theories of health disparities 13–24, *14*;
biological and physiological 14–15;
change 13; conceptual frameworks
for community-level interventions
20–1; Ecologic Model of Physical
Activity 14, 15–16; explanatory 13;
psychosocial and behavioral 17–19;
related to physical activity 13–21,
14; social systems and categories of
difference 21–3; socioenvironmental
19–20
Theory of Planned Behavior *14,* 17
time, as barrier to physical activity 15
tobacco use *see* smoking
Tongans 130
Transtheoretical Model *14,* 17

unemployment: among military veterans
205; among Native Americans 104, *104*
United States Department of Agriculture
(USDA) 160
United States Department of Education
(USDA) 144
United States Department of Health and
Human Services (USDHHS) 144, 181,
190, 277–9
United States Department of Housing and
Urban Development (HUD) 143
urban paradox 149

VA/DoD Millennium Cohort Study 210–11
VA MOVE! Weight Management Program 213
verbal support *72*
veteran identity 203–6; defined 203; factors that serve to influence *203–4,* 203–5
Veterans Health Administration (VHA) 206–7, *207,* 208, 209, 210, 212–13, 215, *216*
video games 4, 70, 86

wearable devices *4,* 95, 193, 215
women: African Americans 49–50; Asian Americans 89–90; cultural 27; Latinos 69
Women's Health and Mindfulness (WHAM) 192, 194
Women's Health Initiative 211
worksite strategies 170
World Bank 244, 246, *248*
World Health Organization (WHO) 1–2, 4, 7; adult physical activity prevalence according to 249–51, *250,* 258; Global Action Plan for the Prevention and Control of Non-communicable Diseases 276, 277, 279; Global Health Observatory 244, 245; Global Recommendations on Physical Activity for Health 2, 246; Global Status Report on Non-communicable Diseases 245, 246, 249, *250*; Global Strategy on Diet, Physical Activity and Health 258, 259, 273; Non-communicable Disease Action Plan 276; on physically disabled populations 226–7; STEPS global surveillance system 244–5

yoga 92, 132
younger adults: Asian Americans *86,* 86–7; LBGT populations 184–5, *185*
youth: African Americans 50; Asian Americans *86,* 86–7; Latinos 69–70; LGBT populations 184, *184,* 187; Native Americans 111; NHPI 131; rural youth 171–3; 2020 target goal for aerobic physical activity among 278–9, *279*
Youth Risk Behavioral Survey (YRBS) 46–7, 131, 279

Zhiiwapenewin Akino'maagewin 113
Zuni high school diabetes prevention program 113